Sucralfate

From Basic Science to the Bedside

Sucralfate

From Basic Science to the Bedside

Edited by

Daniel Hollander, M. D.
University of Kansas Medical School
Kansas City, Kansas

and

G. N. J. Tytgat, M. D.
University of Amsterdam
Amsterdam, The Netherlands

Springer Science+Business Media, LLC

Library of Congress Cataloging-in-Publication Data

On file

DOI 10.1007/978-0-585-32154-7

Originally published by Chugai Pharmaceutical Co. Ltd. in 1995.
MyCopy version of the original edition 1995

10 9 8 7 6 5 4 3 2 1

Contributors

G. Bianchi Porro • Gastrointestinal Unit, L. Sacco Hospital, 20157 Milan, Italy

Robert S. Bresalier • Departments of Medicine, Henry Ford Health Sciences Center and the University of Michigan School of Medicine, Detroit, Michigan 48202

W. Scott Brooks, Jr. • Piedmont Hospital, Atlanta, Georgia 30309

Tomasz Brzozowski • Institute of Physiology, University School of Medicine, Krakow, Poland

Gilles Caillé • Département de Pharmacologie, Faculté de Médecine, Université de Montréal, Montréal H3C 3J7, Canada

W. F. Caspary • Division of Gastroenterology, Department of Internal Medicine, Frankfurt University Hospital Medical Center, D-60590 Frankfurt am Main, Germany

Nicola G. Dahl • Marion Merrell Dow Inc., Kansas City, Missouri 64137

Judah Folkman • Department of Surgery, Children's Hospital, and Harvard Medical School, Boston, Massachusetts 02115

M. Guslandi • Gastroenterology Unit, S. Raffaele Hospital, University of Milan, 20132 Milan, Italy

F. Halter • Gastrointestinal Unit, Inselspital, University Hospital, Bern, Switzerland

Brian A. Hills • Department of Physiology, University of New England, Armidale, NSW 2351, Australia; *present address*: Pediatric Respiratory Research Centre, Mater Children's Hospital, South Brisbane, Queensland, Australia

Daniel Hollander • Dean's Office, University of Kansas School of Medicine, Kansas City, Kansas 66160-7300

Akira Ishimori • Department of Clinical and Laboratory Medicine, Tohoku University School of Medicine, Sendai 982, Japan

Hiroyuki Koba • Chugai Pharmaceutical Co., Ltd., Tokyo 104, Japan

Hans R. Koelz • Department of Medicine, Triemli Hospital, CH-8063 Zurich, Switzerland

Jan W. Konturek • Institute of Physiology, University School of Medicine, Krakow, Poland

Stanislaw J. Konturek • Institute of Physiology, University School of Medicine, Krakow, Poland

Stefano Kusstatscher • Department of Pathology, Brigham & Women's Hospital, and Harvard Medical School, Boston, Massachusetts 02115

Hajime Kuwayama • Department of Medicine, Nihon University School of Medicine, Tokyo, and University of Texas Southwestern Medical School, Dallas, Texas 75216

Shiu Kum Lam • Division of Gastroenterology and Hepatology, Department of Medicine, University of Hong Kong, Queen Mary Hospital, Hong Kong

J. A. Louw • Gastrointestinal Clinic and Department of Medicine, University of Cape Town and Groote Schuur Hospital, Observatory, South Africa

Michael R. Lucey • Department of Internal Medicine, University of Michigan Medical Center, Ann Arbor, Michigan 48109

I. N. Marks • Gastrointestinal Clinic and Department of Medicine, University of Cape Town and Groote Schuur Hospital, Observatory, South Africa

Francois Martin • Division of Gastroenterology, Hopital Saint-Luc, and University of Montreal, Montreal H2X 3J4, Canada

David R. Mathews • Marion Merrell Dow Inc., Kansas City, Missouri 64137

Gerald P. Morris • Department of Biology, Queen's University, Kingston, Ontario K7L 3N6, Canada

Miki Nagata • Department of Pathology, Brigham & Women's Hospital, and Harvard Medical School, Boston, Massachusetts 02115

Kiyoshige Ochi • Development and Technology Division, Chugai Pharmaceutical Co., Ltd., Tokyo 115, Japan

Yoshiyasu Ogihara • Department of Applied Pharmacology, Kyoto Pharmaceutical University, Kyoto 607, Japan

Susumu Okabe • Department of Applied Pharmacology, Kyoto Pharmaceutical University, Kyoto 607, Japan

Roy Charles Orlando • Tulane University School of Medicine, New Orleans, Louisiana 70112

Daniel Rachmilewitz • Department of Medicine, Hadassah University Hospital, Mount Scopus, Hebrew University Hadassah Medical School, Jerusalem, Israel

W. D. W. Rees • Hope Hospital, Salford, and University of Manchester School of Medicine, Manchester, England

Zsuzsa Sandor • Chemical Pathology Research Division, Department of Pathology, Brigham & Women's Hospital, and Harvard Medical School, Boston, Massachusetts 02115; *present address*: Department of Pathology and Laboratory Medicine, Veterans Affairs Medical Center, Long Beach, California 90822

F. Santalucia • Gastrointestinal Unit, L. Sacco Hospital, 20157 Milan, Italy

Y. Shing • Department of Surgery, Children's Hospital, and Harvard Medical School, Boston, Massachusetts 02115

Amelia Slomiany • Research Center, University of Medicine and Dentistry, Newark, New Jersey

Bronislaw L. Slomiany • Research Center, University of Medicine and Dentistry, Newark, New Jersey

Sandor Szabo • Chemical Pathology Research Division, Department of Pathology, Brigham & Women's Hospital, and Harvard Medical School, Boston, Massachusetts 02115; *present address*: Department of Pathology and Laboratory Medicine, Veterans Affairs Medical Center, Long Beach, California 90822

A. Tarnawski • Gastroenterology Section, DVA Medical Center, Long Beach, and Department of Medicine, University of California, Irvine, California 92664

Clifford Tasman-Jones • Department of Medicine, University of Auckland, Auckland, New Zealand

A. B. R. Thomson • Nutrition and Metabolism Research Group, Division of Gastroenterology, University of Alberta, Edmonton T6G 2C2, Canada

Michael Tryba • Department of Anesthesiology, Intensive Care Medicine and Pain Therapy, University of Bochum Bergmannsheil, Bochum, Germany

G. N. J. Tytgat • Department of Gastroenterology–Hepatology, Academic Medical Center, University of Amsterdam, Amsterdam, The Netherlands

Manon Vézina • Département de Pharmacologie, Faculté de Médecine, Université de Montréal, and Centre de Recherche Fernand Seguin, Hôpital Louis-Hippolyte Lafontaine, Montréal, Canada

T. A. Winter • Gastrointestinal Clinic and Department of Medicine, University of Cape Town and Groote Schuur Hospital, Observatory, South Africa

Tadataka Yamada • Department of Internal Medicine, University of Michigan Medical Center, Ann Arbor, Michigan 48109

G. O. Young • Gastrointestinal Clinic and Department of Medicine, University of Cape Town and Groote Schuur Hospital, Observatory, South Africa

Preface

The discovery of hydrochloric acid in the human stomach left an everlasting impression on investigators and physicians concerned with gastrointestinal physiology in general and peptic ulcer disease in particular. In fact, the conclusion was accepted without reservations that acid causes peptic ulcerations. Thus, intragastric acid secretion became the dominant etiological thought in peptic ulcer disease and, not surprisingly, the therapy of peptic disease was directed at either neutralizing or suppressing hydrochloric acid production by the stomach.

Over the past several decades it has been clearly demonstrated that acid hypersecretion is not common in patients with duodenal ulcer disease and is extremely rare in patients with gastric ulcer disease. Therefore, the idea that factors other than hydrochloric acid may be important or even pivotal in the genesis of ulcer disease or in mucosal damage of the upper gastrointestinal tract has gained gradual acceptance. Investigators began looking at the complex factors that normally protect the gastroduodenal mucosa against injury as potential factors in the genesis and in the therapy of peptic disease. These factors have included the mucus and bicarbonate microenvironment at the epithelial surface, the mechanisms of mucosal restitution and surface epithelial cell renewal, the microvascular circulation of the mucosa, and several biochemical, hormonal, and growth factor-like agents that foster mucosal preservation, repair, and renewal. The field of mucosal protection or cytoprotection and the concepts that have arisen from these investigations have provided a new focus of investigation and have added exciting new concepts and working hypotheses to the field of peptic disease. The more recent discovery of the association between colonization of the gastric mucosa with *Helicobacter pylori* and peptic disease has also served to decrease the preoccupation of physicians with acid secretion.

In parallel with the renewed focus on factors other than acid secretion in the genesis of peptic disease, attention has also focused on new therapeutic compounds that may work by mechanisms other than neutralizing acid or suppressing acid secretion. These new series of compounds include sucralfate, prostaglandins, growth factors, cytokines, and antibiotics. The first of this series of compounds to become clinically available was the drug sucralfate.

Sucralfate is a sulfated aluminum salt of sucrose which has little to no acid neutralizing capacity and does not affect acid secretion. The drug was developed in Japan as part of an extensive investigation of short polymers of sucrose. Using animal models of peptic disease, sucralfate was found to promote the healing of experimental ulcers without affecting acid secretion and without systemic absorption. It decreased the activity of pepsin and demonstrated preferential binding to ulcerated surfaces of the stomach. In the initial clinical trials in Japan the drug was found to be safe, devoid of systemic side effects, and as effective as any other agent in the therapy of peptic disease.

Additional excitement about sucralfate was generated when it was discovered that the drug stimulates the synthesis and release of mucosal prostaglandins. In addition, sucralfate was found to require mucosal prostaglandins for its protective action against mucosal injury since its protective activity could be abolished by the preadministration of indomethacin which abolishes the synthesis of mucosal prostaglandins. More recently, sucralfate has also been found to interact with growth factors in the mucosa, opening a new avenue to the understanding of the mechanisms of actions of sucralfate. Also, sucralfate has been shown to be effective in enhancing mucosal circulation and protecting the mucosal microvasculature against injury.

The development of sucralfate, its delineation as a nonsystemic agent capable of successfully treating peptic disease, and its evolving exploration as to the mechanisms of its action demonstrate the great value of international cooperation in the development and exploration of new pharmaceutical agents. In addition, sucralfate was the first drug to clearly demonstrate that agents not having an effect on acid concentration in the stomach can and do have a major role in the therapy of peptic disease. Thus, the clinical experience with sucralfate demonstrates clearly that factors other than acid play a major role in the pathogenesis of peptic disease and that agents that can manipulate factors other than acid secretion are successful in the therapy of peptic disease.

In this book, investigators from many countries have contributed to an elegant summary of our present understanding of peptic disease in general and of the role of sucralfate in peptic disease therapy in particular. Research topics and ideas from the laboratory are presented alongside data from clinical trials and the practice of medicine. Some chapters delineate well-established findings from the laboratory or from patient trials. Other chapters explore areas that are only beginning to be understood and may well form the basis of future investigations in the laboratory or in the clinical arena. Thus, the book attempts to bring together the history of the development of this pharmaceutical compound, its currently known mechanisms of action, the data about its clinical efficacy, and some future directions for research in this exciting and interesting area of gastroenterology and gastrointestinal physiology. The book attempts to bridge the gap between the basic scientists working in their laboratories and clinicians treating patients. Sucralfate serves to form the bridge between these two arenas and should continue to be the nidus of future discoveries in gastrointestinal pathophysiology.

Daniel Hollander
Guido N. J. Tytgat

Kansas City and Amsterdam

Contents

Part I: Introduction

Part II: General Approach to Peptic Disease Therapy

Chapter 3

Ulcer Healing by Strengthening of Mucosal Defense: An Alternative Approach to Inhibition of Acid Secretion

A. Tarnawski

Chapter 4

History of the Development of Sucralfate

Akira Ishimori

Part III: Sucralfate: A Nonsystemic Site Protective Agent

Chapter 5

Chemistry of Sucralfate

Kiyoshige Ochi

Chapter 6

Binding of Bile Acids by Sucralfate

W. F. Caspary

Part IV: Mechanisms of Action of Sucralfate

Chapter 7

Binding of Sucralfate to the Mucosal Surface

Gerald P. Morris

Chapter 8

Stimulation of Mucus Production

Clifford Tasman-Jones

Chapter 9

Gastroduodenal Bicarbonate Secretion and Its Response to Sucralfate

W. D. W. Rees

Chapter 10

Effect of Sucrose Octasulfate on Isolated Gastric Cells

Michael R. Lucey and Tadataka Yamada

Chapter 11

Effect on Gastric Surfactant

Brian A. Hills

Chapter 12

Stimulation of Mucosal Prostaglandins by Sucralfate

Daniel Rachmilewitz

Chapter 16

Sucralfate: Role of Endogenous Sulfhydryls and Basic Fibroblast Growth Factor (bFGF)

Sandor Szabo, Judah Folkman, Y. Shing, Stefano Kusstatscher, Zsuzsa Sandor, and Miki Nagata

Chapter 17

Effects of Sucralfate on Growth Factor Availability

Stanislaw J. Konturek, Jan W. Konturek, Tomasz Brzozowski, Bronislaw L. Slomiany, and Amelia Slomiany

Chapter 18

Duodenal Ulcer Therapy, "Acid Rebound," and Early Relapse

I. N. Marks and G. O. Young

Chapter 19

Effect of Sucralfate on Experimental Ulcers

Susumu Okabe, Yoshiyasu Ogihara, and Hiroyuki Koba

Chapter 20

Effect on Experimental Esophageal Injury

Roy Charles Orlando

Part V: Safety and Drug Interactions

Chapter 21

Safety of Sucralfate

David R. Mathews and Nicola G. Dahl

Chapter 22

Sucralfate Drug Interaction Studies

Gilles Caillé and Manon Vézina

Part VI: Sucralfate and Therapy of Peptic Disease

Part VII: The Preventive Use of Sucralfate

Chapter 33

Future Clinical Development of Sucralfate

G. N. J. Tytgat

I

Introduction

1

Pathophysiology of Peptic Ulcer Disease

F. HALTER

Introduction

Much progress has been achieved in recent years on the understanding of the pathophysiology of peptic ulcer disease (PUD), but a single factor explaining why ulcers occur has not been found. New developments have evolved in waves concentrated on phenomena only partly responsible for the development of peptic ulcers. Every surge has brought new insight but tended to absorb a disproportionate amount of research efforts on mechanisms that can only partially explain the disease. This critique is particularly focused on studies devoted to the role of gastric acid and pepsin, if one considers that the majority of ulcer patients do not secrete excessive amounts of this "aggressive" secretory product. Similarly, the concept of "cytoprotection," albeit of importance, has created a considerable amount of confusion because many have confounded phenomena involved in protection against noxious agents with the considerably more complex field of development and healing of peptic ulcers. The concept of protection has nevertheless helped to better understand the important role of nonsteroidal anti-inflammatory drugs (NSAIDs) in drug-induced ulcer disease. Similarly small is the harvest from the impressive knowledge that has accumulated in recent years on gastrointestinal hormones. The advent of *Helicobacter pylori* is regarded as the breakthrough for the understanding of PUD because the large majority of ulcer patients harbor this infective agent in their stomachs and especially since new therapeutic options have emerged from this discovery. This should, however, not deviate from the fact that the majority of *H. pylori* carriers never develop PUD.

The concept is still valid that a disturbed equilibrium between aggressive and protective factors is responsible for development of peptic ulcers. The interplay between

F. HALTER • Gastrointestinal Unit, Inselspital, University Hospital, Bern, Switzerland.

Sucralfate: From Basic Science to the Bedside, edited by Daniel Hollander and G. N. J. Tytgat. Plenum Press, New York, 1995.

the two phenomena is, however, very complex and this is particularly well exemplified by the profound effect *H. pylori* exerts on both sides of the equation.

Definition

A peptic ulcer is a focal mucosal defect with inflammatory cell infiltration and coagulation necrosis extending through the muscularis mucosae. By contrast, an erosion is a superficial focal lesion characterized by erythema and hemorrhage not extending beyond the boundaries of epithelial structures. Peptic ulcers tend to occur within the section of the gastrointestinal tract that is in contact with gastric juice containing acid and pepsin. Beyond the ligament of Treitz they are only observed in patients suffering from the Zollinger–Ellison syndrome or in postsurgical conditions where unneutralized acid has access to that section of the intestine. Occasionally peptic ulcers are found within the acid-secreting mucosa of the Meckel's diverticulum.

The predilection sites for ulcers are the vicinity of mucosal junctions such as the transitional zone between esophageal and gastric mucosa, the corpus–antral and the gastroduodenal junction. PUD is commonly associated with different types of gastritis. This particularly affects the gastric antrum in patients suffering from duodenal ulcer disease (DU) and tends to extend toward the gastric corpus in patients suffering from gastric ulcer disease (GU). In general, gastritis is more extended the closer the ulcer is located to the cardia. It is now generally accepted that colonization by the bacterium *H. pylori* is causatively related to gastritis associated with PUD.[1,2]

PUD is in general a chronic and recurrent disease and ulcers usually tend to recur at the same site. They may occasionally be confounded with ulcers caused by nonacidic peptic disorders such as Crohn's disease, carcinoma, lymphoma, and sarcoma.

Epidemiology

The 1-year prevalence of PUD amounts to 1 to 2% in the adult population, the lifetime prevalence to 5 to 10%. In recent decades the incidence of DU has decreased while that of GU is stable with a tendency to slightly increase.[3] The latter phenomenon is probably related to the large consumption of NSAIDs. The decrease of DU prevalence started long before the advent of modern acid blockers. Despite the large progress in ulcer therapy, the frequency of complications such as gastric hemorrhage and perforation is stable and rather tends to increase in GU.[3]

Pathogenic Factors of Major Importance

Role of Gastric Acidity

With the advent of the Schwarz dictum "no acid, no ulcer" in 1910, particularly strong attention has been given over many decades to the role of gastric acid in the pathogenesis of PUD. This statement has been corroborated in recent years through the development of potent acid inhibitors such as histamine-H_2-receptor antagonists (H_2RAs) and H^+,K^+-ATPase or proton pump inhibitors (PPIs) with their potential to heal almost all ulcers. Moreover, through these novel drugs important new information has become available on regulation of acid secretion by endocrine, neural, and paracrine pathways. Dysregulation of acid secretion as observed in PUD affects the entire profile of acid secretion such as basal acid output (BAO), maximum acid output (MAO), sensitivity of the parietal cell to exogenous and endogenous stimuli, nocturnal and food-stimulated acid secretion, and a disturbed feedback of antral acidity on gastrin release and gastric acid secretion.[4]

Increase in Maximum Acid Secretory Capacity

Gastric acid activates the inactive pepsinogen produced in the chief cells of the gastric glands into its active form pepsin and the acid/pepsin mixture can promote ulceration through localized self-digestion of the mucosa. In general, patients suffering from DU have an increased parietal cell mass. This observation was first made in a postmortem study on DU patients.[5] Their MAO as measured by the augmented histamine test or the pentagastrin test is directly correlated to the volume of the parietal cell mass. MAO thus reflects parietal cell mass.[6] The concept of the parietal cell mass has indeed revolutionized the understanding of the role of acid in DU disease. The enlarged parietal cell mass was soon linked with the hormone gastrin because this peptide exerts trophic effects on the gastric corpus mucosa and because patients suffering from a gastrinoma (Zollinger–Ellison syndrome) have a substantially enlarged parietal cell mass in conjunction with a particularly aggressive PUD. It was soon noted, however, that only one-third of DU patients have an unequivocal increase in parietal cell mass while this is either normal or decreased in patients suffering from GU and that fasting plasma gastrin is generally normal in DU patients.[7] Only the postprandial gastrin release is slightly exaggerated, when compared with that of healthy subjects. Duodenal ulcers are, however, only occasionally observed in patients with peak acid outputs below 15 mM/hr. This contrasts with patients suffering from GU where peptic ulcers are often found below this threshold and occasionally with acid output values close to zero.[8,9]

Increased Basal Acid Secretion

From all secretory parameters, BAO shows the highest intraindividual variation in health and disease. The amount of acid secreted under fasting conditions is determined by the interaction of the parietal cell mass with hormonal, paracrine, and neural stimulants. In DU patients BAO is in general elevated as a function of an increased parietal cell mass. Basal secretory drive is defined as the ratio of BAO to MAO. In general this factor reflects basal vagal tone. BAO can also rise because of marked hypergastrinemia and a ratio between BAO and MAO greater than 0.6 should raise the suspicion of the presence of a gastrinoma. The overlap between BAO values of healthy subjects and patients suffering from PUD is particularly large and several studies suggest that only 10–20% of all DU patients have elevated BAO levels. In GU BAO levels are generally low and only rarely elevated.[9]

Increased Nocturnal Acidity

Much importance was paid to measurement of nocturnal acid secretion and elevated values were given almost pathognomonic significance in DU patients in the years between 1935 and 1948. It was later denied that extension of measurements of basal acid secretion from the standard 1-hr test to measurements over the entire 12-hr nighttime period would contribute to reduce the overlap between values of DU patients and healthy subjects.[10] Therapeutic trials with H_2RAs have reactivated the interest in nocturnal acidity since it was demonstrated that in DU disease the healing velocity of any preparation correlates best with the percentage of its suppressive effect on nocturnal acidity.[11]

Increased Sensitivity to Gastric Secretagogues

From dose–response studies using pentagastrin as a stimulant it was established that the response curve of patients with DU is shifted to the left of that of normal subjects.[12] This indicates a greater sensitivity of the parietal cell to the respective stimulant, a phenomenon that could be explained by an upregulation of the secretory receptor of the parietal cell. The question is currently at debate whether this phenomenon is related to the exaggerated gastrin response found in DU patients, even though, in general, prolonged application of a hormonal stimulus leads to downregulation of its receptor. New technology and especially the availability of reliable gastrin receptor assays may soon resolve the questions whether DU patients have an increase in the number of gastrin receptors per unit parietal cell or whether this alteration is related to second messengers. An alternative explanation of the enhanced gastrin sensitivity comes from a defect in inhibitory pathways regulated by antral somatostatin. The pathogenic significance of changes in gastrin sensitivity in DU disease should, however, not be overestimated since gastrin ED_{50} values of DU patients representing an index for gastrin sensitivity, considerably overlap with those of healthy subjects[13] (Fig. 1).

Increased Food-Stimulated Acid Secretion

Food intake results in a submaximal acid secretion well proportionate to the peak values obtained with maximum doses of gastric secretagogues. Both the peak meal-stimulated acid response and the duration of the response have been reported to be greater in a fraction of DU patients.[14] This could be related to both the increase in parietal cell mass and/or the increased sensitivity of the parietal cells to endogenous gastrin. The prolonged postprandial acid output results in acid secretion that outlasts the time food is available for buffering and results in an increased duodenal acid load. An additional explanation for the increased postcibal acid secretion is a defect in the ability of low antral pH levels to inhibit gastrin release. The latter phenomenon may be related to defective somatostatin release from antral D cells, and has recently been linked to *H. pylori* colonization.[15]

In addition, a decreased duodenal bicarbonate secretion reported in DU patients may contribute to the excessive duodenal acidification.

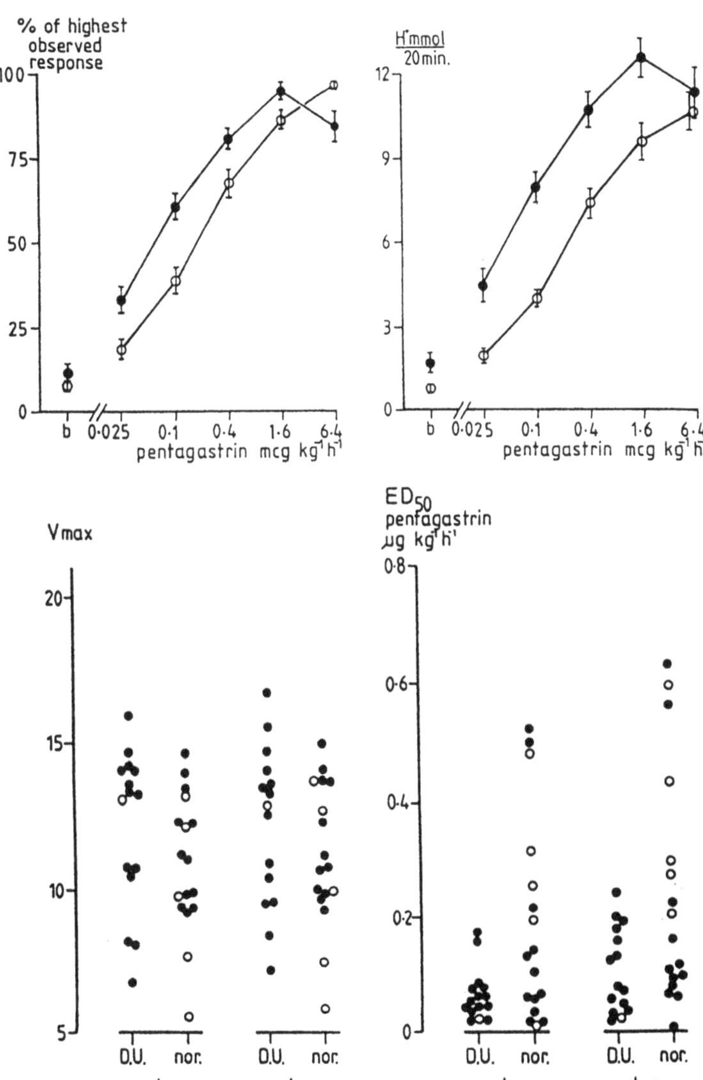

Figure 1. Upper panels: Pentagastrin dose–response results in 17 healthy subjects and 15 duodenal ulcer patients. ○, healthy subjects; ●, DU patients. Lower panels: V_{max} and ED_{50} values in 15 duodenal ulcer patients (D.U.) and 17 healthy subjects (nor.). ●, male subjects, ○, female subjects. n.b.c., non-basal corrected; b.c., basal corrected. V_{max} represents the calculated maximum response to pentagastrin, the ED_{50} values the sensitivity of the parietal cell to the respective peptide. (From Halter F, *et al*: *Scand J Gastroenterol* **17**:539, 1982.)

Disturbed Gastroduodenal Motility

Several studies have reported an accelerated emptying of liquid gastric contents in DU patients.[16] Similar to findings obtained with the acid secretory pattern, emptying rates overlap considerably between DU patients and healthy subjects. The delay may be related to a defective feedback from the duodenal mucosa, whereby intraduodenal acid, fat, and glucose normally inhibit gastric emptying. In GU patients gastric emptying has either been found to be delayed or normal.

Duodenogastric reflux has been held responsible by many as a pathogenic factor for the development of GU. Since this phenomenon occurs commonly in normals, it is unlikely that it plays a crucial role in the pathogenesis of ulcer disease.[17]

Defective Mucosal Defense

The notion that peptic ulcers can only develop when mucosal defense is defective is crucial for the understanding of the pathogenic mechanisms in PUD, even though it is mainly supported by indirect evidence. A particularly important argument comes from the observation that not all patients suffering from Zollinger–Ellison syndrome develop peptic ulcers and that GUs are particularly rare in this syndrome, despite excessive acid production. The mechanisms underlying mucosal protection are multifactorial and include preepithelial and epithelial factors and mucosal blood flow. Prostaglandins play an important role in several of these mechanisms, but it is now well established that mucosal defense can also be activated when prostaglandin synthesis is fully suppressed, e.g., antacids have been shown to retain their protective properties, when prostaglandin synthesis is totally suppressed by indomethacin.[18] It is also of importance to emphasize in this context that mucosal protection cannot be directly translated into acceleration of ulcer healing.

Defective Mucosal Blood Flow

The focal nature of peptic ulcers could best be explained by local ischemia. Many ordinary mucosal gastric arteries have been shown to be functional end-arteries and relatively short time compression of these vessels can produce ulceration.[19] The mucosal blood flow, as measured by reflectance spectrophotometry, which measures relative blood flow, has been shown to be significantly reduced in the antral region of patients suffering from GU and this has been confirmed using the hydrogen clearance method, which measures the absolute blood flow.[20,21] Thus, a generalized decrease in gastric mucosal blood flow and a localized ischemia may be implicated in the pathogenesis of GU but it is questionable whether this applies also to DU.

Role of H. pylori

H. pylori, Gastritis, Duodenitis, and Peptic Ulcer

Virtually all DU patients have antral gastritis which is associated with the almost ubiquitous gastric antral infestation with *H. pylori* in this subset of PUD.[22] In GU disease,

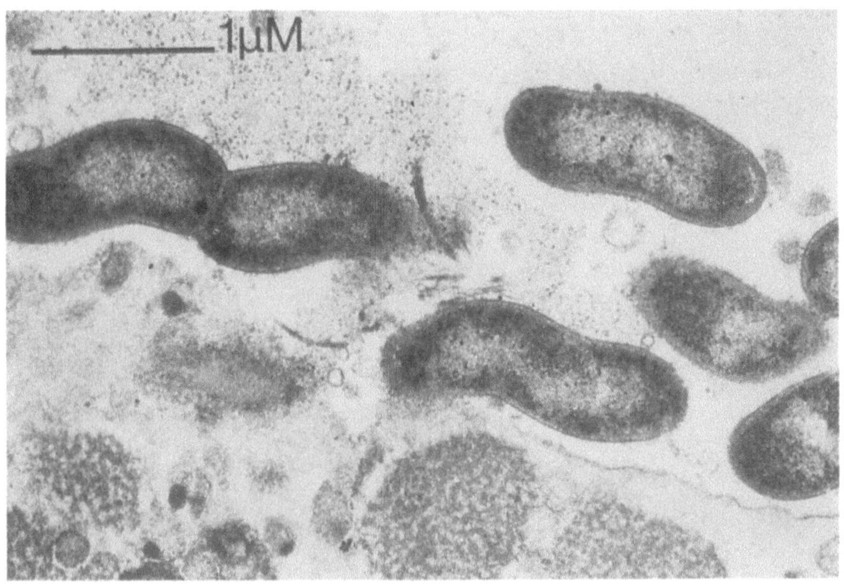

Figure 13.1. *Helicobacter pylori* ultrastructure.

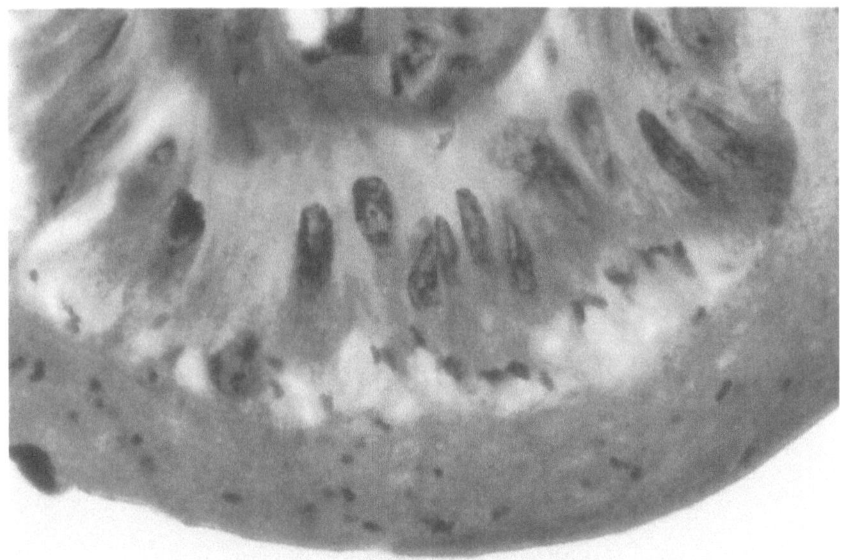

Figure 13.2. *H. pylori* in the mucus layer covering the epithelial cells.

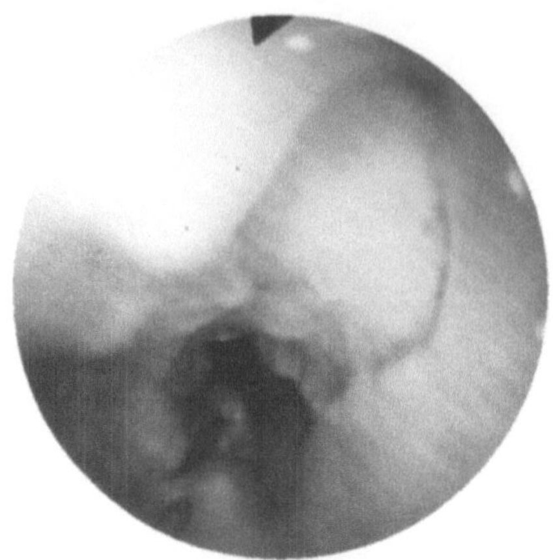

Figure 31.1. Large postsclerotherapy ulceration.

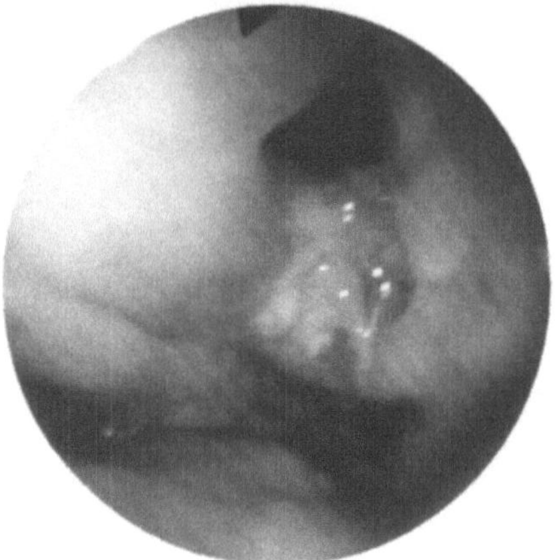

Figure 31.2. Esophageal perforation following variceal sclerotherapy.

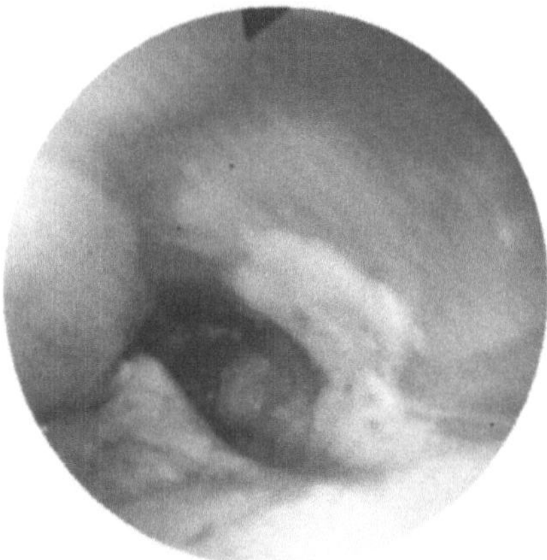

Figure 31.3. Sucralfate coating of postsclerotherapy esophageal ulcerations.

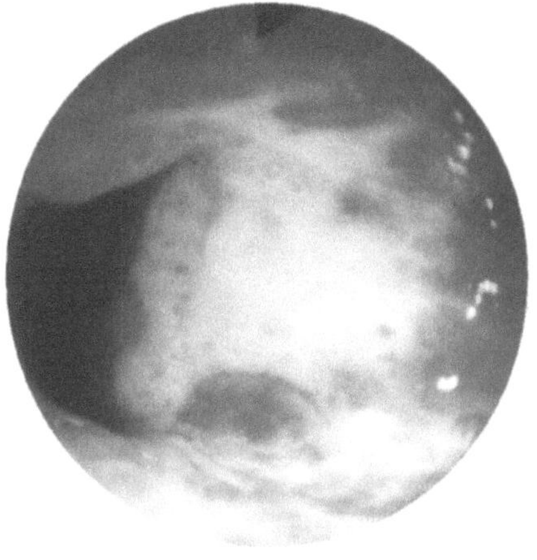

Figure 33.1. Distal rectal postradiation ulceration, selectively coated with sucralfate suspension (2 g/20 ml).

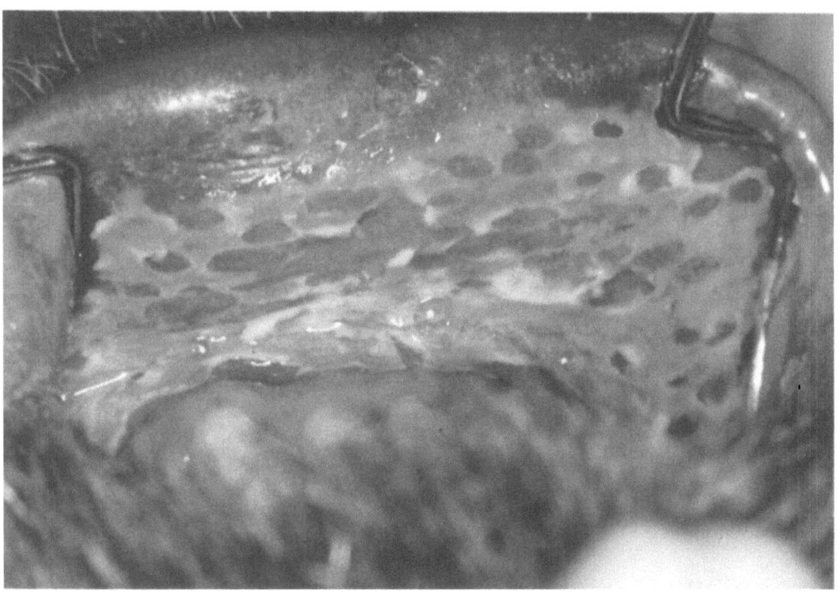

Figure 33.2. Severe oral chemotherapy-induced mucositis.

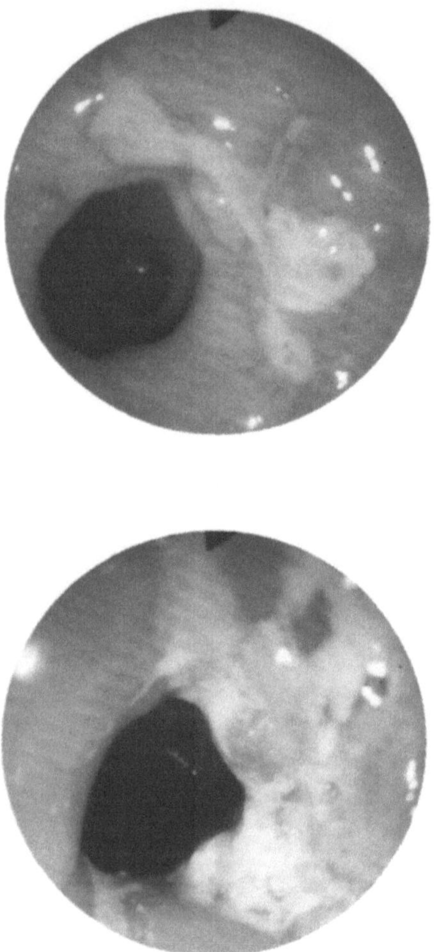

Figure 33.3. Solitary ulcer of the rectum. Coating with sucralfate suspension (p 1 h) 2 g/20 ml enemas.

gastritis is generally more severe and extends from the antrum to the gastric corpus. *H. pylori* colonization is not unequivocally found in GU but some 70–80% patients are infested. When NSAID-induced gastric ulcers are excluded, then over 90% of GU are accompanied by *H. pylori* colonization.

Considerable knowledge has recently accumulated on the mechanisms by which *H. pylori* induces gastritis. *H. pylori* is generally not considered to be an invasive bacterium although occasionally bacteria can be demonstrated within gastric mucosal cells. The vigorous local cellular and humoral immune response suggests, however, that *H. pylori* material gains access to the immune system. Several initiating factors appear to be involved. Release of soluble surface constituents can provoke pepsinogen release from gastric chief cells or trigger local inflammation in the underlying tissue. *H. pylori*'s own urease can recruit inflammatory cells and lead to activation of inflammatory cells. Release of cytokines, such as tumor necrosis factor alpha, interleukins 1 and 6, and oxygen radicals lead to further tissue inflammation accompanied by a potent systemic IgA- and IgG-type immune response.[23] Chronic inflammation and antigens on glandular epithelial cells result in a progressive destruction with loss of the epithelial barrier function. Moreover, it has been postulated that *H. pylori* infection favors backdiffusion of hydrogen ions with subsequent breakdown of the mucosal barrier through alteration in the composition of the mucus glycoprotein. There are indications that the hyperacidity in DU patients induces gastric metaplasia in the duodenal bulb which represents a target for *H. pylori* colonization and ultimately ulcer formation. Most DU patients have foci of gastric metaplasia.[24] *H. pylori* favors the presence of intragastric acid and is generally not found in patients suffering from pernicious anemia. Obviously *H. pylori* needs acid for ulcerogenesis.

The crucial argument that *H. pylori* is actively involved in ulcerogenesis stems from the observations that eradication of the bacterium resolves chronic active gastritis and tends to keep duodenal ulcers healed for up to several years, provided no reinfection occurs.[1,25] The almost compulsory association of *H. pylori* infection with DU disease contrasts fundamentally with the abnormalities of the gastric acid profiles which are only shared by a minority of DU subjects. *H. pylori* is thus considered by many as the highest risk factor in DU disease.

H. pylori, Pepsinogen, Gastrin, and Somatostatin

It is long established that some of the pepsinogen produced by the chief cells of the mucosal glands of the gastric corpus leaks into the plasma and that DU patients have in general elevated plasma pepsinogen I levels.[26] This has recently been linked to *H. pylori* colonization, since plasma pepsinogen levels are at least partly reversible following eradication of *H. pylori*.[27] Similarly, the exaggerated plasma gastrin release of subjects infested with *H. pylori* is normalized once this infective agent is eliminated. The enhanced gastrin release may well result from a disinhibited release of this peptide through a defective somatostatin release since antral somatostatin stores or somatostatin cell density have been reported to be decreased in DU patients. Of special interest are recent observations that in DU patients *H. pylori* colonization induces a reduced somatostatin mRNA expression in D cells, which is reversible once *H. pylori* is eradicated.[15] This could putatively explain both the disinhibited acid secretion and the exaggerated gastrin response in DU disease and, with the known trophic effects of gastrin, possibly also the enhancement of the number of parietal cells and even the upregulation of the receptors of these cells to acid secretory stimulants. This hypothesis is indirectly supported by some studies in which a decrease of acid secretion was observed following *H. pylori* eradication, but this observation has not been confirmed by others. Inhomogeneity of patient groups could well account for the inconsistency of the results (for review see Ref. 7). There is some indication that more acid is secreted in active ulcers as compared with quiescent ulcer disease and that healing with H_2RA treatment produces a short-lived acid rebound, possibly through upregulation of the gastrin receptor.[28] It can thus not be excluded that acid secretion has been modified in some of the patients independently of the *H. pylori* eradication. At the time being the unifying hypothesis that *H. pylori* directly causes peptic ulcers through combined enhancement of acid secretion and breakdown of mucosal protection still contains speculative elements. Indeed the most crucial argument against the dominant role of *H. pylori* in the pathogenesis of this disease stems from the observation that no more than 10–20% of *H. pylori*-infected subjects develop peptic ulcers. Whether or not *H. pylori*-infected patients develop peptic ulcers appears to depend on several factors such as adherence to the gastric surface epithelium, virulence of the *H. pylori* strain, the defense reaction of the individual host, and the age at infection.[29] *H. pylori* attachment to human gastric mucosa is now reported to be mediated by the Lewis^b (Le^b) blood group antigens with fucose at the end of the branched carbohydrate chain.[29a] Gastric tissue lacking Le^b expression or exposure to antibodies for the Le^b antigen results in failure of bacterial bindings.[29b] The affinity of *H. pylori* to Le^b antigens (part of the blood group antigens determining the blood group O) could explain the 1.5 to 2 times higher prevalence of ulcers in people with blood group O. Diversity among *H. pylori* strains is thought to contribute to variability in diseases associated with *H. pylori* infection. Expression of a vacuolating toxin,[29c] production of the Cag A product,[29c] and enhanced activation of neutrophils[29d] are claimed to be bacterial markers for enhanced inflammatory response and peptic ulceration. The age of onset of infection appears to determine the development and intensity of gastritis. *H. pylori* infection in early childhood usually results in advanced atrophic gastritis, gradually reducing the parietal cell mass and preventing DU disease but predisposing to GU and ultimately to gastric cancer. It is well established that severe atrophic gastritis is negatively associated with *H. pylori* because the nonacidic gastric milieu becomes inhospitable to the organism. It appears that individuals with a naturally high acid secretory capacity are relatively resistant to *H. pylori* infection. When infection occurs in hypersecretors the infection is primarily confined to the antrum without or only slow progress toward the gastric corpus and those patients are particularly at risk in developing DU disease.[2,29] In most patients infected with *H. pylori*, infection becomes resilient after a short time and does not lead to progressive destruction of mucosal architecture.

Role of NSAIDs

Aspirin and NSAIDs damage gastric mucosa through local and systemic factors.[30,31] The superficial lesions following topical application are of limited significance, since they usually disappear despite continuation of the therapy. The ulcerogenic effect is most likely attributable to the systemic inhibition of prostaglandin synthesis, since it is not abolished by application of NSAIDs in enteric-coated capsules, prodrugs, or following rectal application.

Epidemiological data leave no doubt that aspirin and related substances are a risk for development of GU and less so for DU. GU is 10- to 20-fold increased in patients who have an aspirin intake of more than 1 g. The risk is smaller in subjects taking NSAIDs such as indomethacin or ibuprofen but is still 2- to 3-fold elevated. NSAID-associated GU appear to be prevented more effectively by cotherapy with prostaglandin analogues than by agents whose effects are only antisecretory.

Based on rather weak evidence it has been postulated that *H. pylori* and NSAIDs are uncomfortable partners (for review, see refs. 32, 32a). In a clinical trial of patients with dyspepsia, however, the use of NSAIDs did not lead to any aggravated damage of the gastric mucosa, even though it had a negative influence on the symptom score.[32b] Development of gastric and duodenal ulcers during chronic NSAID therapy was not found to be influenced by the *H. pylori* status in two controlled studies.[32c,32d] According to these clinical data, NSAIDs appear not to significantly aggravate the mucosal damage inferred by *H. pylori*. Definitive proof of these observations awaits prospective treatment studies and studies on pathogenetic models looking at interactions of both these factors.

Role of Smoking

DU are twice as common in smokers; by contrast, the association between smoking and peptic ulcer is less well established in GU.[33] Smoking has a negative impact both on healing and on ulcer recurrence. In many studies with H_2RAs the prophylactic effect of the medication was fully abolished by smoking.

Additional Factors

Genetic Factors

Familial clustering is well recognized in DU disease. Elevated serum pepsinogen I levels and acid hypersecretion have been described in some DU patients with familial hyperpepsinogenemia I.[34] Recent reevaluation of these sera has revealed that 80% of the subjects with hyperpepsinogenemia have *H. pylori* antibody and it appears more likely that the *H. pylori* colonization is the common denominator. Moreover, hyperpepsinogenemia tends to disappear after *H. pylori* eradication.[27]

Stress, Alcohol

There is very little evidence available that psychological stress or alcohol abuse are causative factors in PUD even though this view is widely accepted both by laypeople and by large sections of the medical profession. Progress in the field of stress and ulcer disease has been hampered by the difficulties in assessing stress itself and the response to stress.

Conclusion

The dictum of Schwarz, "no acid, no ulcer," is still valid and may well, at least in DU disease, be expanded today to "no acid and *H. pylori*, no ulcer." However, since neither acid nor *H. pylori* are sufficient for ulcerogenesis, it is not justified to unconditionally attribute a causative role to either factor. Gastric acid represents a well-defined permissive factor and this also applies for NSAID medication. The role of *H. pylori* is clearly more dominant since its eradication is the only known measure that can cure DU disease without an operation. There is little evidence that many additional factors, long regarded as crucial for development of PUD such as genetic predisposition, psychological stress, and alcohol intake, play a significant role in comparison with the triad acid, *H. pylori* infection, and NSAID medication, but smoking remains an established risk factor. Despite all of the important recent new discoveries, the time has not yet come to remove the black box from its central position within the model of the etiopathogenesis of PUD.

References

1. Rauws EAJ, Langenberg W, Houthoff HJ, *et al*: Campylobacter pyloridis-associated chronic active antral gastritis: A prospective study of its prevalence and the effects of antibacterial and anticulcer treatment. *Gastroenterology* **94:**33–40, 1988. This study showed a strong correlation between chronic active gastritis and the presence of *H. pylori*. It was outlined for the first time that *H. pylori* eradication can improve the gastric mucosa, thus supporting evidence for a true cause–effect relationship in *H. pylori* colonization and chronic active gastritis.
2. Graham DY: Campylobacter pylori and peptic ulcer disease. *Gastroenterology* **96:**615–625, 1989. This study well defines the central role of *H. pylori* in the pathogenesis of duodenal ulcer disease.
3. Sonnenberg A: Geographic and temporal variations in the occurrence of peptic ulcer disease. *Scand J Gastroenterol* **20**(suppl 110):11, 1985. This overview outlines variations in peptic ulcer occurrence between different countries and different age groups. The author suggests that a cohort phenomenon is responsible for the gradual decline of prevalence of peptic ulcer disease.
4. Soll AH: Pathogenesis of peptic ulcer and implications for therapy. *N Engl J Med* **322:**909–916, 1990. In this review the pathogenetic mechanisms of peptic ulcer disease are critically outlined. Special attention is given to the role of mucosal defense factors and the dysregulation of gastric acid secretion.
5. Cox AJ: Stomach size and its relation to chronic peptic ulcer. *AMA Arch Pathol* **54:**407, 1952. The author presents for the first time evidence, based on autopsy studies, that patients with active or healed duodenal ulcers have in general an enlarged stomach with an increased parietal cell mass.
6. Card WI, Marks IN: The relationship between the acid output of the stomach following "maximal" histamine stimulation and parietal cell mass. *Clin Sci* **19:**147–163, 1960. This study showed for the first time that the "maximum acid output" of the human stomach is quantitatively related to the total number of parietal cells. This conclusion was made by measuring maximum acid output before and after partial gastrectomy and relating the difference to the number of parietal cells established by morphometric methodology in the gastric resection specimen.
7. Halter F, Wilder-Smith CH: Gastrin: Friend or foe of peptic ulcer? *J Clin Gastroenterol* **13**(suppl 1):S75–S82, 1991. Gastrin can be regarded as an aggressive or a defensive factor in the pathogenesis of peptic ulcer disease. The aggressive role stems from its regulatory function in acid secretion, the defensive role is based on its trophic function. Both factors are reviewed in detail in this overview.

8. Wormsley KG, Grossman MI: Maximal histalog test in control subjects and patients with peptic ulcer. *Gut* **6**:427–435, 1965. In this fundamental study it was shown for the first time that maximal acid output as induced by histalog considerably overlaps between healthy subjects and the wide spectrum of peptic ulcer disease. This observation was regarded as a potent argument against the dominant role of an increase in parietal cell mass in the pathogenesis of peptic ulcer disease.
9. Baron JH: Pathophysiology of gastric acid secretion, in Domschke W, Wormsley KG (eds): *Magen- und Magenkrankheiten*. Stuttgart, Georg Thieme Verlag, 1981, pp 131–149. Excellent review on value and limitations of measurements of acid output for study of patients suffering from peptic ulcer disease. For the first time threshold values are given below which duodenal ulcers are most unlikely to be encountered.
10. Grossman MI: Dragstedt editorial on gastric acid secretion tests. *Gastroenterology* **53**:681, 1967. In this comment Grossman questions the rationale of measuring basal acid secretion during the nocturnal period as long proposed by Dragstedt and postulates that results obtained with this demanding technique are of no more value than measurement of 1-hr basal secretion.
11. Jones DB, Howden CW, Burget DW, *et al*: Acid suppression in duodenal ulcer: A meta-analysis to define optimal dosing with antisecretory drugs. *Gut* **28**:1120–1127, 1987. In this meta-analysis study a high correlation was observed between duodenal ulcer healing rates obtained within 4 weeks and the suppression of nocturnal hydrogen ion activity.
12. Isenberg JI, Grossman MI, Maxwell V, *et al*: Increased sensitivity to stimulation of acid secretion by pentagastrin in duodenal ulcer. *J Clin Invest* **55**:330–337, 1975. In this study evidence was put forward for the first time that the sensitivity of parietal cells of DU patients to gastrin is higher than in control subjects.
13. Halter F, Bangerter U, Haecki WH, *et al*: Sensitivity of the parietal cell to pentagastrin in health and duodenal ulcer disease: A reappraisal. *Scand J Gastroenterol* **17**:539–544, 1982. This study confirms the enhanced sensitivity of the parietal cells of DU patients to gastrin, but outlines a great overlap between DU patients and healthy controls.
14. Soll AH: Duodenal ulcer and drug therapy, in Sleisenger MH, Fordtran JS (eds): *Gastrointestinal Disease: Pathophysiology, Diagnosis, Management*, Philadelphia, WB Saunders, 1990, pp 814–879. This overview discusses the controversial findings of the disturbances of meal-stimulated acid secretion observed in peptic ulcer disease.
15. Moss SF, Legon S, Bishop AE, *et al*: Effect of Helicobacter pylori on gastric somatostatin in duodenal ulcer disease. *Lancet* **340**:930–932, 1992. In this study somatostatin gene expression was shown to be decreased in DU patients and recovered following *H. pylori* eradication. This indicates that in DU disease gastric secretory function is disinhibited through the decreased expression of mucosal somatostatin.
16. Malagelada JR, Longstreth GF, Deering TB, *et al*: Gastric secretion and emptying after ordinary meals in duodenal ulcer. *Gastroenterology* **73**:989–994, 1977. In this study gastric emptying was measured with a sophisticated technique that allows simultaneous measurement of acid secretion and gastric emptying. It was shown that gastric secretory response to meals in DU disease is prolonged with abnormal high-rate delivery into the duodenum.
17. Müller-Lissner SA, Fimmel CJ, Sonnenberg A, *et al*: Novel approach to quantify duodenogastric reflux in healthy volunteers and in patients with type I gastritis. *Gut* **24**:510–518, 1983. In this study gastric emptying and duodenogastric reflux were measured with a novel technique without trans-pyloric intubation. Neither gastric emptying nor duodenogastric reflux differed between patients with type I gastric ulcer and healthy control subjects.
18. Konturek SJ, Brzozowski T, Drozdowicz D, *et al*: Role of intragastric pH in cytoprotection by antacids in rats. *Eur J Pharmacol* **176**:187–195, 1990. The gastroprotection induced by Maalox or its active component $Al(OH)_3$ requires the presence of luminal acid and this protection does not depend on the mucosal production of endogenous prostaglandins.
19. Piasecki C: Blood flow and ulceration: Localizing mechanisms and ischaemic pathogenesis, in Halter F, Garner A, Tytgat GNJ (eds): *Mechanisms of Peptic Ulcer Healing*. Dordrecht, Kluwer

Academic Publishers, 1991, pp 27–39. Experimental data are presented showing the existence of functional end-arteries in human gastric mucosa. The hypothesis is put forward that stress-induced spasms of such arteries are one of the principal factors in the development of localized peptic ulcers.

20. Kamada T, Kawano S, Sato N, *et al*: Gastric mucosal blood distribution and its changes in the healing process of gastric ulcer. *Gastroenterology* **84**:1541–1546, 1983. Measurements performed by reflectant spectrometry in 24 regions in the stomachs of 42 patients showed a decreased mucosal blood flow in the active phase of a gastric ulcer. This was normalized during the healing process.
21. Murakami M, Inada M, Miyake T, *et al*: Regional mucosal blood flow and ulcer healing, in Koo A, Lam SK, Smaje LH (eds): *Microcirculation of the Alimentary Tract*. Singapore, World Scientific Publishing Co, 1983, pp 293–302. In this study mucosal blood flow, as measured by hydrogen clearance method, was decreased in 23 patients suffering from gastric ulcers.
22. Blaser MJ: Gastric Campylobacter-like organisms, gastritis, and peptic ulcer disease. *Gastroenterology* **93**:371–383, 1987. Highly competent review article on the pathology associated with *H. pylori* infection.
23. Mai UEH, Perez-Perez GI, Wahl LM, *et al*: Soluble surface proteins from Helicobacter pylori activate monocytes/macrophages by lipopolysaccharide-independent mechanism. *J Clin Invest* **87**:894–900, 1991. In this study it is shown for the first time that *H. pylori* is capable of activating human monocytes by a lipopolysaccharide-independent mechanism.
24. Wyatt JI, Rathbone BJ, Sobala GM, *et al*: Gastric epithelium in the duodenum: Its association with Helicobacter pylori and inflammation. *J Clin Pathol* **43**:986, 1990. In this study it is proposed that inflammatory injury of the duodenal mucosa by *H. pylori* may stimulate development of further gastric metaplasia and that the area of duodenum susceptible for colonization with *H. pylori* may increase progressively and mucosal integrity is compromised and ulceration supervenes.
25. Halter F, Hürlimann S, Inauen W: Pathophysiology and clinical relevance of Helicobacter pylori. *Yale J Biol Med* **65**:625–638, 1992. Recent comprehensive review on *H. pylori* containing a broad overview on recent therapeutic modalities applied for eradication of *H. pylori*.
26. Samloff IM, Liebman WM, Panitch NM: Serum group I pepsinogens by radioimmunoassay in control subjects and patients with peptic ulcer. *Gastroenterology* **69**:83–90, 1975. This study shows that the mean pepsinogen I levels of both DU and GU patients are elevated and that the secretory potential of the fundic gland mucosa of the stomach may be reflected by the level of PG I in serum.
27. Chittajallu RS, Dorrian CA, Ardill JES, *et al*: Effect of *Helicobacter pylori* on serum pepsinogen I and plasma gastrin in duodenal ulcer patients. *Scand J Gastroenterol* **27**:20–24, 1992. In this study eradication of *H. pylori* resulted in a fall of pepsinogen I and plasma gastrin levels, indicating a causal relation between *H. pylori* infection and elevation of plasma pepsinogen I and gastrin levels.
28. Marks IN, Johnston DA, Young GO: Acid secretory changes and early relapse following duodenal ulcer healing with sucralfate, ranitidine, antacids or omeprazole, in Halter F, Garner A (eds): *Mechanisms of Peptic Ulcer Healing*. Dordrecht, Kluwer Academic Publishers, 1991, pp 273–282. In this overview it is outlined that ulcer disease-activity or treatment modalities may lead to an increase in parietal cell sensitivity and thus foster early ulcer recurrence.
29. Tytgat GNJ: Does the stomach adapt to *Helicobacter pylori*? *Scand J Gastroenterol* **27**(suppl 193):28–32, 1992. This overview supplies evidence in favor of *H. pylori* being the most important pathogenic factor in peptic ulcer disease.

29a. Borén T, Falk P, Roth KA, *et al*: Attachment of *Helicobacter pylori* to human gastric epithelium mediated by blood group antigens. *Science* **262**:1892–1895, 1993. In this very important paper evidence is put forward that the Le^b antigen mediates *H. pylori* attachment to human gastric mucosa. This supplies a tentative explanation for the increased ulcer prevalence in blood group O subjects.

29b. Cover TL, Blaser MJ: Purification and characterization of the vaculating toxin from *Helicobacter pylori*. *J Biol Chem* **267**:10570–10575, 1992. In this study it is demonstrated that in sera from *H. pylori*-infected persons there is a correlation between toxin-neutralizing activity and recognition of a M_r = 8700 protein.

29c. Crabtree JE, Taylor JD, Wyatt JI, *et al*: Mucosal GI recognition of *Helicobacter pylori* 120-kDa protein, peptic ulceration, and gastric pathology. *Lancet* **338**:332–335, 1991. In this study it was demonstrated that 120-kDa-positive strains of *H. pylori* selectively have pathogenic features associated with active gastritis and peptic ulceration.

29d. Rautelin H, Blomberg B, Fredlund H, *et al*: Incidence of *Helicobacter pylori* strains activating neutrophils in patients with peptic ulcer disease. *Gut* **34**:599–604, 1993. The authors of this study isolated *H. pylori* strains for their ability to induce an oxidative burst in human neutrophils. Strains possessing such activity were more common in patients with peptic ulcer disease than in patients with active chronic gastritis only.

30. Graham DY, Smith JL: Aspirin and the stomach. *Ann Intern Med* **104**:390–398, 1988. This study reviews possible mechanisms through which aspirin damages gastric intestinal mucosa. The authors emphasize that the extent and degree of acute mucosal injury to various NSAIDs has little or no value in predicting the frequency or severity of chronic gastric ulcer or gastrointestinal bleeding.

31. Graham DY: The relationship between nonsteroidal-antiinflammatory drug use and peptic ulcer disease. *Gastroenterol Clin North Am* **19**:171–183, 1990. Excellent overview dealing with the role of NSAID in ulcer pathogenesis.

32. MCarthy DN: *Helicobacter pylori* infection and gastroduodenal injury by nonsteroidal-anti-inflammatory drugs. *Scand J Gastroenterol* **26**(suppl 187):91–97, 1991. This paper deals with the interrelationship between *H. pylori* infection and damage induced by NSAID. The hypothesis is put forward that *H. pylori* infection may represent an additive risk factor for development of GU during NSAID therapy.

32a. Taha AS, Russell RI: *Helicobacter pylori* and non-steroidal anti-inflammatory drugs: Uncomfortable partners in peptic ulcer disease. *Gut* **34**:580–583, 1993. In this widely quoted review paper the authors supply some indirect, weak evidence for a synergistic action between *H. pylori* and NSAIDs. It is mainly based on the fact that *H. pylori* prevalence is higher in elderly subjects, where NSAID consumption is high.

32b. Goggin PM, Collins DA, Jazrawi RP, *et al*: Prevalence of *Helicobacter pylori* infection and its effect on symptoms and non-steroidal anti-inflammatory drug induced gastrointestinal damage in patients with rheumatoid arthritis. *Gut* **34**:1677–1680, 1993. The authors studied 52 patients with rheumatoid arthritis requiring long-term NSAID treatment for dyspeptic symptoms. *H. pylori* infection was associated with increased dyspeptic symptoms in patients receiving NSAIDs but did not potentiate NSAID gastropathy.

32c. Kim JG, Graham DY, The Misoprostol Study Group: *Helicobacter pylori* infection and development of gastric or duodenal ulcer in arthritic patients receiving chronic NSAID therapy. *Am J Gastroenterol* **89**:203–207, 1994. The authors prospectively evaluated development of gastric or duodenal ulcers in 181 arthritics followed for up to 3 months while receiving an NSAID chronically and with no active antiulcer medications. Stepwise logistic regression analysis indicated none of the variable factors of age, gender, alcohol consumption, type of arthritis, or *H. pylori* status were significantly associated with development of peptic ulceration.

32d. Laine L, Sloane R, Ferretti M, *et al*: The influence of *H. pylori* on gastric injury and prostaglandin concentration with NSAID therapy: A prospective double-blind evaluation. *Gastroenterology* **104**:A118, 1994. In a prospective study of 52 healthy volunteers, *H. pylori* infection did not increase the risk of developing gastric injury during 1 month of NSAID therapy.

33. Ainley CC, Forgcas JC, Keeling PW, *et al*: Outpatients endoscopic survey of smoking and peptic ulcer. *Gut* **27**:648–651, 1986. In a study on 1100 outpatients undergoing upper gastrointestinal endoscopy a dose–response effect was observed between the number of cigarettes smoked and duodenal and gastric ulceration.

34. Rotter JI, Sones JQ, Samloff IM, *et al*: Duodenal ulcer disease associated with elevated serum pepsinogen I. An inherited autosomal dominant disorder. *N Engl J Med* **300**:63–66, 1979. The hypothesis is put forward that an elevated serum pepsinogen I concentration could be a subclinical marker of the ulcer diathesis in families with an autosomal dominant form of peptic ulcer disease. This study was published before it was established that *H. pylori* infection may be the cause for enhanced release of pepsinogen I into blood circulation.

2

Decreased Intragastric Acid Concentration as an Approach to Peptic Disease Therapy

A. B. R. THOMSON

Introduction

Recent research has focused on the pathophysiology of peptic ulcer disease (Fig. 1), and this includes factors such as the changing demographics of ulcer disease, modern methods of ulcer diagnosis, natural history, and the current status of surgery in patients with peptic ulcer disease. The importance of the gastric mucosal barrier has been examined, as has the role of prostaglandins in mucosal protection in health and disease.

Why do physicians treat patients with peptic ulcer disease? The therapeutic goals should be the elimination of symptoms, ulcer healing, prevention of ulcer recurrence and complications. From the patient's perspective, the disappearance of symptoms is most important. While the duodenal hydrogen ion (H^+) load after meals is greater in patients with duodenal ulcer disease (DU) than in healthy volunteers, it is unproven that acid is the major factor in the pathogenesis of pain.

Surgery used to be performed on patients with chronic peptic ulcer disease since medical therapy was generally inadequate in past years. Medical therapy at that time was limited to antacids, ineffective dietary manipulation, and anticholinergics. Then came the family of H_2-receptor antagonists (H_2RA), the mucoprotective agents (also known as the "cytoprotective" agents), specific M_1 anticholinergics, and the H^+/K^+-ATPase proton "pump blockers." With so many medications available for the treatment of peptic disorders, has the problem of peptic ulcer disease been solved? No, since none of these agents changes the natural history of this recurrent disorder, and there are still many unanswered questions regarding the management of these patients.

A. B. R. THOMSON • Nutrition and Metabolism Research Group, Division of Gastroenterology, University of Alberta, Edmonton T6G 2C2, Canada.

Sucralfate: From Basic Science to the Bedside, edited by Daniel Hollander and G. N. J. Tytgat. Plenum Press, New York, 1995.

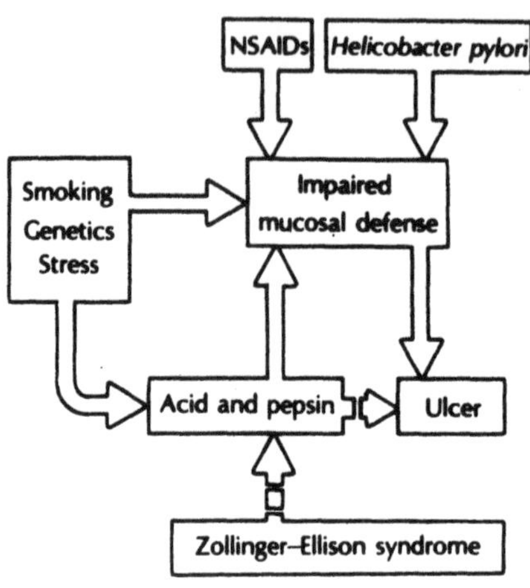

Figure 1. A model of the pathogenesis of peptic ulcer. Acid and peptic ulcer activity overpower mucosal defense to produce ulcers, most commonly when mucosal defense is impaired by exogenous factors. Two factors, nonsteroidal anti-inflammatory drugs (NSAIDS) and *Helicobacter pylori* infection, appear to be linked to the impairment of mucosal defense. The hypersecretion of gastric acid in the Zollinger–Ellison syndrome (dotted arrow) is one exception in which ulcers occur in the absence of *H. pylori* infection. In ordinary peptic ulcer disease, other risk factors are also important (e.g., smoking, genetic factors, and psychological stress), but the evidence is conflicting about whether these factors impair mucosal defense, modulate the secretion of acid, or both (reprinted from Kurata, *Curr Op Gastroenterol* **6**:894–897, 1990, with permission).

The Patient

Peptic ulcer disease is still a major health care problem. The number of patients admitted to hospitals for duodenal (DU) or gastric (GU) ulcer disease is declining, and the age-adjusted mortality rate is also falling. However, community-based studies show that the prevalence of peptic ulcer disease is remaining stable in men and is increasing in women to the point that approximately equal numbers of men and women are now developing DU. Thus, there is a shift away from patients coming to hospitals for treatment of their peptic ulcer disease and fewer patients dying of DU and GU. However, many individuals are still suffering from these disorders, and there remains a considerable morbidity from recurrent pain, and ulcer complications such as hemorrhage, obstruction, or perforation.

There are certain reasonable and prudent approaches to life-style. It is helpful to inquire about life-style, including the nature and hours of work; habits of eating, sleeping, smoking, and drinking; worries and concerns; sources of relaxation and pleasure; and hopes and aspirations. Bland diets, milk therapy, or frequent feedings do not heal ulcers, but diets may improve symptoms. Coffee, tea, juices, and alcohol may be taken in moderation, and should be avoided only if these fluids aggravate symptoms. If pain is relieved by small amounts of milk or snacks, enjoy that relief! Unless normal-sized meals cause a bloated feeling, there is no special need to ritualistically consume six small meals a day. A reasonable exercise program for purposes of general well-being is to be advised. Sedatives should not be used unless clearly indicated for health-related purposes other than dyspepsia or ulcer disease. Whenever possible, the patient should avoid aspirin-containing drugs, nonsteroidal anti-inflammatory agents (NSAIDs), and perhaps glucocorticosteroids. The patient–physician relationship is important, as the physician's sympathy for, and understanding of the patient and the patient's interpersonal relationships and current life situation are all important. Caring and compassion must continue to play a major role in the management of patients with any chronic recurrent illness.

Pathogenesis

What causes peptic ulcer disease? These conditions are likely related to an imbalance of the so-called "aggressive" and "defensive" factors. Traditional physiology focused on the cephalic, gastric, and intestinal phases of acid secretion, with the parietal cell secretion of acid being stimulated by acetylcholine, histamine, and gastrin. Now we must direct our attention to the cellular and molecular levels, with the parietal cell and/or the adjacent mast cell having receptors for gastrin, histamine-2 (H_2), and acetylcholine. Intracellular events are also important, including the influx of calcium, activation of cyclic AMP, and the final step of acid secretion, the H^+/K^+-ATPase ("proton pump").

Patients with DU may, as a group, secrete more acid than do healthy individuals (Table I). In addition, DU patients may have impaired acid-controlled inhibition of gastrin release and/or impaired mucosal defense. There are also numerous abnormalities in gastric physiology in patients with GU (Table II). The basal and peak acid output is higher in patients with quiescent DU as compared with normal subjects. When endoscopic biopsy specimens of the antrum are grown in tissue culture, basal gastrin and somatostatin secretion are less in DU than in the controls. Also, in DU, cAMP-stimulated release in response to gastrin is greater and the response to somatostatin is less than in healthy persons. This raises the possibility of disordered hormonal control of acid secretion in DU.

Approximately one-third of patients with DU have an affected family member. Subgroups of patients have been identified with rapid gastric emptying, G-cell hyperplasia or hyperfunction, or have associated genetic syndromes such as multiple endocrine

Table I. Pathophysiological Abnormalities in Duodenal Ulcer Patients[a]

- Increased parietal cell mass
- Increased sensitivity of parietal cells to secretagogues
- Increased parietal cell stimulation by increased gastrin release
- Increased numbers of antral G cells
- Decreased sensitivity of parietal cells to inhibitory factors
- Increased drive to secrete acid and pepsin
- Increased gastric emptying
- Decreased pancreatic bicarbonate secretion
- Increased duodenal acid load
- Impaired duodenal mucosal synthesis of prostaglandin

[a]Reproduced from: Mahachai V, Bedard B: Update in peptic ulcer therapy. *Med North Am* **19 March**: 3628–3642, 1988, with permission.

Table II. Pathophysiological Abnormalities in Gastric Ulcer Patients[a]

- Decreased acid secretion and increased H^+ backdiffusion
- Chronic superficial and atrophic gastritis
- Increased concentration of bile acids and pancreatic juice in stomach (duodenogastric reflux)
- Delayed gastric emptying
- Inappropriately decreased pyloric sphincter pressure under basal conditions and in response to stimuli

[a]Reproduced from: Mahachai V, Bedard B: Update in peptic ulcer therapy. *Med North Am* **19 March**:3628–3642, 1988, with permission.

neoplasia type I (pituitary, parathyroid, pancreas, pancreatic adenomas), systemic mastocytosis, or the rare tremor–nystagmus–ulcer syndrome.

Finally, environmental agents such as smoking, stress, and ethanol abuse may play a role in the development or chronicity of peptic diseases. These are factors that the patient has control over, but unfortunately all too often may ignore her/his physician's advice.

Prediction of Healing, and Problems

There is a highly significant and predictable relationship between the primary determinants of antisecretory therapy and duodenal ulcer healing,[1] namely the degree and duration of suppression of intragastric acidity and the duration of treatment (Fig. 2A,B). The optimum intragastric pH threshold to obtain 100% healing at about 4 weeks is pH 3 or above for 18–20 hr of the day (Fig. 3). A recent meta-analysis[2] has shown that DU healing not only correlates with the degree of acid suppression but also with the duration of acid suppression and the length of treatment.

If we can predict ulcer healing so well from the degree of acid inhibition achieved by some form of therapies, then are there any unanswered questions? The treatment of patients with peptic disorders has several problems: (1) the reduction in ulcer-related pain is not invariably superior with active agents; (2) some patients fail to heal even after high doses of acid inhibitory agents given for prolonged periods; (3) ulcers frequently recur when patients are off therapy, and even sometimes recur when patients remain on maintenance therapy; (4) the prevention of the development of gastric lesions in patients in an intensive care unit setting, or following the use of NSAIDs, remains fraught with difficulty. Finally, while there is now a host of medications that are useful for the treatment of acute ulcer disease, none of these agents alters the natural history of the disease, and none of them prevents recurrence unless maintenance therapy is utilized. The tendency to recur persists independently of the number of courses of ulcer-healing therapy. Is there any difference between ulcers recurring when the patient is on or off maintenance therapy? Compared with ulcers recurring during maintenance treatment, recurrences during periods of no treatment tend to be more frequent and more rapid; the recurrences are more likely to be associated with symptoms; and recurrences are more likely to be associated with complications such as hemorrhage. Finally, if one extrapolates the relationship between suppression of 24-hr or nocturnal acidity (%) against healing rate at 4 weeks

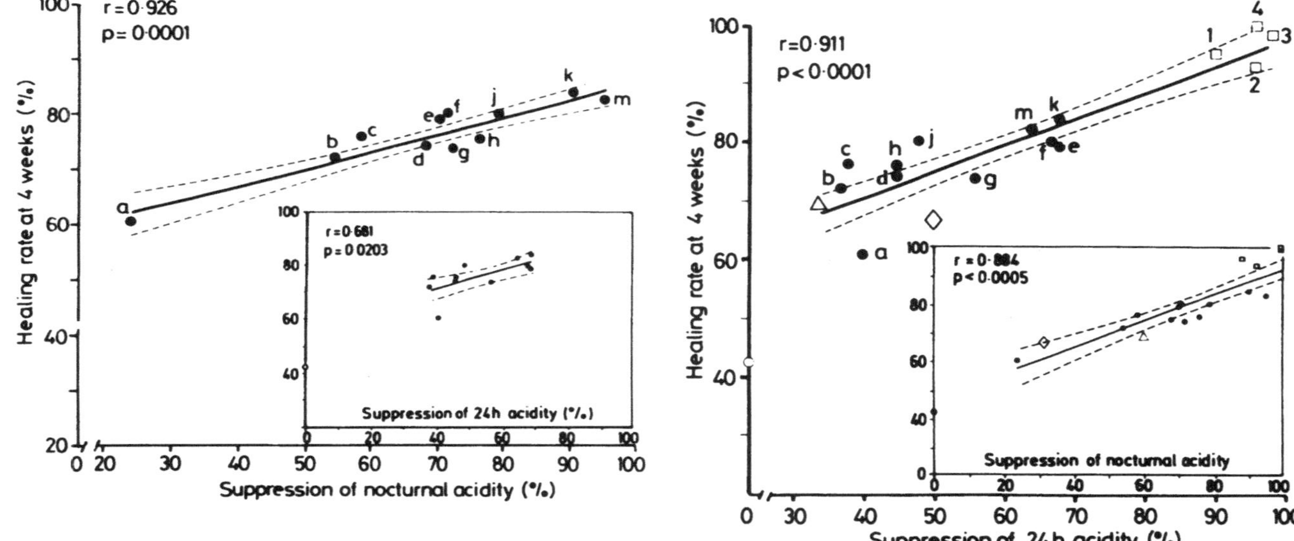

Figure 2. Regression line and 95% confidence limits between suppression of acidity (%) and healing rate (%) at 4 weeks for 11 dose regimens of H_2-receptor antagonists (A) and all drugs (B).

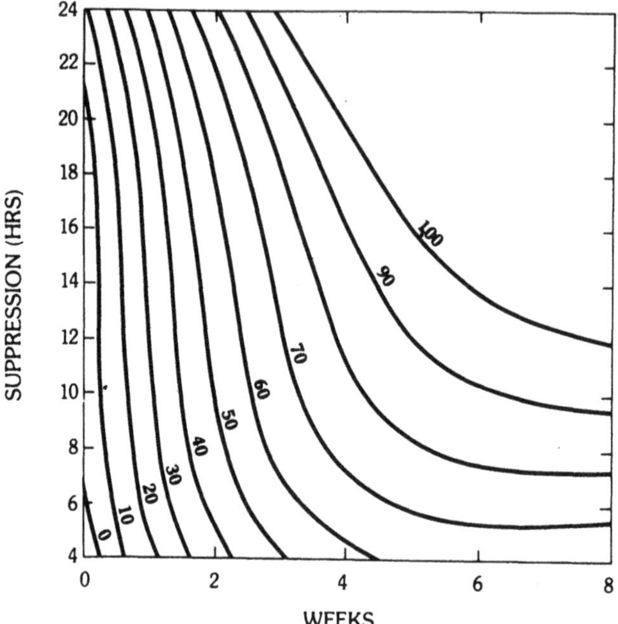

Figure 3. Contour plot of duodenal ulcer healing rate predicted by the duration of suppression above a fixed pH threshold of pH 3.0 and duration therapy.

(Fig. 1), to zero (0%) suppression of acidity, it is predicted that about 50% of patients will heal with no acid inhibition! Yes, there must be important factors other than acid suppression that are important in the healing of ulcers. Thus, it must be stressed that peptic ulceration is a chronic illness for which a variety of medications are a treatment, not a cure.

Resistance

Some patients with peptic ulcers do not heal after an appropriate dose of an H_2RA given for an adequate period. These ulcers are said to be resistant or "refractory." For example, Bardhan and his colleagues defined cimetidine resistance as "a symptomatic, endoscopically proven ulcer that does not heal with at least two months' treatment with 1 gm or more of cimetidine per day." Differences in clinical and endoscopic features between refractory and nonrefractory ulcer patients are few: patients who tend to be cimetidine-resistant are younger and have a longer ulcer history or a family history of ulcer disease. Their ulcers tend to be larger and have a more severe surrounding duodenitis. Acid and pepsin secretion are similar, gastrin concentrations are normal, blood levels of the drug and suppression of acid secretion are both satisfactory. Patients with DU may have a vagal hyperfunction that might be related to defective inhibitory mechanisms, although evidence for excessive vagal tone, as reflected by plasma levels of pancreatic polypeptide (PP) in patients with duodenal ulcer, is contradictory.

Refractoriness may occur at any time during the course of the disease: previous treatment with cimetidine may have resulted in rapid ulcer healing, with subsequent relapses becoming refractory to H_2RA treatment. Refractoriness probably indicates a change in the natural history of the disease and in some patients may reflect a poor prognosis. This means that identification of refractory ulcer patients at the start of treatment is not possible, and we really do not know for certain at this point why resistance occurs.

What should be done with the 15–20% of patients who do not heal on H_2RAs? Assuming that the diagnosis of peptic ulcer disease is correct, then it is appropriate to consider treatment with a proton pump inhibitor, or with a mucosal protective agent if acid suppression is considered the therapy of choice.

Tolerance and Rebound

Depending on the duration of therapy with various H_2RAs, there may be greater acid secretion in, for example, the fourth as compared with the first week of treatment. With discontinuation of H_2RAs, there may be acid hypersecretion in healthy volunteers without known ulcers, as well as in persons with a recent history of DU. This may be the case regardless of whether the measurement is basal acid output, responses to low-dose pentagastrin or histamine, modified sham feeding, or maximal pentagastrin or histamine stimulation. This possible "acid rebound" may be related to upregulation of the H_2 and gastrin receptors, with increased responsiveness to physiological stimuli once treatment is withdrawn; transient hypergastrinemia would not appear to be the mechanism. The full clinical significance of tolerance and rebound needs to be established. Of note, acid secretion in ulcer patients may fall after the ulcer has healed,[2,4] and does not occur with all acid-lowering therapies.[5]

Better Healing–Fewer Recurrences

The recurrence is well recognized as part of the natural history of DU. In fact, the chance of a recurrence of a DU is about 80%, but when the patient is placed on maintenance therapy—with sucralfate, an H_2RA, a proton pump inhibitor, or adequate doses of antacids—the recurrence rate falls to about 20%. The risk of recurrence tends to be lower with greater acid suppression, but the rates with sucralfate are as low as with all but the most extreme acid inhibition. Colloidal bismuth subcitrate may slow the rate of relapse of ulcers after discontinuation of acute treatment as compared with an H_2RA. Sucralfate may slow the time to ulcer recurrence. This effect lasts for the first 12 months after healing. We do not yet know the extent of acid inhibition required to achieve a given rate of maintained healing [as we know, for example with acute DU (Fig. 3)]. Nor do we understand why not inhibiting acid secretion with a mucosal protective agent achieves the same goal. But factors other than acid may be important in ulcer recurrence, such as smoking, infection with *Helicobacter pylori* (Hp), or psychological factors. Polycyclic antidepressants may relieve ulcer pain and help to heal ulcers. Psychological group counseling does not influence the tendency of DU to relapse, whereas hypnotherapy may delay relapse in patients who have received ranitidine to heal their ulcers and then continued on this drug for a further 10 weeks.

We know of the importance of pH in causing ulcers; what about Hp? The presence of Hp in the antral and duodenal mucosa is very common in patients with DU, and eradication of Hp is associated with lower rates of ulcer recurrence, much the same as stopping smoking appears to improve maintenance rates. However, individuals who are Hp-positive do not necessarily develop an ulcer or have an ulcer recurrence, whereas ulcers can recur after Hp eradication especially when taking NSAIDs. Yet, if infection with Hp is eradicated, the ulcers may remain in remission for over a year. It is therefore likely that both gastric juice (pH) and Hp are involved in ulcerogenesis. Single therapy with acid-inhibiting agents does not eradicate Hp, and if acid inhibition is discontinued, the ulcer will likely recur. Sucralfate also does not eradicate Hp, so it remains a puzzle just why the ulcer recurrence takes longer off therapy after healing with sucralfate versus an H_2-blocker.

Does acid secretion change with healing of DU? Some authors have suggested that acid secretion is lower or unchanged in patients with healed "inactive" DU than when the ulcer is active. There is a drug effect, however, with peak acid output (PAO) falling after healing of the DU with sucralfate, but no fall when the DU is healed with ranitidine. Others have also suggested that acid secretion may fall after DU healing with sucralfate, and may rise after treatment with nizatidine.

There is the possibility that agents that enhance mucosal defense may give a "better heal" of DU. While the 6-week healing of DU is similar with cimetidine and with colloidal bismuth subcitrate (72 and 86%, respectively), the regenerating mucosa of healed ulcers is histologically good in 60% of those healed with bismuth, compared with only 31% healed with cimetidine ($p = 0.027$), and thus was associated with a lower rate of recurrence in the former than in the latter (4 versus 20%, respectively; $p = 0.044$). All recurrent ulcers in both treatment groups had fair or poor patterns of regenerating mucosa. This greater histological maturity of the regenerating mucosa may contribute to the lower recurrence rate in bismuth- than in cimetidine-treated patients.

Summary

Peptic ulcer disease is common, and is effectively treated by primary care physicians. In about three-quarters of patients the ulcer will heal after a 4-week course of agents that enhance defense or inhibit aggression such as acid and pepsin. Recurrence rates of ulcers are high when patients are not on maintenance therapy, but the natural history of peptic ulcer disease is not altered by simply healing the active ulcer. pH, Hp, and mucosal protective factors are all important in the pathogenesis of ulcer disease and the approach to therapy must address the two sides of the aggressive/defensive factor equation.

References

1. Burget DW, Chiverton SG, Hunt RH: Is there an optimal degree of acid suppression for healing of duodenal ulcers: A model of the relationship between ulcer healing and acid suppression. *Gastroenterology* **99**:345–351, 1990. It is the duration that the intragastric pH is above 3 that is important for DU healing: it is not necessary to achieve more potent acid inhibition.
2. Johnston DA, Marks IN, Young GO, *et al*: Duodenal ulcer healing and acid secretory responses to modified sham feeding and pentagastrin stimulation. *Aliment Pharmacol Ther* **4**:403–410, 1990. DU healing with sucralfate results in decreased acid secretory responses to vagal and pentagastrin stimulation.
3. Jones DB, Howden CW, Burget DW, *et al*: Acid suppression in duodenal ulcer: A meta-analysis to define optimal dosing with antisecretory drugs. *Gut* **28**:1120–1127, 1987. The duration of acid suppression is important to predict the rate of DU healing after varying periods of treatment.
4. Kummer AF, Johnston DA, Marks IN, *et al*: Changes in nocturnal and peak acid outputs after duodenal ulcer healing with sucralfate or ranitidine. *Gut* **33**:175–178, 1992. Acid secretion in DU patients falls after ulcer healing is achieved by healing with either of these medications.
5. Savarino V, Mela GS, Zentilin P, *et al*: Lack of gastric acid rebound after stopping a successful short-term course of Nizatidine in duodenal ulcer patients. *Am J Gastroenterol* **86**:281–284, 1991. Acid rebound may not be the problem that it was once thought to be—at least not with this H_2-receptor antagonist.

II

General Approach to Peptic Disease Theory

3

Ulcer Healing by Strengthening of Mucosal Defense

An Alternative Approach to Inhibition of Acid Secretion

A. TARNAWSKI

Peptic ulcer is a defect in the gastric wall involving the entire mucosal thickness and penetrating through the muscularis mucosae. Involvement of the muscularis mucosae is crucial for distinguishing ulcers from erosions where necrosis is confined only to the mucosa.[1,2]

An ulcer develops as a result of imbalance between aggressive factors (e.g., hypersecretion of H^+ ions, pepsin, lysolecithin, nonsteroidal anti-inflammatory agents. *H. pylori*-derived toxins)[3] and mucosal defensive mechanisms shown in Fig. 1.[4]

Mucosal Defensive Mechanisms

Unstirred Layer of Mucus and Bicarbonate

The first line of mucosal defense is an unstirred layer formed by mucus gel and bicarbonate, which covers the mucosal luminal surface maintaining a neutral microenvironment at the surface epithelial cells. In addition to being a part of the unstirred layer, mucus serves as a lubricant, retards diffusion of H^+ ions and pepsin, inhibits pepsinogen activation, and exerts antibacterial actions. A range of GI hormones, including gastrin, secretin, prostaglandin E_2, and cholinergic agents, stimulate mucus secretion.[5]

Bicarbonate is secreted into the lumen by surface epithelial cells in addition to bicarbonate originating from stimulated parietal cells ("alkaline tide"). While gastric

A. TARNAWSKI • Gastroenterology Section, DVA Medical Center, Long Beach, and Department of Medicine, University of California, Irvine, California 92664.

Sucralfate: From Basic Science to the Bedside, edited by Daniel Hollander and G. N. J. Tytgat. Plenum Press, New York, 1995.

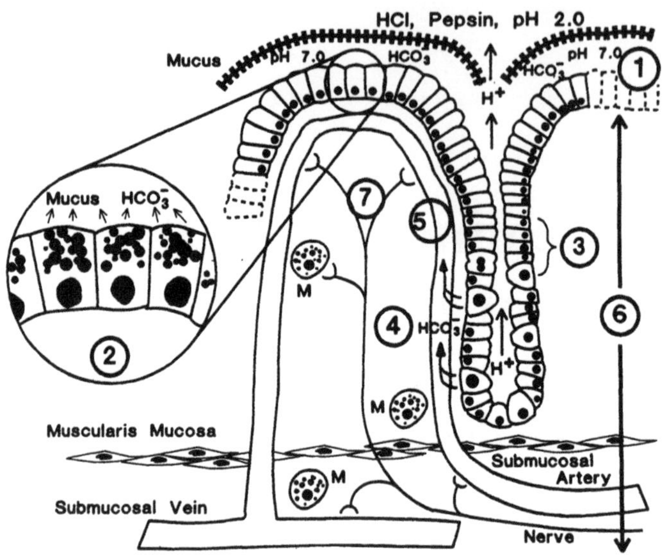

Figure 1. Mucosal defensive mechanisms. (1) Unstirred layer of mucus and bicarbonate maintains a "neutral" microclimate at the luminal surface of the surface epithelial cells. (2) The surface epithelial cells are capable of mucus, bicarbonate, and prostaglandin secretion. (3) Continuous mucosal cell renewal from the progenitor cells in the mucosal proliferative zone. (4) "Alkaline tide"—parietal cells secrete HCI into the gastric gland lumen and concurrently secrete bicarbonate into the lumen of adjacent microvessel. (5) Mucosal microvessels. (6) Continuous generation of prostaglandin E_2 and prostacyclin by the mucosa is crucial for the maintenance of mucosal integrity. Most mucosal defensive mechanisms are stimulated or facilitated by endogenous or exogenous prostaglandins. (7) Sensory nerve stimulation leads to the release of neurotransmitters such as calcitonin gene-related peptide and substance P in nerve terminal. (Reprinted from Tarnawski A, Erickson R: Sucralfate—24 years later: Current concepts of its protective and therapeutic action. *Eur J Gastroenterol Hepatol* **3**:795–810, 1991.)

bicarbonate secretion amounts to only 10% as compared with gastric acid secretion rate, the mucus gel minimizes luminal loss of bicarbonate, thus maintaining a neutral microclimate at the mucosal surface. Bicarbonate secretion is stimulated by prostaglandins and aluminum ions.[6]

Surface Epithelial Cells

The second line of mucosal defense is formed by a continuous layer of surface epithelial cells which secrete mucus and bicarbonate (contributing to the unstirred layer) and generate prostaglandins. Because of the presence of phospholipids on their surfaces, these cells are hydrophobic, repelling acid- and water-soluble damaging agents. Interconnected by tight junctions, surface epithelial cells for a "barrier" preventing backdiffusion of acid and pepsin.[4]

Cell Renewal

Continuous cell renewal from progenitor cells in the mucosal proliferative zone enables replacement of damaged or aged surface epithelial cells. Usually it takes 3–5 days to completely replace the surface epithelium. It takes longer (months) to replace the glandular cells. Superficial injury to the surface epithelium is restituted within several hours by migrating cells from the neck area.[7]

"Alkaline Tide"

Parietal cells secreting HCl into the gastric gland lumen concurrently secrete bicarbonate into the lumen of adjacent microvessels. The bicarbonate is transported upward, contributing to the neutral microclimate at the luminal surface.

Microcirculation

Mucosal circulation in microvessels delivers oxygen and nutrients to the entire mucosa and removes toxic substances. The microvascular endothelium generates vasodilators such as prostacyclin and nitric oxide, which protect the gastric mucosa against injury and oppose the mucosal damaging action of vasoconstrictors such as leukotriene C_4, thromboxane A_2, and endothelin. When the microvasculature is damaged, endothelial cells lining microvessels in the periphery of injured areas initiate repair and reconstruction of the microvascular network through angiogenesis.[8]

Prostaglandins

Continuous generation of prostaglandin E_2 and prostacyclin by the mucosa is crucial for maintaining mucosal integrity. Almost all of the mucosal defensive mechanisms are stimulated or facilitated by endogenous or exogenous prostaglandins. Inhibition of prostaglandin synthesis by nonsteroidal anti-inflammatory agents or neutralization of endogenous mucosal prostaglandins with specific antibodies results in formation of gastric and intestinal ulcerations.[9]

Sensory Nerves

Stimulation of gastric sensory nerves leads to the release of neurotransmitters such as calcitonin gene-related peptide (CGRP) and substance P in the nerve terminals, located within or close to the large submucosal vessels. CGRP exerts a mucosal protective action most likely through vasodilation of submucosal vessels mediated by nitric oxide generation. Mucosal macrophages secrete a range of cytokines which affect cell growth and proliferation.

Disruption of the mucosal defenses permits ulcerogenic agents and aggressive factors to penetrate into the mucosa, initiating release of proinflammatory and vasoactive mediators (serotonin, leukotriene C_4, platelet-activating factor, endothelin) and directly digesting cellular and connective tissue components of the mucosa. This chain of events culminates in formation of mucosal erosions or, if submucosal vessels are involved, in ulcerations.

Ulcer Development

Recent studies have demonstrated that ligation of gastric submucosal arteries or their prolonged occlusion by contraction of muscularis mucosae and/or muscularis propria result in ulcer formation.[10] In studies of gastric ulcer formation in rats, we found that within 5–15 min after acetic acid application, thrombi develop in submucosal vessels and collecting venules leading to microvascular stasis and ischemic mucosal necrosis.[2]

These studies clearly demonstrated that vascular and microvascular changes are the earliest events in the development of experimental gastric ulcer. These vascular changes cause mucosal ischemia, free radical formation, and cessation of nutrient delivery, all resulting in mucosal necrosis.

During the acute stage of ulceration, the mucosa and submucosa become necrotic, attracting polymorphonuclear leukocytes and macrophages. Necrotic portions of the mucosa detach and/or are removed by scavenging macrophages within 24 hr. By 48 hr, necrosis involves the muscularis mucosae. By 72 hr, the ulcer undergoes transition into the "chronic" stage, characterized histologically by the presence of granulation tissue at the ulcer base and appearance of a distinct ulcer margin at the adjacent nonnecrotic mucosa[2] (Fig. 2).

Ulcer Healing

Ulcer healing is a very complex process, requiring interaction of different tissue and cellular systems. It involves filling the mucosal defects with proliferating and migrating

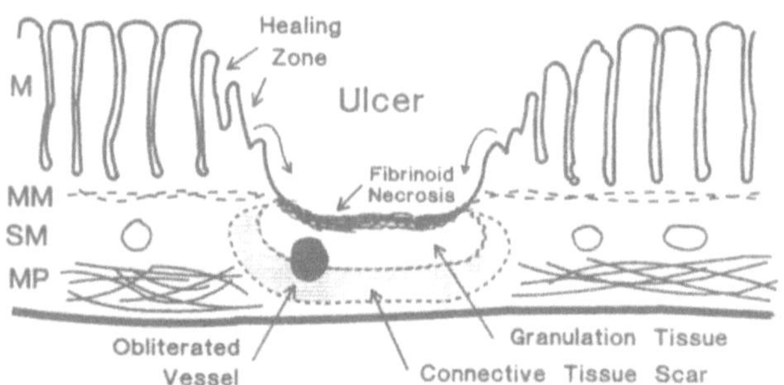

Figure 2. Diagrammatic presentation of ulceration in the gastric or duodenal mucosa. M, mucosa; MM, muscularis mucosae; SM, submucosa; MP, muscularis propria. (Reprinted from Tarnawski A, *et al*: in Garner A, O'Brien P (eds): *Mechanisms of Injury, Protection and Repair of the Upper Gastrointestinal Tract*. New York, John Wiley & Sons, 1991, pp 521–531.)

epithelial cells, reconstructing glandular structures, and reepithelializing the mucosal surface with connective tissue components (cells, microvessels, and extracellular matrix for the lamina propria and the microvascular network). The following factors and/or morphologic structures play an important role in ulcer healing[11] (Fig. 3).

Luminal Factors

Inhibiting secretion of aggressive factors as hydrochloric acid and pepsin accelerates ulcer healing. Reduction of acid secretion is the basis for the therapeutic actions of H_2-receptor antagonists and proton pump inhibitors. Mucus and bicarbonate secretion may also be important in ulcer healing because the mucus/bicarbonate layer may protect newly formed cells from further acid and pepsin digestion.

Mucosa at the Ulcer Margin

Mucosa at the ulcer margin forms a characteristic "healing" zone. The glands become cystically dilated, the cells lining these dilated glands become dedifferentiated and proliferate. Proliferation of mucosal cells at the ulcer margin is important for ulcer healing because it supplies cells for reepithelializing the mucosal surface and reconstructing the gastric glands. These cells migrate from the ulcer margin onto the granulation tissue to cover (reepithelialize) the ulcer base. In addition, the poorly differentiated cells

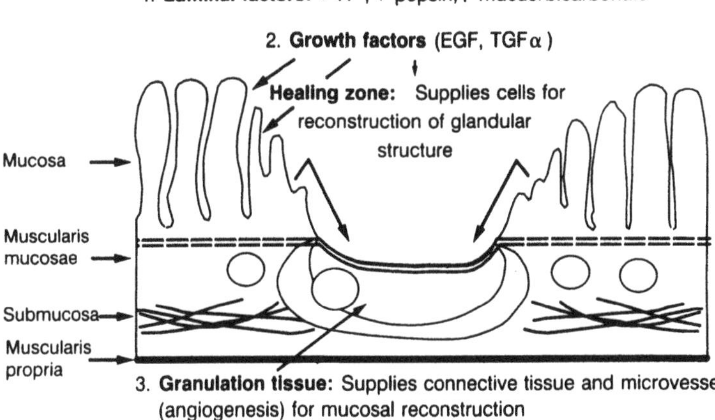

Figure 3. Diagrammatic presentation of ulcer healing process and factors affecting ulcer healing. Healing of the ulcer is accomplished by filling the mucosal defect with: (1) cells migrating from the healing zone and replicating [under the influence of epidermal growth factor (EGF) and transforming growth factor alpha (TGFα)] and (2) connective tissue cells including microvessels originating from the granulation tissue. [Reprinted from Tarnawski A, *et al*: *J Clin Gastroenterol* **13**(suppl 1):S42–S47, 1991.]

from the base of the ulcer margin sprout into the granulation tissue forming tubules, which undergo transformation into gastric glands. The stimulus for increased cell proliferation is most likely initiated by epidermal growth factor (EGF) and/or transforming growth factor alpha (TGF_{α}) which are mitogenic peptides for gastric epithelial cells. Immunohistochemical studies demonstrated that cells lining dilated gastric glands at the ulcer margin display an enormous increase in expression of EGF and its receptor at the initial stage (1–7 days) after ulcer induction.[12] The source of EGF is either luminal, secreted with saliva, or it is locally synthesized by the cells of regenerating glands. Thus, EGF and its receptor (which is also shared by TGF_{α}) play an important role in ulcer healing. It should be noted that exogenous EGF and TGF_{α} accelerate healing of experimental gastroduodenal ulcers, while removal of salivary glands (a major source of EGF present in the gastric lumen) delays ulcer healing.

Granulation Tissue—Role of Extracellular Matrix

During the chronic stage of ulceration, granulation tissue develops at the ulcer base. Granulations consist of proliferating connective tissue cells, i.e., macrophages, fibroblasts, and endothelial cells which form microvessels through the process of angiogenesis. Granulation tissue is an important component of the ulcer healing process because it supplies connective tissue cells and extracellular matrix for restoring the lamina propria and microvessels for reconstituting microvasculature within the mucosal scar. Granulation tissue undergoes continuous remodeling and changes in cellular composition. Initially, inflammatory cells and macrophages are abundant while in later stages, fibroblasts predominate.[11]

The extracellular matrix components such as fibronectin, laminin, and collagens facilitate cell migration, proliferation, differentiation, and attachment. Fibronectin is the key component of the extracellular matrix, because it is a link between cells and the extracellular matrix. It has extensive codistribution with collagen type III, affecting formation and maturation of connective tissue, including granulation tissue. Laminin and collagen type IV are two major basement membrane proteins. They serve as adhesive proteins promoting the attachment of various types of cells to the extracellular matrix. In a recent study we sequentially analyzed the distribution of fibronectin, laminin, collagen type III and IV in the gastric mucosa and granulation tissue during healing of experimental gastric ulcers.[13] This study demonstrated that expression of extracellular matrix components is significantly increased during ulcer healing and persists after the ulcers have healed. A strong expression of the extracellular matrix components at the base of the ulcer margin indicates a close interaction between granulation tissue and epithelial cells at the ulcer margin in the process of reepithelialization during healing. A strong expression of extracellular matrix components in and around regenerating capillary vessels in granulation tissue suggests their participation in angiogenesis. The growth of granulation tissue and generation of new microvessels by angiogenesis is stimulated by the fibroblast growth factors and possibly by other growth factors and cytokines including platelet-derived growth factor, transforming growth factors, prostaglandins and/or interleukin-1 and tumor necrosis factors.

Angiogenesis in Granulation Tissue

Formation of a new microvascular network—angiogenesis—is a major component of wound healing and tissue regeneration. It is important for repair of acute gastric mucosal injury and is essential for healing chronic gastroduodenal ulcers. The *in vivo* and *in vitro* studies, including our own data, indicate that angiogenesis occurs by a series of steps that include: (1) degradation of basement membranes, (2) endothelial cell migration and proliferation into the perivascular space, (3) formation of microvascular tubes followed by anastomoses, (4) establishment of lumina and basement membranes, and ultimately (5) formation of a capillary network. By forming a capillary network, angiogenesis in granulation tissue enables nutrient and oxygen delivery to the ulcer base and thus facilitates the healing process. It has been demonstrated that increasing the oxygen tension in wounds doubles or triples collagen production and epithelial cell growth.[14]

Folkman *et al.* reported that stimulating angiogenesis in granulation tissue with basic fibroblast growth factor dramatically accelerates the healing of experimental (cysteamine-induced) duodenal ulcer in rats. In our previous study we showed that chronic indomethacin administration (1 mg/kg i.p., daily) inhibits angiogenesis in granulation tissue and delays healing of experimental gastric ulcers in rats.[15]

The final outcome of the healing process reflects a dynamic interaction between the epithelial component from the "healing" zone at the ulcer margin (under EGF and TGF_{α} control) and the connective tissue component (including microvessels) originating from granulation tissue and regulated by fibroblast growth factors.

Factors Affecting Ulcer Healing—Focus on Agents Strengthening Mucosal Defense

As discussed above, a number of factors appear to influence ulcer healing, namely luminal factors (H^+ secretion, pepsin, mucus, bicarbonate) as well as prostaglandins, growth factors, angiogenic factors, oxygen and nutrient supply.

The previous chapters discussed etiologic factors of peptic ulcer disease and therapy aimed at reduction of gastric acid secretion. While reducing acid secretion has been the mainstay in the therapeutic approach to ulcer healing, it is aimed at only one side of the ulcer equation, namely the aggressive factors. Recent clinical and experimental data indicate that healing of gastroduodenal ulcers can be successfully accomplished without inhibition of acid secretion by topically active agents such as prostaglandins, low-dose aluminum-containing antacids, sucralfate, colloidal bismuth, and basic fibroblast growth factor. Compounds that inhibit the cyclooxygenase enzymes, such as aspirin and other nonsteroidal anti-inflammatory drugs, cause gastroduodenal damage and ulceration, and the damage could be prevented or diminished by pretreatment with exogenous prostaglandins, suggesting that prostaglandins play a role in maintaining normal mucosal integrity and healing peptic ulceration. Prostaglandins could be expected to offer a therapeutic potential in ulcer disease. In fact, numerous studies have shown efficacy for prostaglandin analogues in treatment of both gastric and duodenal ulcers. In general, prostaglandins are effective (usually in doses inhibiting acid secretion), but no more effective than traditional antiulcer therapies, such as H_2-receptor antagonists, antacids, and sucralfate. Some studies suggest that prostaglandins may have special efficacy in treating "resistant" duodenal ulcers. A meta-analysis of published data indicated that duodenal ulcer recurrence rate following prostaglandin therapy may be lower than that observed after treatment with H_2-receptor antagonists. However, there are very limited data to support a greater efficacy for prostaglandins in treating peptic ulcer disease. Although several prostaglandin analogues are available for routine antiulcer therapy in several countries, including Canada, they were not approved for treatment of peptic ulcer in the United States.[16]

It has been demonstrated that low-dose antacid treatment (which does not significantly affect gastric luminal pH) is effective in accelerating the healing of gastric and duodenal ulcers. This means that ulcer healing can be accomplished without inhibition of acid secretion or its neutralization.

Another antiulcer drug—sucralfate—does not inhibit gastric acid secretion and has only a minimal acid-neutralizing capacity, but is as effective as H_2-receptor antagonists in healing gastroduodenal ulcers.[4] Similarly, colloidal bismuth and basic fibroblast growth factors do not reduce acid secretion but promote effective ulcer healing.[15] The mechanisms for the healing action of these drugs are entirely different from the H_2-receptor antagonists and proton pump inhibitors, and are related to stimulation of mucosal defensive factors. Postulated mechanisms for the ulcer healing action of topically active drugs are presented in Table I.

Aluminum-containing antacids and sucralfate stimulate mucus, bicarbonate, and prostaglandin secretion, thus enhancing mucosal defense. More recent data indicate that in addition they stimulate nitric oxide production and angiogenesis, and promote the binding of EGF and basic fibroblast growth factor (bFGF) to the ulcer base.[15]

Folkman, Szabo, and co-workers treated rats with chronic DU with acid-stable bFGF over a period of 3 weeks. This stimulated angiogenesis in granulation tissue more than ninefold as compared with controls and significantly accelerated ulcer healing.[15] Effective ulcer repair was accomplished despite the fact that this regimen of bFGF treatment increased gastric acid and pepsin secretion. The ability of angiogenic growth factor to accelerate the healing of duodenal ulcers despite high concentrations of gastric acid and pepsin stresses the importance of mucosal defense in ulcer healing. bFGF is a direct mitogen for vascular endothelial cells, fibroblasts, smooth muscle cells, and certain epithelial cells. These properties are most likely responsible for its healing abilities.

Table I. Postulated Mechanisms for the Ulcer Healing Action of Topically Active Drugs

1. Increased delivery of EGF to the ulcer margin (binding of luminal EGF or stimulation of its local synthesis) enhances cell proliferation, migration, reepithelialization, and reconstruction of glandular structures.
2. Increased delivery of bFGF to the ulcer base (by its binding and protection against acid degradation) stimulates angiogenesis and collagen formation in granulation tissue.
3. Stimulation of mucus, bicarbonate, and prostaglandin secretion in the mucosa at the ulcer margin protects cells from acid and pepsin digestion, allowing reepithelialization of the ulcer crater.

Sucralfate, which is structurally related to heparin, binds bFGF, protects it from acid degradation, and increases its concentration locally in granulation tissue at the ulcer base. Sucralfate has been previously shown to bind luminal gastric EGF to the ulcer base. More recent studies indicate that chronic sucralfate administration induces increased expression of EGF, TGF_{α}, and their common receptor in the gastric mucosa.[17] Increased local concentration of these growth factors facilitates ulcer healing.

Quality of Ulcer Healing

Assessment of gastric ulcer healing is usually based on endoscopic visualization or experimentally on measurements of ulcer size. Neither method involves histologic or ultrastructural assessment of subepithelial mucosal reconstruction. These approaches have resulted in the assumption that the mucosa of grossly "healed" gastric and/or duodenal ulcers returns to normal, either spontaneously or following treatment.[11] In previous studies we demonstrated that reepithelialized mucosa of grossly "healed" experimental gastric ulcer has prominent histologic and ultrastructural abnormalities which include: reduced height, marked dilation of gastric glands, poor differentiation and/or degenerative changes in glandular cells, increased connective tissue, and disorganized microvascular network. In clinical studies prominent histologic abnormalities were found in the mucosa of healed duodenal ulcers.[11] It is possible that the marked abnormalities found in the subepithelial mucosa of grossly "healed" gastric ulcers might interfere with mucosal defenses and may predispose these areas to subsequent ulcer recurrence when ulcerogenic factors are present.[11] This hypothesis is supported by clinical observations indicating that gastric ulcers tend to recur at the same location.[18]

Therefore, the quality of mucosal restoration may be an important factor in determining whether ulcers will recur. If this is the case, then many therapeutic regimens may be in need of reevaluation. Although a number of pharmacologic agents are known to accelerate the rate of gastric ulcer healing, it is unknown what effect these agents might have on the quality of ulcer healing and reconstruction of mucosal architecture. The lower ulcer recurrence rate after treatment with sucralfate and colloidal bismuth may indicate that these drugs provide better quality of ulcer healing.

References

1. Cotran RS, Robbins SL, Kumar V (eds): Healing and repair, in *Robbins Pathologic Basis of Disease*. Philadelphia, WB Saunders, 1989, pp 71–86. The basic morphology of the peptic ulceration is presented.
2. Tarnawski A, Hollander D, Stachura J, *et al*: Vascular and microvascular changes—Key factors in the development of acetic acid-induced gastric ulcers in rats. *J Clin Gastroenterol* **12**(suppl 1):S148–S157, 1990. This paper presents a sequential analysis of the development of acetic acid-induced gastric ulcers in rats. It demonstrates the important role of vascular and microvascular factors in ulcer formation.
3. Richardson CT: Pathogenic factors in peptic ulcer disease. *Am J Med* **79**(2C):1–7, 1985. Summary of the pathogenetic factors playing a role in peptic ulcer disease.

4. Tarnawski A, Erickson RA: Sucralfate—24 years later: Current concepts of its protective and therapeutic actions. *Eur J Gastroenterol Hepatol* **3**(11):795–810, 1991. Review of the current knowledge of pharmacologic and therapeutic actions of sucralfate. Also, the general principles of gastric mucosal defense and injury, as well as ulcer healing are presented.
5. Allen A, Hunter AC, Mall A: Mucus secretion, in Hollander D, Tarnawski A (eds): *Gastric Cytoprotection*. New York, Plenum Press, 1989, pp 75–90. Review of the role of mucus in gastric mucosal defense.
6. Shorrock CH, Rees WDW: Bicarbonate secretion and alkaline microclimate, in Hollander D, Tarnawski A (eds): *Gastric Cytoprotection*. New York, Plenum Press, 1989, pp 91–108. Review of bicarbonate's role in gastric mucosal defense.
7. Eastwood GJ: Epithelial cell renewal in cytoprotection, in Hollander D, Tarnawski A (eds): *Gastric Cytoprotection*. New York, Plenum Press, 1989, pp 109–124. An excellent chapter discussing epithelial cell renewal and its role in mucosal protection.
8. Szabo S, Folkman J, Morales RE, *et al*: Vascular factors in mucosal injury, protection and ulcer healing, in Garner A, O'Brien PE (eds): *Mechanisms of Injury, Protection and Repair of the Upper Gastrointestinal Tract*. New York, John Wiley & Sons, 1991, pp 447–454. An excellent chapter discussing the role of vascular factors in injury, protection, and healing of gastroduodenal mucosa.
9. Wilson DE: Cytoprotective therapy: Prostaglandins in cytoprotection, in Hollander D, Tarnawski A (eds): *Gastric Cytoprotection*. New York, Plenum Press, 1989, pp 169–186. An excellent review of the role of prostaglandins in mucosal defense and ulcer healing.
10. Piasecki C: Evidence for an infarctive pathogenesis of acute and chronic gastroduodenal ulceration. *J Physiol Pharmacol* **43**:99–112, 1992. A demonstration that ligation of small gastric arteries produces ulcerations.
11. Tarnawski A, Stachura J, Krause WJ, *et al*: Quality of gastric ulcer healing: A new emerging concept. *J Clin Gastroenterol* **13**(suppl 1):S42–S47, 1991. Experimental basis for hypothesis regarding the quality of ulcer healing (i.e., quality of mucosal restoration) as an important factor in determining ulcer recurrence.
12. Tarnawski A, Stachura J, Durbin T, *et al*: Increased expression of epidermal growth factor receptor during gastric ulcer healing in rats. *Gastroenterology* **102**:695–698, 1992. A study demonstrating increased expression of EGF receptors in the margin of experimental gastric ulcer and in the mucosal scar.
13. Lu S-Y, Tarnawski A, Stachura J, *et al*: Sequential expression and distribution of fibronectin, laminin and collagen III and IV during experimental gastric ulcer healing. *Gastroenterology* **A116**:192, 1992. This study demonstrated increased expression of extracellular matrix components during healing of experimental gastric ulcer.
14. Hunt TK: The principles of wound healing, in Halter A, Garner A, and Tytgat GNT (eds): *Mechanisms of Peptic Ulcer Healing*, Falk Symposium No. 59. Dordrecht, Kluver Academic Publishers, 1991, pp 1–12. This paper describes general principles of wound healing.
15. Folkman J, Szabo S, Stovroff A, *et al*: Duodenal ulcer. Discovery of a new mechanism and development of angiogenic therapy that accelerates healing. *Ann Surg* **214**:414–427, 1991. Landmark paper demonstrating that basic EGF accelerates the healing of experimental duodenal ulcer by inducing angiogenesis.
16. Wilson DE: Role of prostaglandins in gastroduodenal mucosal protection. *J Clin Gastroenterol* **13**(suppl 1):S65–S71, 1991. This paper reviews the role of prostaglandins in mucosal protection and ulcer healing.
17. Tarnawski A, Stachura J, Durbin T, *et al*: Sucralfate treatment induces increased expression of EGF, TGF_{α} and their common receptor in the gastric mucosa. A key to the ulcer healing and trophic action? *Gastroenterology* **102**:A175, 1992. This study showed that chronic administration of sucralfate to rats increases expression of EGF, TGF_{α} and their receptors in the gastric mucosa.
18. Litman A, Hanscom DH: The course of recurrent ulcer. *Gastroenterology* **61**:585–591, 1971. A demonstration that recurrent gastric ulcers recur usually in the same location as the previous ulcers.

4

History of the Development of Sucralfate

AKIRA ISHIMORI

Introduction: Research and Development of Sucralfate

Sucralfate was introduced in Japan as a selective ulcer-protecting agent in 1968 and it is currently accepted worldwide as a nonsystemic site protector. This agent has an unusual developmental history among the drugs for peptic ulcer disease (PUD). The development of sucralfate is a true reflection of international collaboration.

The rapid progress in medicine in recent years cannot be fully appreciated without considering the worldwide research collaboration. The long-cultivated tradition that exchange of information through printed literatures contributes to the progress in medicine is definitely exemplified by sucralfate.

The history of sucralfate can be divided roughly into two terms; the first term is its development and clinical application in Japan, and the second term is its subsequent worldwide development.

The Developmental History of Sucralfate in Japan

Antipepsin Agents and Sucralfate

Sucralfate was developed initially as an antipeptic agent (Table I). In 1932, Babkin and Komarov[1] discovered the pepsin-suppressing activity of chondroitin sulfate contained in gastric mucus and suggested that this moiety might be one of the defensive factors. They also pointed out the possibility that drugs capable of enhancing defensive factors could be useful when applied to the treatment of PUD.

AKIRA ISHIMORI • Department of Clinical and Laboratory Medicine, Tohoku University School of Medicine, Sondai 982, Japan.

Sucralfate: From Basic Science to the Bedside, edited by Daniel Hollander and G. N. J. Tytgat. Plenum Press, New York, 1995.

Table I. History of Antipeptic Drugs

1907	Deklug	Theory of mucosal protection by gastric mucus
1931	Fogelson	Clinical application of gastric mucin
1932	Babkin and Komarov	Discovery of antipeptic effect of gastric mucus
1954	Levey and Sheinfeld	Antiulcerogenic effect of chondroitin sulfate
1959	Anderson	Antiulcerogenic effect of carrageenan
1960	Bonfils	Clinical application of carrageenan
1963	Cook	Synthesis of antipeptic preparations
1967	Cayer	Clinical application of amylopectin sulfate
	Hino Nao	Clinical application of aluminum sucrose sulfate (sucralfate)
1968	Ishimori	Clinical application of sorbitol sulfate, carboxymethyl dextran, dextran sulfate, amylopectin sulfate, and aluminum dextran sulfate
	Ishimori	Theory of local protection of ulcer lesion

The development of antipeptic agents starting with polyanionic carbohydrate had a slow start (Table I). However, the development of synthetic antipeptic agents by Cook and co-workers[2] in 1963 opened up the clinical application of antipeptic agents. Amylopectin sulfate[3] was developed by G. D. Searle in the United States and dextran sulfate was developed in Sweden, and some clinical trials as to their antipeptic activity were conducted.

Although a number of synthetic antipeptic agents were investigated clinically in Japan as well, sucralfate was the only drug that became clinically useful as an antiulcer agent.

The local protection by binding of antipeptic agents to the surface of ulcers had already been proposed as a mechanism and the administration of these drugs on an empty stomach had also been recommended based on the proposed mechanisms of action.

At that time, we synthesized a number of antipeptic agents and investigated them clinically in patients with peptic ulcers. Results are shown in Table II. Some agents accelerated ulcer healing and this provided good prospects for future development of those drugs as antiulcer agents.

Globally, the subsequent development of antipeptic agents took different paths in Japan and other countries. The reasons for the difference may be attributed to two factors. The first was related to drug side effects and the second was the difference in clinical applications, based on differences in mechanisms of action.

The major side effect of antipeptic agents was intestinal and cecal ulcerations in animal experiments. Whereas amylopectin sulfate, the most promising antipeptic agent at that time, caused ulcerative lesions,[4] sucralfate was quite harmless.

It was confirmed by electrophoresis that crystalline pepsin can bind to sucralfate although the binding was weak. It was also demonstrated that similar to the effect of antacids, the suppression of peptic activity in gastric juice by sucralfate was transient.[5]

An antipeptic agent, pepstatin, which is a more specific pepsin inhibitor, can also suppress pepsin activity in the stomach but only transiently. Studies of PUD patients showed that pepstatin was not very effective in accelerating ulcer healing. This suggested

Table II. Therapeutic Effect of Synthetic Antipeptic Drugs in Peptic Ulcer[a]

Antipeptic preparations	No. of cases	Healing ratio: Gastric ulcer	Healing ratio: Duodenal ulcer	Average time required for healing
Sorbitol sulfate	5	1/5 (20%)	0/1 (0%)	21 days
Carboxymethyl-dextran	11	5/7 (71%)	3/5 (60%)	63.5
Dextran sulfate	18	10/19 (53%)	0/2 (0%)	56.4
Amylopectin sulfate	28	16/23 (70%)	6/10 (60%)	52.5
Aluminum dextran sulfate	30	21/25 (84%)	8/9 (89%)	56.3

[a]Data from Ishimori A: *Jpn J Gastroenterol* **66**:753–755, 1968.

that suppression of pepsin activity in gastric juice cannot provide sufficient beneficial effects to allow ulcer healing.

Those findings suggested that the remarkable effects of sucralfate in accelerating ulcer healing were to be attributed to other mechanisms than its sole efficacy in suppression of pepsin activity.

Subsequently, attention was directed to sucralfate's strong protective effects on substrate proteins. The binding of antipeptic agents to substrate proteins was extremely strong and this binding was considered to play an important role in indirect suppression of peptic activity. From this viewpoint, it was suggested that antipeptic agents contributed to accelerating ulcer healing through enhancing defensive factors.[5]

Selective Ulcer Protection of Sucralfate

The white coating covering ulcerous lesions observed endoscopically is considered to contain protein components, capable of binding to antipeptic agents. Immunoelectrophoresis of specimens of white coating obtained from the surface of ulcerations was conducted using antibodies to serum proteins. As shown in Fig. 1, it was observed that the white coating contained components corresponding to serum proteins.[5] In a similar examination using antiserum to fibrinogen, the component reactive with the antibody was also observed in the white coating but it moved to the opposite side of the plasma fibrinogen. This suggested that the protein component in the white coating had been somewhat altered chemically.

Namely, it was considered that the white coating covering the ulcer base contained proteins derived from blood and that these proteins were somewhat altered chemically through reactions with gastric juice. All of those proteins were perceived to bind strongly to sucralfate.[5] On the other hand, it was noted that the binding of sucralfate to gastric mucus was not as strong. Thus, sucralfate is thought to bind to ulcerated lesions in a concentration-dependent manner.

In this connection a clinical experience is worth mentioning supporting the adhesion mechanism of sucralfate. In a 58-year-old woman, endoscopic examination revealed a posterior gastric ulcer with marginal scarring and mucosal fold convergence covered with white coating. Treatment with sucralfate alone for 2 months provided some contraction of

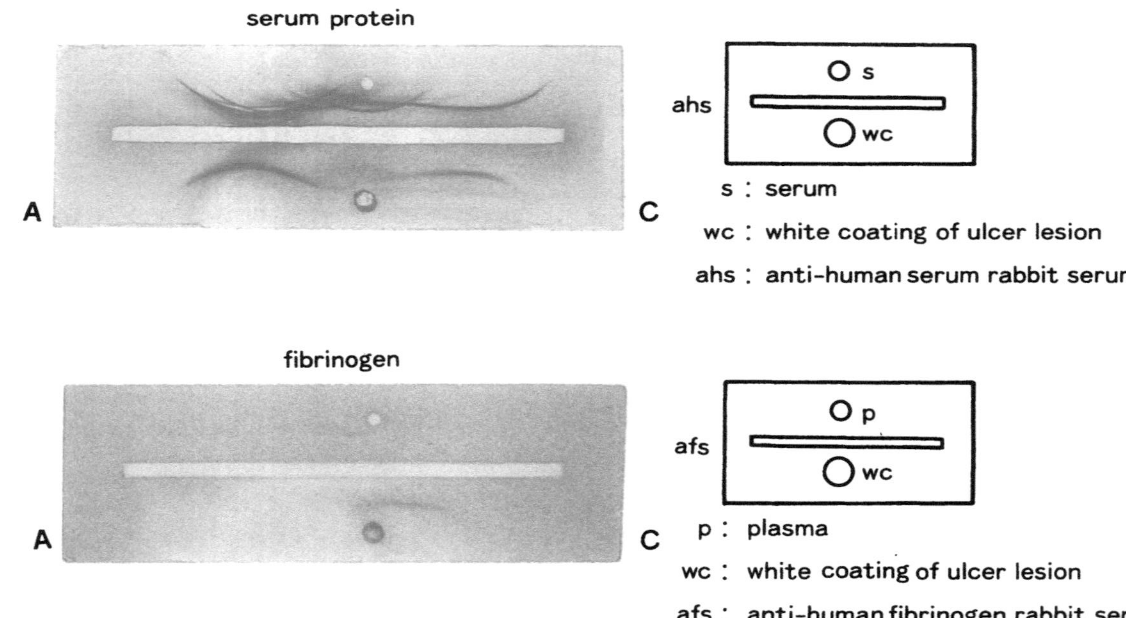

Figure 1. Immunoelectrophoresis of white coating obtained from the surface of ulcer lesion by biopsy, using anti-human serum and antifibrinogen.

the ulcer area, but no further improvement was observed. Rotation therapy immediately following oral administration of sucralfate was then employed so that the preparation could gain access to the ulcer lesion. Subsequently, complete healing of the lesion accompanied by disappearance of the white coating was achieved in a very short period of time.

This clinical observation suggested that sucralfate may exert its ulcer healing effect topically by binding to the exposed ulcer base, thereby protecting the ulcer from strong proteolytic action of gastric juice. In other words, although the protective action of sucralfate requires topical adherence, the antipeptic activity is also required to counteract the strong peptic activity of gastric juice. Thus, sucralfate is more than a classic antipeptic agent because of its selective ulcer adherence.[5]

In clinical use, it is essential to administer the drug based on its mechanisms of action in order to obtain the maximal efficacy. It is inadequate to administer sucralfate after meals when food proteins still reside in the stomach because the formation of a protective layer is interfered with, which is the principal mechanism of action of sucralfate by binding to substrate proteins at the ulcer base. Thus, the administration of sucralfate on an empty stomach before meals and at bedtime has been employed in Japan.[5] This time schedule enables sucralfate to exert its protective effects for a long time unlike the short-acting effects of antacids. In contrast, postmeal administration was employed for amylopectin sulfate. This dosing schedule may have been responsible for the lack of amylopectin efficacy observed in clinical trials.

Twenty years ago, a double-blind, placebo-controlled trial was conducted in Japan on gastric ulcer patients to investigate the efficacy of sucralfate administered alone on an empty stomach.[6] Evaluation was made mainly by endoscopy supplemented with radiography. As shown in Fig. 2, the results demonstrated significantly better efficacy of sucralfate in accelerating ulcer healing than placebo. Since then, sucralfate has been recognized as a major drug for ulcer therapy in Japan.

Globalization of Research on Sucralfate

Confirmation of Clinical Efficacy and Mechanism of Action of Sucralfate

Clinical Efficacy

It was around 1978 that sucralfate was introduced overseas after its 10-year experience of clinical application in Japan. At first, evaluation was slow since endoscopic examination of the duodenum was still in its infancy. In addition, sufficient information regarding the mechanisms of action of sucralfate was not available. Furthermore, it seemed that the failure of amylopectin sulfate's development in the United States created a negative image for the clinical evaluation of sucralfate.

About that time cimetidine was launched as the first H_2RA and this drug established its position firmly. In addition, endoscopic examination of the duodenum became widespread. This helped to establish the concept of controlled clinical trials to investigate antiulcer agents making it easier to evaluate the clinical efficacy of sucralfate.

In 1979, sucralfate was found to be as effective as cimetidine in accelerating the healing of gastric and duodenal ulcers.[7]

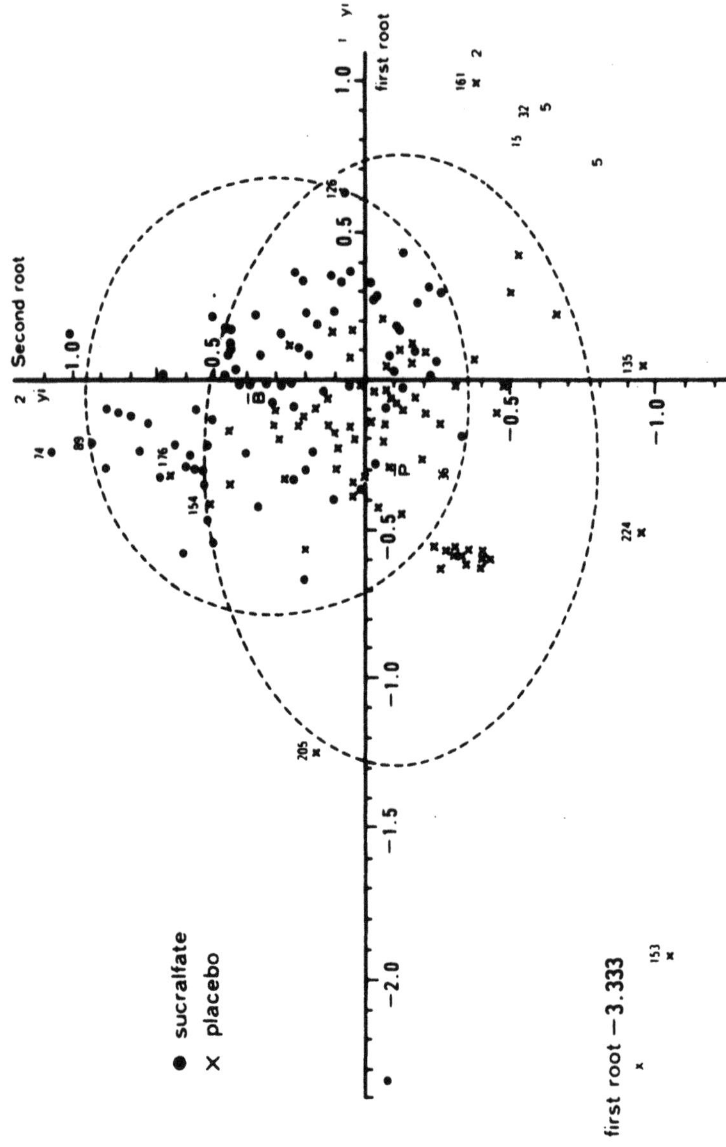

Figure 2. Results of double-blind controlled clinical trials of sucralfate (●) and placebo (×) in Japan (1973).

In 1982, it was revealed that the group of patients healed with sucralfate had a lower recurrence rate than that of patients healed with cimetidine[8] and that sucralfate was better than placebo in the maintenance treatment for preventing ulcer relapse.[9] In Japan, sucralfate had been considered to be more effective in the treatment of gastric ulcer than duodenal ulcer. Clinical studies performed in Europe and the United States, however, showed a reverse trend and gave the impression that sucralfate was mainly effective in the treatment of duodenal ulcer. The more widespread use of duodenoscopes at that time was considered as one of the reasons for the difference, since previous studies in Japan relied mainly on radiography. However, aside from differences in methodology, it is possible that sucralfate may be more effective in the treatment of duodenal rather than gastric ulcerations as it is expected that sucralfate will bind to duodenal ulcerations more firmly than to gastric lesions because of the high acidity in patients with duodenal ulcers. Moreover, the narrow duodenal lumen facilitates access of sucralfate to the ulcer crater when it passes through the lumen.

Mechanisms of Action

As for the mechanisms of action, it has been confirmed by a number of studies that sucralfate binds to the ulcer base.[10–14] This concept of selective ulcer-protecting agents, which was proposed in Japan, became recognized internationally. As shown in Fig. 3, histoautoradiographs of experimental ulcers showed that sucralfate binds to surface proteins and forms a protective layer that covers the ulcer base.[15]

The selective binding of sucralfate to the ulcer base has also been confirmed clinically. In an examination of resected specimens obtained from gastric ulcer patients given sucralfate orally 16 hr before the operation, it was shown (Fig. 4) that sucralfate had bound more to the ulcer base than to the normal mucosa surrounding the ulcer.[16] Thus, sucralfate has become recognized as a local or site protective agent.

New Developments in Sucralfate Research

What is noteworthy in the global sucralfate research is that the studies have become varied and the targeted area for investigations, widespread.

Clinical Application

It is quite natural that, following the internationalization of sucralfate research, its clinical application to different problems has widened concomitantly with an increase in numbers of institutes involved in sucralfate research. For example, the efficacy of sucralfate for reflux esophagitis and hemorrhagic ulceration or gastritis have been reported and of particular note is its effect in the prophylaxis of stress ulcer bleeding. No significant difference of effect exists among sucralfate, antacids, and H_2RAs regarding prevention of bleeding. However, it should be noted that patients treated with antacids or H_2RAs developed nosocomial pneumonia significantly more often than those treated with sucralfate.[17] This fact confirmed the expectation that drugs that do not affect gastric acidity and do not foster bacterial overgrowth in the stomach, would be more appropriate for

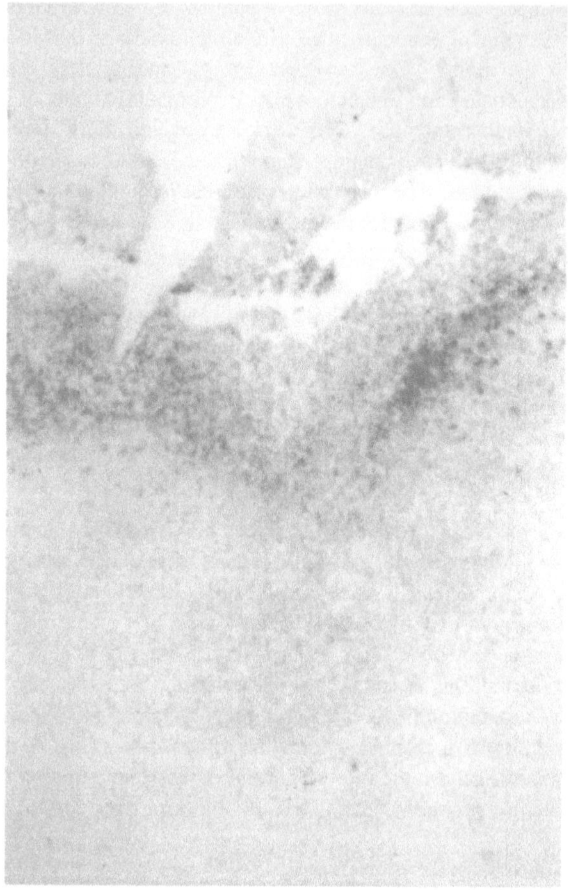

Figure 3. Histoautoradiograph showing sucralfate binding to the base of an experimental ulcer.

mechanically ventilated patients than antacids and H_2RAs. Considering that nosocomial infection of methicillin-resistant *S. aureus* has been gradually increasing, the above fact attests to the great clinical significance of sucralfate.

Mechanisms of Action

As the therapeutic efficacy of sucralfate was established, additional mechanisms of action were discovered. Investigation has centered on the mechanisms of enhancing gastric mucosal defenses, i.e., cytoprotection. Binding of sucralfate to ulcerated lesions is based on physicochemical interactions. It has been established that sucralfate changes the viscosity of gastric mucus and that the drug can adhere to nonulcerated mucosal surfaces.

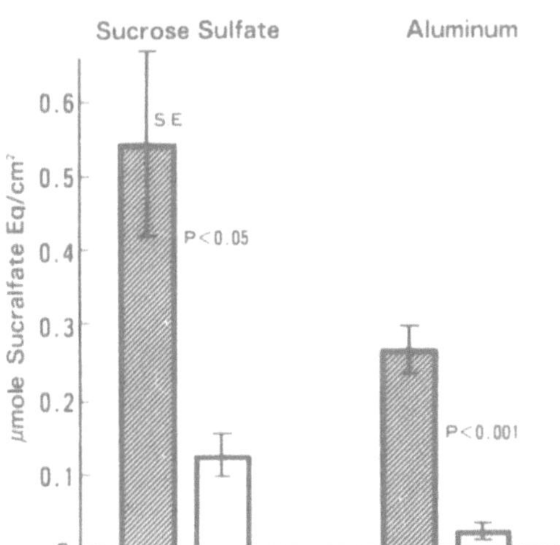

Figure 4. Selective binding of sucralfate to ulcer lesions (gastrectomized specimens) (shaded bars, gastric ulcer; open bars, nonulcer; $n = 6$).

Thus, sucralfate can exert its various effects on the normal mucosa diffusely as well as on ulcerated lesions. Thus, sucralfate's cytoprotective mechanisms include: (1) antipeptic activity and bile acid adsorption, (2) promotion of sodium bicarbonate secretion, (3) augmentation of mucous resistance by promotion of mucus secretion and change in mucous components, (4) stimulation of prostaglandin secretion, (5) protection of blood vessels, (6) promotion of epithelial regeneration by protection and stimulation of the mucosal proliferative zone, and (7) stimulation of growth factors such as epidermal growth factor.

The various effects of sucralfate are exerted at its contact sites in the stomach and duodenum. Considering that the binding of sucralfate at the ulcer crater is much stronger than the adhesion to the normal mucosa, it is postulated that those effects would be magnified at the ulcerated area. Thus, the actions of sucralfate seem to be divided into two groups: one is a group of local or site protective actions selectively directed to the ulcerated area as initially emphasized in Japan[5] and the second group consists of stimulation of mucosal defenses, i.e., cytoprotection. However, the difference between the two groups of actions is modulated by the strength of binding.

Conclusion

Selective ulcer binding and protection was the new concept proposed in Japan at the time of the development of sucralfate. This concept has been widely accepted internationally. At this point, the defensive and cytoprotective mechanisms of sucralfate have also been accepted internationally. It must be emphasized that research about the cytoprotective mechanisms of sucralfate has greatly advanced the overall understanding of cytoprotection in general. In the first 10 years or so, sucralfate research was done primarily in Japan. Since then, research into the mechanisms of action of sucralfate has become global. It should be pointed out that the history of sucralfate has taken steps of unique internationalization. I remember that the following question was raised at the press conference at the First International Sucralfate Symposium in Hamburg, 1980, and no one was able to provide an answer: "What is the reason for the commencement of full-scale international investigations at this point whereas the drug with the unique mechanism of actions has been in clinical use for more than 10 years in Japan? It is hard to understand!" It is easy to say "internationalization" but I realize that it can't be accomplished in a day.

References

1. Babkin BP, Komarov SA: The influence of gastric mucus on peptic digestion. *Can Med Assoc J* **27**:463–469, 1932. The pepsin-suppressing activity of chondroitin sulfate in mucus is described.
2. Cook DL, Eich S, Cammarata PS: Comparative pharmacology and chemistry of synthetic sulfated polysaccharide. *Arch Int Pharmacodyn* **144**:1–19, 1963. This paper gives a detailed description of synthetic antipeptic agents.
3. Cayer D, Raffin JM: Effect of Depepsin in the treatment of peptic ulcer. *Ann NY Acad Sci* **140**:744–746, 1967. The first evaluation of amylopectin sulfate, developed in the United States, in PUD patients.
4. Watt J, Marcus R: Ulceration of the colon in rabbits fed sulfated amylopectin. *J Pharm Pharmacol* **24**:68–69, 1972. A major side effect of antipeptic agents is intestinal, especially colonic ulceration.
5. Ishimori A: Mechanism of the antipeptic action of anionic carbohydrate and its clinical application for the treatment of peptic ulcer. *Tohoku J Exp Med* **103**:141–157, 1971. The suppression of peptic activity in gastric juice by sucralfate is transient.
6. Yamagata S, Ishimori A, *et al*: Clinical evaluation of pharmacotherapy for peptic ulcer with antipepsin agents by double blind technique. *Tohoku J Exp Med* **110**:377–404, 1973. Gastric ulcer healing is improved after sucralfate therapy.
7. Marks IN: A skeptical view of medical treatment, in Truelove SC, Willoughby CP (eds): *Topics in Gastroenterology*. Oxford, Blackwell, vol 7, pp 111–129, 1979. Sucralfate has comparable efficacy to cimetidine in healing gastroduodenal ulcers.
8. Marks IN, Weight JP, Lucks W, *et al*: Relapse rates after initial ulcer healing with sucralfate and cimetidine. *Scand J Gastroenterol* **17**:429–432, 1982. Relapse rates after sucralfate-induced healing are lower compared with cimetidine-induced healing.
9. Moshal MG, Spitaels J-M, Manion GL: Double-blind placebo-controlled evaluation of one year therapy with sucralfate on healed duodenal ulcer. *Scand J Gastroenterol* **18**(suppl 83):57–59, 1983. Sucralfate is superior to placebo in keeping DU in remission.
10. Bigley LD, Giesing D: Studies on acting mechanism of sucralfate, in Caspary WF (ed): *Duodenal Ulcer, Gastric Ulcer: Sucralfate*. Munich, Urban & Schwarzenberg, 1981, pp 3–12.
11. Harrington SJ, Schlegel JF, Code CF: The protective effect of sucralfate on the gastric mucosa in rats. *J Clin Gastroenterol* **3**(suppl 2):129–134, 1981.
12. Steiner K, Garbe A: Specific binding of ^{14}C-sucralfate to acetic acid-induced gastric and duodenal ulcers of the rat, in Caspary WF (ed): *Duodenal Ulcer, Gastric Ulcer: Sucralfate*. Munich, Urban & Schwarzenberg, 1981, pp 19–21.
13. Sasaki H, Hinohara Y, Tsunoda Y, *et al*: Binding sucralfate to duodenal ulcer in man. *Scan J Gastroenterol* **18**(suppl 83):13–14, 1983.
14. Quinton A: Binding duration of sucralfate assessed at different doses. International update: GL therapy, Maui, 1987. References 10–14 discuss binding of sucralfate to the base of peptic ulcers.
15. Nagashima R, Hirano T: Selective binding of sucralfate to ulcer lesion. *Arzneim Forsch* **30**:80–83, 1980. This study illustrates the selective binding of sucralfate to an ulcer base.

16. Nakazawa S, Nagashima R, Samloff IM: Selective binding of sucralfate to gastric ulcer in man. *Dig Dis Sci N S* **26**:297–300, 1981. This is a fundamental study indicating selective binding of sucralfate to gastric ulcers in man.
17. Driks MR, Craven DE, Celli BR, *et al*: Nosocomial pneumonia in intubated patients given sucralfate as compared with antacids or histamine-type 2 blockers. *N Engl J Med* **317**:1376–1382, 1987. Nosocomial pneumonia was thought to occur more often after H_2RA therapy of intubated patients.

III

Sucralfate: A Nonsystemic Site Protective Agent

5

Chemistry of Sucralfate

KIYOSHIGE OCHI

Introduction

Sulfated polysaccharides possess antiulcer effects in experimental ulcer models and antipeptic activity *in vitro*. The efficacy of natural polysaccharide is closely related to the degree of the sulfation rather than the length of the sugar chain. Therefore, Namekata and co-workers investigated the antiulcer activities of the oligo- and monosaccharide sulfates whose sugar chain structures are well-known.[1]

They synthesized sodium salts of the sulfates of glucose, sorbitol, and glucosamine as monosaccharide, sucrose, lactose, and maltose as disaccharide, raffinose as trisaccharide, and stachyose as tetrasaccharide and investigated their antiulcer and antipeptic effects using Shay rat preparations. They found that antiulcer effects were greater as the degree of sulfation increased.[2,3] The length of the saccharide portion was also related to the antiulcer efficacy of the compounds. Longer sugar chains could provide more hydroxyl groups to be sulfated, but possible steric hindrance could cause difficulties in sulfating all of the hydroxyl groups. Taking into consideration activity, stability of the sulfated compound, maximum degree of sulfation in a molecule, availability as raw material, quality, and cost, they finally selected sucrose as the most promising saccharide.

In a comparison of antiulcer effects between the sodium sucrose sulfate obtained through the reaction of sodium hydroxide with the pyridinium sucrose sulfate prepared by the reaction of sucrose with sulfur trioxide in pyridine and the sucrose sulfate–aluminum hydroxide complex (sucralfate) obtained through the reaction of the sodium sucrose sulfate with basic polyaluminum chloride, sucralfate showed greater promise.[4]

The stability of the sulfate moieties introduced into sucrose was studied. The sodium sucrose sulfate is amorphous and undergoes gradual hydrolysis with adhering water at room temperature to generate sulfuric acid which forms a strong acidic milieu and accelerates decomposition per se. The aluminum complex is also amorphous but does not undergo hydrolysis and is stable during prolonged storage.

KIYOSHIGE OCHI • Development and Technology Division, Chugai Pharmaceutical Co., Ltd., Tokyo 115, Japan.

Sucralfate: From Basic Science to the Bedside, edited by Daniel Hollander and G. N. J. Tytgat. Plenum Press, New York, 1995.

Sucralfate was successfully developed as an antiulcer medication. It was marketed in Japan in 1968 and is currently available worldwide as an antiulcer agent that stimulates the defense mechanisms of the mucosa.

This chapter reviews the chemistry of sucralfate, particularly its synthetic and analytical chemistries. Even at the present time, however, several chemical issues regarding sucralfate remain unclear.

Synthetic Study of Sulfate and Its Aluminum Complex

Preparation of Sucrose Sulfate

Sucrose sulfate is usually obtained by the reaction of sucrose with either sulfur trioxide or chlorosulfonic acid in the presence of an organic base, e.g., pyridine. The organic base of pyridine affords pyridine–sulfur trioxide complex (Py-SO_3) with either sulfonation agent. Py-SO_3 reacts with primary and secondary hydroxyl moieties to provide a pyridinium salt of the sulfate. Since the solubility of sucrose, the raw material, in the solvent differs from that of the pyridinium sulfate produced, it is important to select proper reaction conditions in order to achieve persulfation.

Since a sucrose molecule possesses eight hydroxyl moieties consisting of three primary and five secondary ones, alteration of the molar ratio of the sulfur trioxide versus sucrose leads to products with varied compositions. In the two solvents of pyridine and dimethylformamide (DMF) possessing comparatively low and high dissolubility, respectively, the correlation between the molar ratio of Py-SO_3 against sucrose and the composition of produced compounds, particularly regarding the degree of sulfation, was investigated.[5]

In DMF, the reaction of sucrose with more than 9 molar ratios of Py-SO_3 yielded sucrose sulfate with a mean number of 7.9 sulfated hydroxy groups (*N*), indicating complete persulfation. In pyridine, on the other hand, an *N* value of 7.9 was attained using only 5 molar ratios (Table I). These findings suggested that the sucrose mass surface participated in the reaction in the presence of excess sulfating agent. The persulfated product, pyridinium sucrose sulfate, was converted to crystalline potassium salt subjected to the following structural analyses, conforming to an octasulfate structure with elemental analysis, X-ray diffraction analysis,[6] FTIR analysis, and ^{13}C-NMR analysis, respectively (Figs. 1–3).

Characterization of Basic Poly Aluminum Chloride

Sucralfate is synthesized by the reaction of aqueous sodium sucrose sulfate with basic poly aluminum chloride (PAC). PAC is usually prepared by dissolving aluminum metal into heated aqueous aluminum chloride solution. Methods consisting of adding either aqueous alkali or aluminum hydroxide to aqueous aluminum chloride and, in a particular case, of subjecting aqueous aluminum chloride to electrolysis are also known.

In aqueous aluminum chloride, trivalent aluminum ion (Al^{3+}) forms an aquo complex $[Al(H_2O)_6]^{3+}$ by the coordination of 6 moles of water molecules, with a tetrahedral structure as shown in Fig. 4a.

Table I. Analysis Data for the Sodium Salts of Sucrose Polysulfates

Molar ratio Py-SO_3[a]	Solvent[b]	Analysis results C %	Analysis results S %	S/C	N[c]
3	DMF	24.16	13.04	0.54	2.4
5	DMF	19.21	16.37	0.85	3.8
9	DMF	12.21	21.55	1.76	7.9
11	DMF	12.46	21.87	1.76	7.9
15	DMF	12.37	21.12	1.71	7.7
5	Py	12.08	21.33	1.77	7.9
9	Py	12.21	21.64	1.77	7.9

[a]Molar ratio to sucrose molecule.
[b]DMF, dimethylformamide; Py, pyridine.
[c]Calculated from $N = 4.5 \times$ S/C.

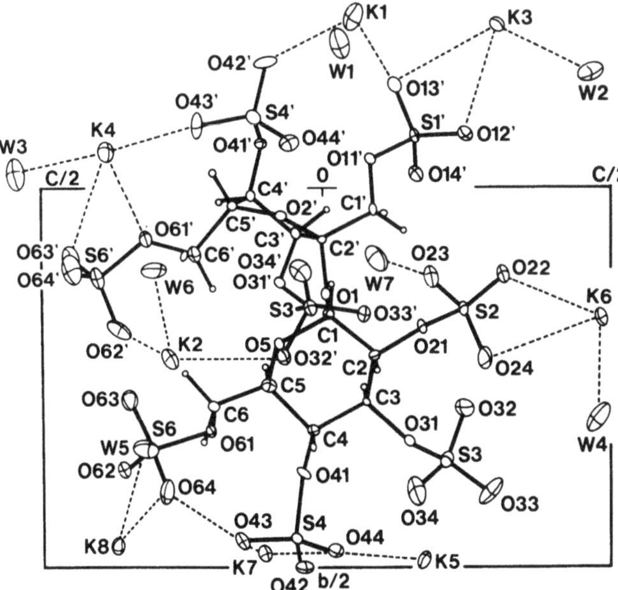

Figure 1. Three-dimensional drawing of potassium sucrose octasulfate heptahydrate molecule by X-ray diffraction analysis, showing the numbering of the atoms and 15% probability thermal ellipsoids for the non-hydrogen atoms in the asymmetric unit. Dotted lines indicate some of the $K^+ \cdots$ O bonds and hydrogen bonds.

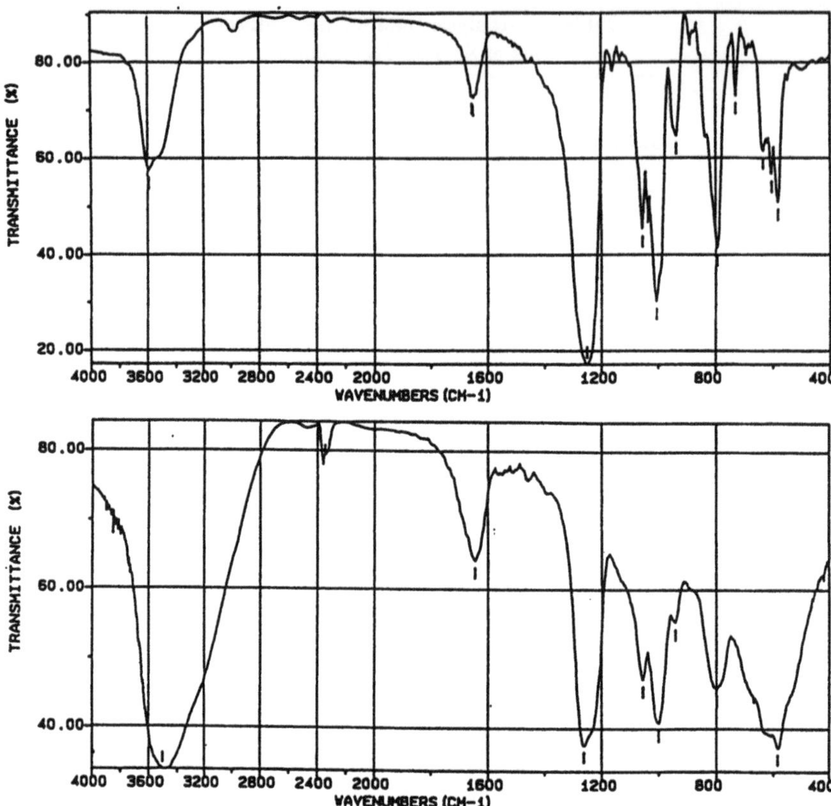

Figure 2. Fourier transform infrared (FTIR) spectra of crystalline potassium sucrose octasulfate (top) and dry sucralfate (bottom), showing the existence of similar characteristic absorption bands corresponding to sulfate groups. From these spectra, the sucrose sulfate structure of water-insoluble sucralfate is very similar to that of the water-soluble potassium salt.

When the coordinating water molecules are dissociated as hydrogen ion, new coordinating bonds form between the hydroxyl moiety generated and that of another aquo complex ion to provide a dimer cross-linked between the molecules. Further progress of the dissociation and the resultant increase in the number of hydroxyl moieties lead to increased intermolecular bonds to produce oligomers, such as trimer and tetramer, and polymer with higher molecular weights. These mixtures are generally referred to as "bridged complex."

Alkalinity is employed as an index representing the extent of dissociation. It is expressed as $m/3n \times 100\%$ when basic PAC has the general formula: $[Al_n(OH)_mCl_{3n-m}] \cdot (H_2O)_{6n-m}$ which represents aluminum chloride for $n = 1$ and $m = 0$ and aluminum hydroxide for $n = 1$ and $m = 3$ where basicities are 0 and 100%, respectively. Arbitrary values are theoretically allowed for n and m.

Binding forms of the bridged complex exist: the monohydroxo bridge (point–
having one hydroxyl moiety between the molecules, the dihydroxo bridge (line
having two hydroxyl moieties, and trihydroxo bridge (face–face) having three hy
moieties[7] (Fig. 4b).

In the above-mentioned manufacturing procedure of basic PAC, elevation
alkalinity caused by an increase in the content of hydroxyl moiety within the aquo
of aluminum chloride leads to an increase in the number of cross-links between of
ions. This phenomenon has been confirmed by instrumental analyses such a
centrifugation and gel filtration and a chemical analysis consisting of the color
method employing extraction with oxine salt.

In the HPLC analysis, three peaks with different relative retention time from aluminum chloride were observed and peaks attributable to compositions with higher molecular weights intensified with increase of basicity[8] (Table II).

Preparation of Sucralfate

Sucralfate is manufactured as a complex by the reaction of the aqueous sucrose octasulfate obtained by sulfation of sucrose with aqueous basic PAC. The water-soluble salts of sucrose sulfate, such as sodium, potassium, and ammonium salts, are employed for this reaction. These salts dissociate in water to form polyvalent ions and the sucrose sulfates behave as octavalent polyanions. Basic PAC, on the other hand, dissociates in water and behaves as polycations having valences of the general formula $Al_2(OH)_n^{(6-n)xm+}$

Generally, when a polyvalent anion is present in a solution of basic PAC, the charge on the aluminum portion is neutralized by the simultaneous formation of a new coordinate bond, where the polyvalent anion molecule plays the role of a cross-linking agent between the aluminum portions. The aqueous solubilities of the polymers are generally poor, so that intermolecular aggregations take place resulting in water-insoluble precipitate.

The octavalent polyanion of sucrose sulfate was aggregated by basic PAC to afford complexes as water-insoluble precipitates. The complexes are usually obtained as a solid, but sometimes as an oily deposit or a solution in a large amount of water without precipitating. The complexes with a low degree of sulfation sometimes possess comparatively high water-solubilities and solids can be obtained either by the concentrating operation of water or by adding alcohols.[8]

The factor most responsible for the physical properties of the complex produced is PAC, whose properties are considered to depend especially on the extent of the hydroxo cross-linking (degree of polymerization).

Chemical Structure of Sucralfate

The structural formula of sucralfate is generally presented as indicated in Fig. 5.[9] This is an average representation as the rational formula and not considered to represent the actual structure of the aluminum portion. Accordingly, this representation should be understood to be an average model reflecting difficulties in indicating its genuine structure.

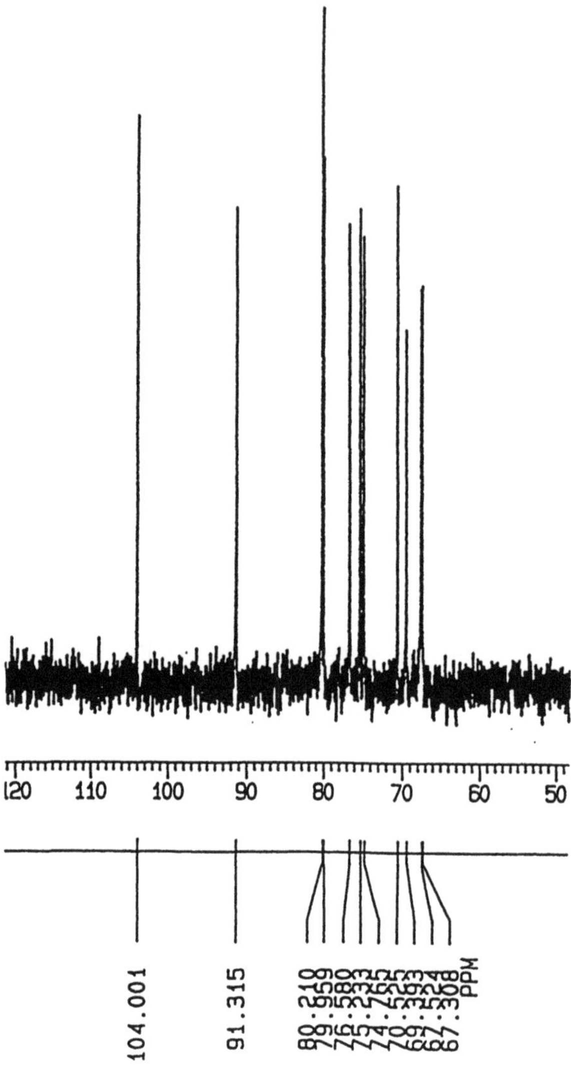

position	Glucose *	Fructose *
C 1	9 1. 3	6 9. 3
C 2	7 6. 5	1 0 3. 9
C 3	7 5. 1	8 0. 2
C 4	7 4. 7	8 0. 2
C 5	7 0. 4	8 0. 2
C 6	6 7. 3	6 7. 3

*ppm

The portion y(H_2O) represents total moisture, the total moles of which is represented by y, consisting of the adsorbed water and water of constitution. The wet powder immediately after production contains about 40w% of water on the basis of sucralfate. The water content of sucralfate depends on separation and storage conditions, and is decreased by drying to reach a minimum value of approximately 5% of the dried powder.[10]

The water content can be increased by suspending the dried powder in water or storing it under wet conditions. Hence, there exists an equilibrium between the water content of sucralfate and the moisture content (humidity) in the production/storage environments.

Heating to over 200°C can break the reversibility where the water contents cannot return to their previous values. The cause is presumed to be change of the hydroxy cross-linking [Al–$(OH)_2$–Al] to the oxo one [Al–O–Al] through thermal dehydration of the aluminum hydroxide moiety.

Sucralfate exists not as crystalline but as amorphous forms judging from the fact that the powder X-ray diffraction pattern analysis does not afford distinct analysis peaks.[11] This finding does not contradict the assumption that the average rational formula rather than the structural formula given in a single expression is a valid representation of the chemical structure of sucralfate.

Analysis and Characterization of Sucralfate

Behavior with Addition of Acid

Nagashima and co-workers investigated the acid-neutralizing actions of sucralfate including changes in its physical properties induced by acid.

When hydrochloric acid was added to a suspension of sucralfate, the changes in the physical properties of sucralfate were different from those of aluminum hydroxide. As dilute hydrochloric acid was added to a water suspension of sucralfate with vigorous stirrings, interparticle aggregation took place to produce a coarse dispersion when more than a certain amount (approximately 0.06 meq/meq sucralfate) of acid was added. Further addition of acid (approximately 0.08 meq) increased the number of particles, softened them, and finally produced a paste at the bottom of the container.[9]

When excess hydrochloric acid is added, sucralfate gradually dissolves into the aqueous solution, and the aluminum hydroxide portions dissociate from the sucrose sulfate. The resulting sucralfate paste can attach to the gastric mucosa and retard the permeation of hydrochloric acid into it.[12]

Detailed changes of the chemical structure have yet to be described. However, it is presumed that changes of the physical properties of sucralfate result from structural

←

Figure 3. ^{13}C nuclear magnetic resonance (NMR) spectrum of potassium sucrose octasulfate, yielding clearly separated peaks corresponding to 12 carbons, assigned successfully to the respective positions of glucose and fructose moieties (see table), suggesting the absence of contaminants (isomers) related to a diminished number of sulfate groups, introduced by insufficient sulfation reaction condition in the eight hydroxyl groups in the sucrose molecule.

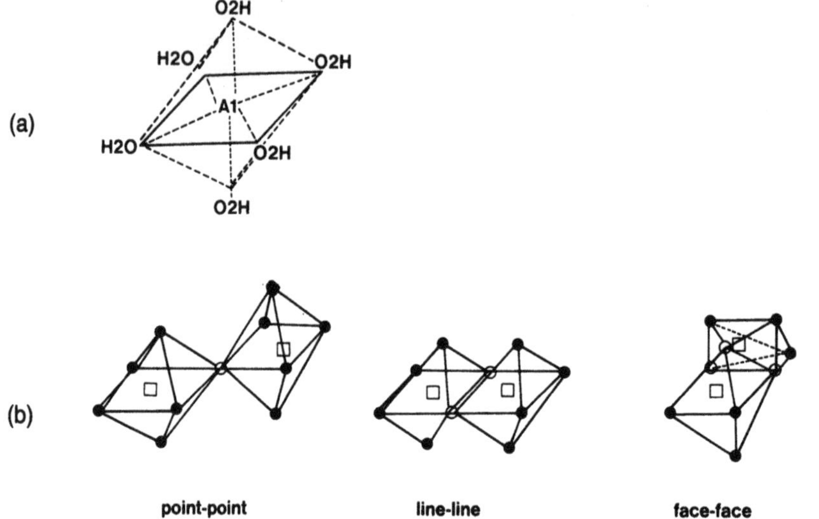

Figure 4. Structure of hexaaquo complex of trivalent aluminum ion (a), and structural models of hydroxodimer (b), showing intermolecular dimerization between two hydroxyl groups caused by dissociation of coordinating water. Each model represents the intermolecular dimerization between the two same molecules having one hydroxyl group, those having two hydroxyl groups, and those having three hydroxyl groups, respectively. The ratio of components of dimers or higher oligomers are varied by the number of hydroxyl groups in the solution, determined mainly by basicity desired. (□, trivalent aluminum ion; ○, hydroxyl group (binding position); ●, coordinated water.

Table II. Peak Area Ratios as a Function of Alkalinity

	Peak area ratio (%)		
Alkalinity	Peak 1[a]	Peak 2	Peak 3
50%	2.05	4.59	93.4
67%	35.19	14.4	50.39
75%	62.9	14.9	22.2
80%	70.25	21.8	7.97
83%	75.72	24.3	0

[a]Relative retention time to aluminum chloride (1.00): peak 1 0.76, peak 2 0.83, peak 3 0.96.

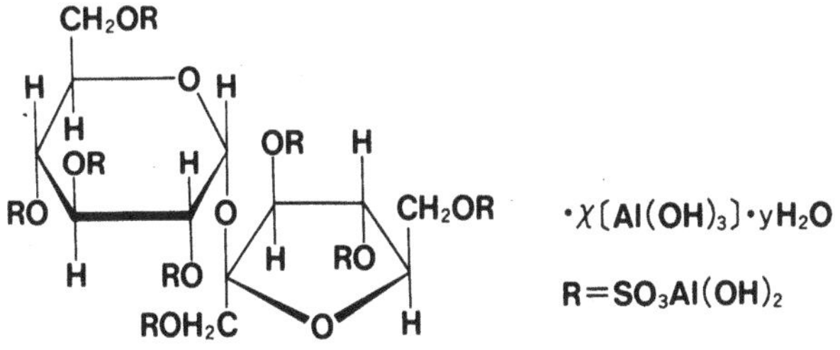

$\cdot \chi [Al(OH)_3] \cdot yH_2O$

$R = SO_3Al(OH)_2$

$C_{12}H_{30}Al_8O_{51}S_8 \cdot \chi Al(OH)_3 \cdot yH_2O$

Figure 5. Structure of sucralfate.

changes between the sulfate anion and the bridged complex cation, induced by changes in the charge of the bridged complex.

Recovery of the Sucrose Sulfate Moiety from Sucralfate

The sucrose sulfate moiety is recovered from sucralfate by breaking the bond between the sulfate and aluminum. The cleavage is carried out by treating sucralfate with a large excess of strong acid such as sulfuric or hydrochloric acid (Method A) or with strong alkali such as sodium or potassium hydroxide (Method B), while cooling the solution to prevent the degradation of the sulfate moieties.

While either procedure will recover sucrose sulfate, Method A may be preferred because it does not require special removal of the aluminum hydroxide.

The sulfuric acid–sodium hydroxide reagent is more efficient in cleaving the bond, ensuring satisfactory solubility of sucralfate in salt solutions and allowing the determination of sucrose octasulfate by HPLC ion-exchange mode. The sodium sucrose sulfate produced by this method can be analyzed without recovery procedures, by direct injection into a chromatography apparatus.[5] Crystals of potassium sucrose octasulfate are used as the standard and permit the accurate determination of the sucrose sulfate content in sucralfate.[13]

Solubility in Inorganic Salt Solution

Sucralfate is insoluble in water and organic solvents, but, in the presence of aqueous cations and anions, it can be ionized because of the amphoteric nature of the aluminum hydroxide moiety. When a large excess of amphoteric ions is present, some ionized sucralfate molecules move into the aqueous solution. The amount of sucralfate depends on the kind of salt, concentration, and temperature.

The transparent solution is obtained by stirring sucralfate with aqueous sodium chloride at room temperature followed by the removal of excess sucralfate by centrifugation; subjected to HPLC analysis, the peak attributable to the sucrose octasulfate was obtained. The peak patterns obtained from HPLC analyses did not show an increase in the number and amount of peaks corresponding to sucrose sulfate containing less than eight sulfate moieties, indicating that hydrolysis of the sulfate moiety did not occur.

Aluminum assay of the deposit produced by the removal of excess sodium chloride by dialysis yielded a lower value than that for sucralfate and this indicated that the hydroxy cross-linking aluminum hydroxide were partially dissociated.

It was presumed from the above experiments that the presence of neutral salts provides a kind of equilibrium between solid and solution of sucralfate in their aqueous solutions.

Using sodium chloride as an example, sodium ion intervenes in the hydroxo bridges between the aluminum molecules and an equilibrium of the partial structures of the complex ion formed moves from [–Al–OH–Al–] to [–Al–ONa + Cl–Al–] depending on the concentration of sodium chloride, where ionization of sucralfate is promoted and its solubility is increased. When sucralfate mass excess to this salt concentration is present, the ionization of the aluminum moiety does not proceed and most of the sucralfate remains as solid, where a small amount of the ionized sucralfate is transferred to the aqueous solution.

In salt solutions with higher salt concentrations or larger amount, the ionization proceeds from the aluminum hydroxide moiety to the bond between the sulfate and aluminum which formed sucralfate, so that a new equilibrium could be produced where the coordinate bond [–O–SO–O–Al–] is converted to the ionized [–SO–ONa + Cl–Al–]. Alteration of the concentration and amount of salt solutions forces sucralfate to participate in the equilibriums with varied elements.

This method has been applied to the sulfuric acid–sodium hydroxide reagent for the pretreatment in the HPLC analysis for measuring the sucrose octasulfate content of sucralfate.[13]

Detailed quantitative investigations of the equilibrium mechanisms and dependences on temperature and concentration have not been carried out.

Adsorbent Characteristic with Protein

Sucralfate binds to damaged mucosa in the stomach and the duodenum *in vivo*.[14] It also adsorbs and deactivates pepsin, a major aggressive factor secreted in the stomach together with the gastric juice. These actions are mediated by the protein-adsorbing activity of sucralfate.

Aqueous sucrose octasulfate has an antipeptic activity, and this protein-adsorbing activity is principally derived from the structure of the sucrose sulfate moieties. The basic aluminum hydroxide moieties bound to the sulfate moieties are helpful in protein adsorption.

As described above, sucrose sulfate behaves as the cross-linking agent between the basic aluminum hydroxide molecules and plays a role in determining the steric structure of the bridged complex. Accordingly, it affects the steric structure of sucralfate together with the intermolecular structure of the basic aluminum hydroxide moiety derived from raw material, basic PAC. The structure of the poly aluminum hydroxide moiety surrounding the sulfate permits adsorption of macromolecular protein.

Various functional moieties existing around the sucrose molecule, which can form the hydrogen and coordinate bonds, prevent the approach of substrate protein and also decrease the enzymatic activity of pepsin. These moieties can also prevent reversible release of protein by desorption.

Since sucralfate is insoluble in water, increasing the surface area by pulverizing the solid to particles as much as possible is one of the factors required to further increase the adsorption activity. While the dried powder is conventionally employed for the pulverization to particles by milling, the wet-milling of sucralfate wet powder with addition of water is also possible. In either case, it is possible to prepare fine particles below 50 μm in average diameter. An aqueous suspension prepared by adding water to the particles maintains the suspension state at high concentrations ranging from 1 to 1.5 g/ml where neither sedimentation nor aggregation occurs even at or above room temperature. As a result, this property has provided for the wet-milled powder a promising possibility of its direct use as the original solution for preparation of sucralfate suspension. A suspended state of sucralfate particles in dilute suspensions can be maintained by adding thickening agents.

The adsorption activity of protein can be measured by means of an experimental system *in vitro* using bovine serum albumin (BSA). Namely, the BSA dissolved in a buffer solution is adsorbed by the milled sucralfate and the adsorbed amount is determined by the difference between the initial amount and the residual amount remaining in the solution. Similarly, antipeptic activity of sucralfate can be confirmed by measuring the activity of pepsin remaining in the solution.[15]

When protein adsorption is measured using sucralfate compounds prepared with several kinds of basic PAC differing in acid-neutralizing capacity (alkalinity), preparation procedures, and conditions, some sucralfate compounds have only 70–80% of the activity of the original sucralfate.

These sucralfate compounds with lower activities in protein adsorption also show lower activity in *in vivo* experimental systems examining the suppressive activity against an ethanol-induced gastric mucosal injury.[16]

Thus, the preparative procedures for the basic PAC, affecting the steric structure of the basic aluminum hydroxide moiety of sucralfate, and the preparation of the polymerized complex are both important factors regarding sucralfate's therapeutic activity. Hence, excellent manufacturing and quality controls are required for the satisfactory activity and quality of sucralfate.

References

1. Namekata M: Proteolytic action of pepsin: Studies on oxidised starch sulfates for medical purpose. III. Inhibition of the proteolytic action of sulfates of oxidised starch and its reduced products. *Chem Pharm Bull* **10**:171–176, 1962. Ibid. IV. Protective effect of sulfates of oxidised starch and its reduced products on experimental peptic ulceration. Ibid. **10**:177–181, 1962.
2. Namekata M, Matsuo A, Momose A, *et al*: Studies on oligo saccharide sulfates and monosaccharide sulfates for medical purpose. I. Antipeptic and antiulcerogenic properties of the disaccharide sulfates. *Yakugaku Zasshi* **87**:376–380, 1967.
3. Namekata M, Sakamoto N, Yokoyama Y, *et al*: Ibid. II. Antipeptic and antiulcerogenic properties

of the tri, tetra-saccharide sulfates, monosaccharide sulfates and sulfates of its reduced products. *Yakugaku Zasshi* **87**:778–780, 1967.

4. Namekata M, Tanaka T, Sakamoto N, *et al*: Ibid. III. Antiulcerogenic properties of the sucrose sulfates aluminium complex. *Yakugaku Zasshi* **87**:889–893, 1967.
5. Ochi K, Watanabe Y, Okui K, *et al*: Preparation of sucrose sulfate by pyridine-sulfur trioxide complex and its structure: Crystalline salts of sucrose octasulfate. *Chem Pharm Bull* **28**:638–641, 1980.
6. Nawata Y, Ochi K, Shiba M, *et al*: Structure determination of octasulfate crystal by X-ray diffraction analysis: Structure of potassium sucrose octasulfate heptahydrate. *Acta Crystallogr* **B37**:246–249, 1981.
7. Ban S, Hatano S, Kobayashi T: Research reviews on structure and behavior of poly aluminum chloride: Basic research for poly aluminum chloride as an aggregation agent. *Suido Kyokai Zasshi* **404**:18–29, 1968.
8. Ochi K, Sasahara K, *et al*: Determination of components of basic poly aluminum chloride by HPLC method: Sucrose sulfate–poly aluminium hydroxide complex prepared from highly basic poly aluminum chloride. Japan Patent Kokai 1983:943–945 (Kokai No. S58-208, 294).
9. Nagashima R, Yoshida N: Acid neutralizing behavior in artificial gastric juice: Sucralfate, a basic aluminum salt of sucrose sulfate. I. Behaviors in gastroduodenal pH. *Arzneim Forsch* **29**:1668–1676, 1979.
10. Ushio H, Shiba M: Water determination analysis with several methods: Behavior of water containing in sucralfate molecule. 102nd Annu Meet Jpn Pharm Soc Abstr Pap 645, 3Y11-1, 1982.
11. Morikawa M, Miyake M, Iwai S, *et al*: Radial distribution analysis by X-ray diffraction method suggests the existence of main dimer component of aluminum hydroxide moiety in sucralfate molecule: Structural analysis of the amorphous sodium salt and aluminium hydroxide salt of sucrose sulfate. *J Chem Soc Faraday Trans 1* **77**:629–639, 1981.
12. Nagashima R, Hinohara Y, Hirano T, *et al*: Selective binding of sucrose sulfate to ulcer lesion. II. Experiments in rats with gastric ulcer receiving 14C-sucralfate or potassium 14C-sucralfate or potassium 14C-sucrose sulfate. *Arzneim Forsch* **30**:84–88, 1980.
13. Criteria of test items and test methods of bulk sucralfate. *Pharmacopoeia of Japan XII* pp 514–516.
14. Sakai H, Hinohara Y, Tsunoda Y, *et al*: Binding of sucralfate to duodenal ulcer in man. *Scand J Gastroenterol* **18**(suppl 83):13–14, 1983.
15. Ochi K, Sasahara K, *et al*: Experimental adsorption activity of bouvine serum albumin and the method of preparation of suspension formulation: Stock solution of sucralfate suspended in water and production thereof. Japan Patent Kokai 1993 (Kokai No. H5-9122, PCT No. WO 92/4030).
16. Nagashima R, Hoshino E, Hinohara Y, *et al*: Effect of sucralfate on ethanol-induced gastric mucosal damage in the rat. *Scand J Gastroenterol* **18**(suppl 83):17–20, 1983.

6

Binding of Bile Acids by Sucralfate

W. F. CASPARY

Introduction

The gastric mucosal barrier is considered to play an important role in protecting the gastric mucosa from the destructive effects of several luminal agents.[1,2] The breakdown of the gastric mucosal barrier has been associated with erosive mucosal injury and ulceration induced by such factors as stress and endogenous compounds including bile salts and urea.[2–5]

Bile acids were one of the factors considered to be of importance in the pathogenesis of gastric ulcer disease.[6] Binding of bile acids to antacids has been considered to play an important role regarding the beneficial therapeutic action in the treatment of peptic ulcer disease.[7,8]

Sucralfate is a complex salt of sucrose sulfate and aluminum hydroxide. It is very poorly soluble in water, a property that greatly limits experiments aimed at determining its mode of action.[9–11] It is minimally soluble in dilute acid and in alkali. When dissolved it breaks down into its aluminum salt and sucrose sulfate, forming a polyanion gel-like substance.

In the presence of acid, sucralfate releases aluminum, acquires a strong negative charge, and binds electrostatically to any positively charged chemical groups in its environment, including proteins, peptides, drugs, metals, and large molecules such as mucins (glycoprotein, glycolipoproteins); with mucins it may form complex gels with various types of cross-linkages. Its physical, mechanical, adsorbent, ion-exchange, and buffering properties may contribute to mucosal protection.[11]

W. F. CASPARY • Division of Gastroenterology, Department of Internal Medicine, Frankfurt University Hospital Medical Center, D-60590 Frankfurt am Main, Germany.

Sucralfate: From Basic Science to the Bedside, edited by Daniel Hollander and G. N. J. Tytgat. Plenum Press, New York, 1995.

Binding of Bile Acids by Sucralfate

Binding of Bile Acids in Vitro—Use of Pure Bile Acids

Bruusgaard *et al.*[12] and Caspary[13,14] were the first authors to demonstrate that sucralfate has potent bile acid binding properties. Bruusgaard *et al.* used bile acids in gastric aspirates mixed with duodenal aspirates obtained after stimulation of the gallbladder with cholecystokinin (CCK), whereas Caspary examined binding of pure bile acids to sucralfate and cholestyramine.

Sucralfate bound effectively glycocholic acid and chenodeoxycholic acid (Fig. 1) with increasing concentrations of sucralfate (20–1000 mg/5 ml). Binding to cholestyramine was, however, more effective (Fig. 2): Sucralfate (50 mg/ml) bound 19 μmole (38%) CDCA (10 mM), whereas cholestyramine (20 mg/ml) bound 43 μmole (86%) CDCA at a CDCA concentration of 10 mM.

Graham *et al.*[15] investigated the *in vitro* adsorption of bile sales and aspirin to sucralfate in environments simulating the stomach (pH 1.5), small intestine (pH 7), and colon (pH 7.8).

Bile salts were rapidly adsorbed by sucralfate. Adsorption was linearly related to the concentration of sucralfate except when the binding capacity was greater than 300 μmole/g.

Sucralfate adsorbed all bile salts tested (except taurocholic acid at pH 1.5), but was less effective than cholestyramine. Bile salt binding of sucralfate was much less effective at neutral pH, whereas cholestyramine did bind bile salts very effectively at neutral and acid pH (Tables I and II).

Aspirin was minimally adsorbed by sucralfate [7.5 μmole (1.4 mg)/g sucralfate, pH 1.5]. The authors concluded that adsorption of aspirin to sucralfate does not explain the protective effect of sucralfate against aspirin injury.

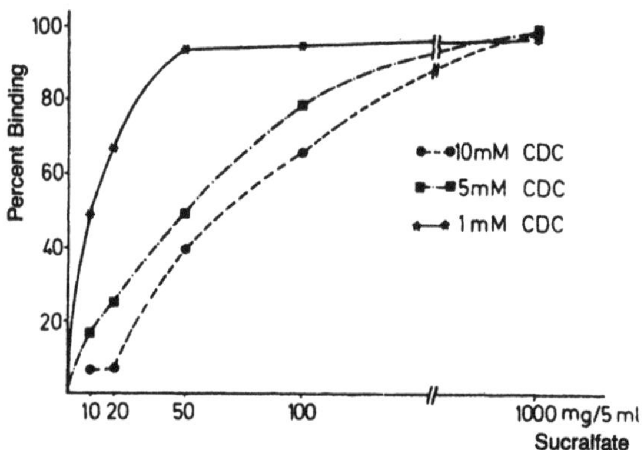

Figure 1. "Binding" of chenodeoxycholic acid (CDCA) to sucralfate. Binding was assessed *in vitro* at different concentrations of CDCA (1, 5, 10, mM) by increasing concentrations of sucralfate (10, 20, 50, 100, 1000 mg/5 ml). Results are expressed in percent binding. (After Caspary and Graf.[14])

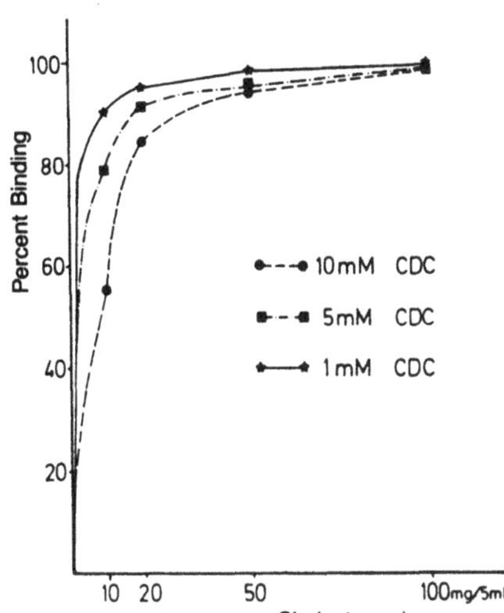

Figure 2. "Binding" of chenodeoxycholic acid (CDCA) to cholestyramine. Binding was measured *in vitro* at different concentrations of CDCA (1, 5, 10, mM) by increasing concentrations of cholestyramine (10, 20, 50, 100 mg/5 ml). Results are expressed in percent binding. (After Caspary and Graf.[14])

Another bile salt binding study compared the bile salt binding properties of commonly used gastrointestinal drugs: Maalox, Carafate (sucralfate), and cholestyramine.[16] Binding of sodium taurocholate was measured in calcium-free phosphate buffer adjusted to pH 2.0 or 7.0.

When Maalox (850 mg) was added to 10 ml of the test solution with an initial pH of 2.0, the pH increased to 8.82. Sucralfate acted differently. When sucralfate was added to the test solution with an initial pH of 2.0, the pH increased to 4.17; when added to the test solution with an initial pH of 7.0, the pH was lowered to 4.8. Thus, sucralfate had a weak buffering capacity.

The total bile salt binding by Maalox was proportional to the amount of Maalox added. The binding of taurocholate by sucralfate was determined by the pH of the test

Table I. Binding Capacity of Sucralfate for Bile Salts from a 5 mM Solution at Neutral and Acid pH[a]

	Binding capacity (μmole/g)				
pH	GC[b]	GCDC	TC	TDC	TCDC
7.0	51	41	20	33	7
1.5	ins	ins	0.1	447	380

[a]After Graham *et al.*[15]
[b]GC, glycocholate; GCDC, glycochenodeoxycholate; TC, taurocholate; TDC, taurodeoxycholate; TCDC, taurochenodeoxycholate; ins, insoluble.

Table II. Percentage of Bile Acids Adsorbed from a 5 mM Bile Salt Solution by Sucralfate (1 g/dl) and Cholestyramine (1 g/dl) at Neutral and Acid pH[a]

		% adsorbed from a 5 mM bile salt solution				
Binding agent	pH	GC[b]	GCDC	TC	TDC	TCDC
Sucralfate	7.0	10	8	4	6	1
Cholestyramine	7.0	80	77	87	91	85
Sucralfate	1.5	ins	ins	0	67	76
Cholestyramine	1.5	ins	ins	76	86	90

[a]After Graham *et al.*[15]
[b]GC, glycocholate; GCDC, glycochenodeoxycholate; TC, taurocholate; TDC, taurodeoxycholate; TCDC, taurochenodeoxycholate; ins, insoluble.

solution: at an initial pH of 7.0, total bile salt binding increased in proportion to the amount of sucralfate added to the solution, but a hyperbolic pattern of the binding curve was observed when the initial pH of the solution was 2.

The bile salt binding by sucralfate was much greater at the lower pH (<4.3) than at the higher pH (>4.3). The bile salt property of cholestyramine was 20- to 40-fold higher than that of sucralfate and 40-fold higher than that of Maalox.

In an *in vitro* study, Lipsett and Gadacz[17] compared bile salt binding by cholestyramine, Maalox, sucralfate, and Meciadanol (flavonoid) at pH 7.0 (Table III). Significant bile salt binding for sucralfate was not found in this study except for taurocholate and taurodeoxycholate. The authors doubt that binding of bile acids may occur at all at low pH values. They stress that at a pH less than 3, the free forms and glycine conjugates of bile salts will precipitate because the pH is lower than the pK_a. Thus, at a low pH, the concentration of bile sales in the supernatants is low primarily because of precipitation rather than adsorption of the bile salts.

Bile Acid Binding in Vitro— Use of Natural Bile Acids in Gastric and/or Duodenal Juice

Bruusgaard *et al.*[12] used for their binding studies bile acids obtained from gastric and duodenal juice after stimulation of the gallbladder by CCK at different pH values. At pH 2 and 3 binding of total bile acids to sucralfate did not differ from binding to cholestyramine; at higher pH values binding of bile acids to sucralfate was, however, considerably less than binding by cholestyramine. In other words, bile acid binding by sucralfate was pH-dependent, whereas binding of bile acids to cholestyramine was as effective at pH 9 as at pH 2.

In a study from Finland[18] total bile acid binding from aspirated gastric juice was tested using sucralfate as binding agent. In addition, binding properties of sucralfate were compared with those of cholestyramine (Questran) and antacids composed of aluminum hydroxide (Neutragel), magnesium hydroxide (Magnesiamaito), and aluminum–

Table III. ***In Vitro*** **Binding of Bile Salts of Cholestyramine Resin, Antacid, Sucralfate, and Meciadanol**[a]

	Percentage of bile salt binding at pH 7								
	C	DC	CDC	GC	GDC	GCDC	TC	TDC	TCDC
Cholestyramine	94	97	91	94	97	96	95	96	94
Maalox	10	47	25	26	29	22	33	15	17
Sucralfate	0	0	0	30	37	22	48	61	4
Meciadanol	84	0	0	60	61	64	53	69	80

[a]After Lipsett and Gadacz.[17]

magnesium hydroxide plus magnesium carbonate (Novaluzid). The pH value of the gastric aspirate was 4, and the total bile acid concentration 1.5 μmole/ml. To 10-ml samples the following additions were made: 0.5 g sucralfate in 2 ml water, 1 g cholestyramine in 2 ml water, and 2 ml of the antacids.

Sucralfate adsorbed bile acids significantly better than the antacids composed of magnesium hydroxide or aluminum–magnesium hydroxide plus magnesium carbonate (Table IV). Binding was equivalent to binding by aluminum hydroxide, but was significantly less than by cholestyramine.

Time-response measurements showed that bile acid adsorption by each of the test drugs reached its maximum in 10 or 15 min. Study of the pH-dependence (pH 2, 4, 6, 8) of bile acid adsorption revealed that sucralfate adsorbed bile acids significantly better at the more alkaline pH values of 6 and 8 than at pH 2. Aluminum hydroxide behaved differently: its adsorptive capacity markedly decreased with increasing pH.

Binding of bile acids to sucralfate and antacids was tested in a "quasiphysiological" reflux mixture obtained from nonstimulated gastric juice and hepatic bile.[19] In this study bile acid adsorption was measured by the HPLC technique. The bile acid concentration of the reflux mixture was about 2 μmole/liter. Five milliliters of the reflux mixture was incubated with 1 ml of sucralfate or antacids for 60 min at 37°C. Bile acids were determined after centrifugation in the supernatant.

The pH values observed and the percentage of adsorption are given in Table V.

Addition of sucralfate to the "quasiphysiological" reflux mixture resulted in the lowest pH. Since different antacids were used, this study cannot clearly demonstrate a pH-dependence of bile acid adsorption. Total bile acid adsorption was highest with aluminum-

Table IV. Bile Acid Adsorption Rates (%) at pH 4 Using Bile Acids in Gastric Juice Aspirates[a]

Sucralfate	Cholestyramine	$Al(OH)_3$	$Mg(OH)_2$	Al-Mg hydroxide plus Mg carbonate
54	94	59	31	25

[a]After Stahlberg *et al.*[18]

Table V. Bile Acid Adsorption and pH Achieved by Adding Sucralfate or Antacids to a "Quasiphysiological" Reflux Mixture[a]

Substrate	pH	TUDC[b]	TC	GC	TCDC	TDC	GCDC	GDC	TLC	TBA
Sucralfate	3.72	100	40	67	82	100	100	100	100	76
Aludrox	4.50	100	80	94	100	100	100	100	36	90
Maalox	4.96	100	79	100	100	100	100	100	27	90
Gelusil	6.64	100	27	22	62	66	74	38	59	45
Solugastril	7.59	100	44	35	60	51	75	50	45	53

[a]After Kurtz *et al.*[19]
[b]TUDC, tauroursodeoxycholic acid; TC, taurocholic acid; GC, glycocholic acid; TCDC, taurochenodeoxycholic acid; TDC, taurodeoxycholic acid; GCDC, glycochenodeoxycholic acid; GDC, glycodeoxycholic acid; TLC, taurolithocholic acid; TBA, total bile acids.

containing antacids with relatively lower neutralizing capacity (Aludrox, Maalox), decreased by adding antacids with more potent neutralizing capacity (Gelusil, Solugastril). Total bile acid adsorption by sucralfate was intermediate (76%).

There was a marked difference of adsorption for the different bile acids. The nontoxic and polar TUDC is adsorbed by all antacids and sucralfate completely, but the strong nonpolar and toxic TLC is only adsorbed effectively by sucralfate.

In a later study the same authors[20] showed that bile acid adsorption was pH-dependent to the same antacids used. The highest total bile acid adsorption was observed at pH 3. The degree of bile acid adsorption correlated with the lipophilicity of bile acids, i.e., the most lipophilic and toxic bile acids were bound most effectively.

Effect of Sucralfate on Bile Acid Absorption in Vivo

Tanghöj *et al.*[21] measured serum bile acid (SBA) concentrations in healthy volunteers after a standard test meal and after oral bile acid administration of 1 g chenodeoxycholic acid (CDCA). On a separate occasion the tests were repeated by addition of 2 g sucralfate or 8 g cholestyramine. Sucralfate did not influence postprandial levels of SBA, but significantly reduced SBA after CDCA loading. Cholestyramine lowered SBA both after the test meal and after CDCA loading.

Protective Effect of Sucralfate against Bile Acid-Induced Damage of Gastric Mucosa

Since the binding capacity of sucralfate is pH-dependent, Danesh *et al.*[22] tested in rats whether an acid pH medium is required for the protective effect of sucralfate against mucosal injury. The effect of sucralfate (300 mg/kg) at an acidic pH of 1.5 and a near-neutral pH of 6.5 was examined following mucosal damage induced in rats by aspirin alone and aspirin combined with bile acids [taurodeoxycholic acid (TDCA)].

Since the erosive activity of aspirin and bile acids is pH-dependent,[23] a threefold greater amount of aspirin and a twofold higher concentration of bile acids were required for the induction of mucosal lesions at pH 6.5.

Sucralfate significantly reduced mucosal damage induced by aspirin alone and aspirin combined with bile acids at pH 1.5 and 6.5 (Table VI). Thus, the protective effect of sucralfate against mucosal injury induced by aspirin and bile acid was not dependent on an acidic medium. This suggested that sucralfate retains its mucosal protective effects when gastric acid secretion is inhibited.

An *in vitro* study[24] on the effect of sucralfate on recovery of chambered rat gastric mucosa from taurocholate-induced damage revealed that addition of 100 mg of sucralfate in 50 mM HCl reduced the average lesion area induced by Na-taurocholate from about 15% to 3% under conditions of nonstirring of the medium.

The ability of sucralfate to accelerate the recovery process after damage was abolished by indomethacin pretreatment. This study demonstrated that sucralfate is capable not only of prevention or attenuation of acute damage when administered prior to damaging agents, but also of arresting the sequence of events that produces hemorrhage in the previously inflamed or damaged stomach.

Romano *et al.*[25] examined the effect of sucralfate and its components on taurocholate-induced damage to rat gastric mucosal cells in tissue culture. They found that sucralfate, but not its components (sucrose octasulfate, aluminum hydroxide), protected rat gastric mucosal cells against taurocholate-induced damage under conditions independent of systemic factors and in a neutral environment. In addition, sucralfate significantly stimulated prostaglandin production by cultured cells, but the protection by sucralfate *in vitro* did not seem to depend on its stimulatory effect on endogenous prostaglandin synthesis.

Another group[26] had earlier observed that sucralfate provided protection against taurocholate-induced gastric mucosal damage and speculated that sucralfate-induced stimulation of endogenous gastric mucosal prostanoid formation may at least in part explain its effective protective properties.

Sucralfate decreased H^+ disappearance induced by taurocholate in rat stomach and significantly reduced the index of mucosal damage.[27]

Since it has been shown *in vitro*[15] (Table I) that binding of taurocholate to sucralfate is only minimal at pH 1.5, it is very unlikely that the protective effect of sucralfate against taurocholate-induced gastric mucosal damage was the result of adsorption of taurocholate to sucralfate.

Transmural gastric potential difference (PD) has been used by several groups as a parameter for the integrity of the gastric mucosal barrier.[5,8,13] Intragastric instillation of 10 mM glycocholic acid in 100 ml water induced a significant decrease of transmural gastric PD from 41.7 mV to 27 mV after 18 min. Addition of 1 g of sucralfate reduced the drop of transmural PD significantly from 41.9 mV to only 33 mV ($p < 0.05$).[13]

Bile Acid Adsorption of Sucralfate in Alkaline Reflux Gastritis

Alkaline reflux gastritis is a chronic symptom complex occurring in patients after surgical treatment of peptic ulcer disease and is characterized primarily by epigastric pain, which is frequently associated with nausea and vomiting.[28] The presumption is that an increased reflux of duodenal contents into the stomach leads to mucosal damage and the resultant symptoms. Cholestyramine has failed to be of any benefit for patients with clinical symptoms of alkaline reflux gastritis in two double-blind trials.[29,30]

Table VI. Effect of Sucralfate on Aspirin- and Bile Acid-Induced Gastric Mucosal Erosions at pH 1.5 and pH 6.5[a]

pH1.5						
Erosions	ASA[b]	ASA + SF	ASA + TDCA	ASA + TDCA + SF		
Scores	6.6	1.2	15.5	2.2		
p value	<0.001		<0.001			
pH 6.5						
Erosions	ASA + TDCA	ASA + TCA	ASA + TCA + GCA	ASA + GCA + SF	ASA + SF	ASA + TDCA + SF
Scores	4.9	0.2	4.1	0.2	2.3	0.2
p value	<0.001		<0.001		<0.01	

[a]After Danesh *et al.*[22]

[b]ASA, aspirin; SF, sucralfate; TCDA, taurochenodeoxycholic acid; TCA, taurocholic acid; GCA, glycocholic acid.

The therapeutic effect of sucralfate (6 g/day) and placebo was compared on symptoms, endoscopic findings, and gastric mucosal histology in 23 patients with symptoms of alkaline reflux gastritis who had undergone Billroth I, Billroth II, gastric resection, or vagotomy and pyloroplasty.

After 6 weeks of treatment the two treatment groups did not differ significantly with respect to symptom score or endoscopic findings.[28] However, after the 6-week, double-blind phase, the inflammatory cell score of the sucralfate-treated group was significantly lower than that of the placebo-treated group. Thus, we may conclude that sucralfate lowered the inflammatory cell score of patients with symptoms of alkaline reflux gastritis. This reduction, however, was not associated with an improvement in symptoms.

In experimental esophagitis induced in a rabbit model, sucralfate was not able to prevent the mucosal permeability defect observed after exposure to taurocholate, but did significantly diminish the degree of esophagitis and permeability changes caused by pepsin.[20]

A clinical study in intensive care unit patients demonstrated that Maalox, sucralfate, and Meciadanol reduced bile salt concentration in gastric aspirates significantly.[17]

Effect of Sucralfate on Fecal Bile Acid Excretion and Potential Use in the Treatment of Cholerrheic Enteropathy

The relative ability of the resin cholestyramine and sucralfate to bind bile acids in the gastrointestinal tract and increase fecal bile acid excretion has been studied in normal rats on a standard diet.[31] Both drugs increased fecal bile acid excretion with a definitely higher effect of cholestyramine [from μmole/day to 85.7 μmole on 1% cholestyramine for 21 days versus an increase from 23.8 to 36.8 μmole/day on sucralfate (1 g/100 g food)].

The resin, however, produced a higher fecal bile acid excretion after 1 week than after 3 weeks, whereas sucralfate-induced fecal bile acid excretion increased with time of administration. *In vitro* cholesterogenesis was clearly increased by cholestyramine and moderately by sucralfate although [^{14}C]acetate incorporation into cholesterol was not quantitatively correlated to the amount of bile acids excreted in feces.

Two anecdotal reports[32,33] suggested the use of sucralfate for the treatment of cholerrheic enteropathy. The first observation[33] was confirmed[32] by another case report on a patient with cholerrheic enteropathy and severe perirectal pain after partial ileal bypass. After treatment with 2 g of sucralfate for 4 days, the patient's perirectal burning pain was totally relieved for the first time in 9 months, whereas cholestyramine and loperamide were without any effect.

The speculation that sucralfate may be used in the treatment of cholerrheic enteropathy or as a cholesterol-lowering agent like cholestyramine has, however, not been confirmed by controlled clinical trials.

Summary

Bile acids may be one of the aggressive factors to play a role in the pathogenesis of peptic ulcer. Since especially aluminum-containing antacids possess potent bile acid properties, adsorption of bile acids to sucralfate has been examined thoroughly. Sucralfate has potent bile acid binding properties which are pH-dependent: at the low pH of the stomach bile acid adsorption is very effective, but decreases with increasing pH. Addition of sucralfate to media containing mucosa-damaging bile acids decreased gastric mucosal damage. Whether the bile acid binding properties or the direct action of sucralfate on the gastric mucosa are responsible for the protective action of sucralfate is, however, still not clear.

References

1. Davenport HW: Destruction of mucosal barrier by detergents and urea. *Gastroenterology* **54:**175–182, 1968. Classical paper on definition and properties of the gastric mucosal barrier.
2. Ritchie WP: Bile acids, the "barrier", and reflux-related clinical disorders of the gastric mucosa. *Surgery* **82:**192–200, 1977. Paper with original data suggesting that bile acid reflux may be responsible for gastritis and barrier-breaking.
3. Duane WC, Wiegand DM, Siebert CE: Bile acid and bile salt disrupt gastric mucosal barrier by different mechanisms. *Am J Physiol* **242:**G95–G99, 1982. *In vitro* study demonstrating effects of bile acids on the gastric mucosal barrier.
4. Black RB, Hole D, Rhodes J: Bile damage to gastric mucosal barrier: The influence of pH and bile acid concentration. *Gastroenterology* **61:**178–184, 1971. Paper showing gastric mucosal injury by bile, as well as concentration- and pH-dependence of the damaging effect.
5. Geall MG, Phillips SF, Summerskill WHJ: The profile of gastric potential difference in man: Effect of aspirin, alcohol, bile and exogenous acid. *Gastroenterology* **58:**437–442, 1970. Original paper demonstrating effects of aspirin on transmural gastric potential difference in humans.
6. DuPlessis DJ: Pathogenesis of gastric ulceration. *Lancet* **1:**974–978, 1965. Classical hypothetical paper stressing the importance of bile acids in the pathogenesis of gastric ulcers.
7. Clain JE, Malagelada JR, Chadwick VS, *et al*: Binding properties in vitro of antacids for conjugated bile acids. *Gastroenterology* **73:**556–560, 1977. One of the first papers on *in vitro* bile acid binding properties of antacids.
8. Caspary WF: Einfluß von Aspirin, Antacida, Alkohol und Gallensäuren auf die transmurale elektrische Potentialdifferenz des menschlichen Magens. *Dtsch Med Wochenschr* **100:**1263–1266, 1975. Original paper on the effect of various gastric mucosal barrier breakers on transmural gastric potential difference in humans.
9. Nagashima R: Development and characteristics of sucralfate. *J Clin Gastroenterol* **3**(suppl 2)**:**105–110, 1981. Excellent review article on the properties of sucralfate.
10. Nagashima R: Mechanism of action of sucralfate. *J Clin Gastroenterol* **3**(suppl 2)**:**117–127, 1981. Review article with emphasis of the mechanism of action of sucralfate.
11. McCarthy DM: Sucralfate. *New Engl J Med* **325:**1017–1025, 1991. Most recent comprehensive review article on sucralfate, its mechanism of action, and results of clinical trials.
12. Bruusgaard A, Elsborg L, Reinecke V: Bile acid binding properties of sucralfate, in Caspary WF (ed): *Duodenal Ulcer, Gastric Ulcer: Sucralfate, a New Therapeutic Concept*. Munich, Urban & Schwarzenberg, 1981, pp 28–31. Original data of bile acid binding by sucralfate and antacids using natural bile.
13. Caspary WF: Einfluß von Glykocholsäure und Sucralfat auf die transmurale elektrische Potentialdifferenz des menschlichen Magens, in Caspary WF (ed): *Ulcus duodeni, Ulcus ventriculi. Sucralfat, eine neue therapeutische Konzeption*. Munich, Urban & Schwarzenberg, 1980, pp 22–27. Clinical study in humans testing the effect of sucralfate on glycocholic acid-induced decrease of gastric transmural potential difference.
14. Caspary WF, Graf S: Binding of bile acids by sucralfate and cholestyramine, in Caspary WF (ed): *Duodenal Ulcer, Gastric Ulcer: Sucralfate, a New Therapeutic Concept*. Munich, Urban &

Schwarzenberg, 1981, pp 32–38. Comparative *in vitro* study testing bile acid binding properties of cholestyramine and sucralfate.

15. Graham DY, Sackman JW, Giesing DH, *et al*: In vitro adsorption of bile salts and aspirin to sucralfate. *Dig Dis Sci* **29**:402–406, 1984. Original data of a careful *in vitro* study on bile acid binding properties of sucralfate and aspirin.
16. Shiau Y-F, Schenkein JP, Liu H-J, *et al*: Bile salt binding properties of commonly used gastrointestinal drugs: Maalox, Carafate, and questran. *J Pharm Sci* **77**:527–530, 1992 (Abstract). *In vitro* study comparing bile salt binding properties of Maalox, sucralfate (Carafate) and cholestyramine.
17. Lipsett P, Gadacz TR: Bile salt binding by Maalox, sucralfate, and Meciadanol: In vitro and clinical comparisons. *J Surg Res* **47**:403–406, 1989. *In vitro* study comparing bile salt properties at various pH values of Maalox, sucralfate and the flavonoid, Meciadanol, using pure bile acids.
18. Stahlberg M, Jalovaara P, Laitinen S, *et al*: Adsorption of bile acids by sucralfate, antacids and cholestyramine. *Clin Ther* **9**:615–621, 1987. Bile acid binding by sucralfate, antacids, or cholestyramine using natural bile acids obtained from gastric or duodenal aspirates.
19. Kurtz W, Güldütuna S, Leuschner U: Gallensäurebindung durch Antazida in "quasi-natürlichem" Refluxmilieu. *Z Gastroenterol* **27**:370–373, 1989. Binding of bile acids by antacids and sucralfate using reflux mixtures from nonstimulated gastric juice and hepatic bile.
20. Kurtz W, Güldütuna S, Leuschner U: Einfluß von pH und Antazidummenge auf die Gallensäurenbindung in quasinatürlichem Refluxmilieu. *Z Gastroenterol* **29**:237–241, 1991. Degree of bile acid adsorption correlated with the lipophilicity of the bile acids used: the most lipophilic and toxic bile acids were bound most effectively.
21. Tanghöj H, Stenstam H, Tobiasson B: Effects of sucralfate and cholestyramine on bile acid absorption. *Gastroenterology* **88**:1699, 1985 (Abstract). This study demonstrates that administration of sucralfate did not reduce postprandial serum bile acid concentration, but serum bile acid concentration was reduced by sucralfate after a loading dose with chenodeoxycholic acid. Cholestyramine, however, reduced serum bile acids postprandially.
22. Danesh BJZ, Duncan A, Russel RI: Is an acid pH medium required for the protective effect of sucralfate against mucosal injury? *Am J Med* **83**(suppl 38):11–13, 1987. In this paper evidence is presented that sucralfate reduced in rat gastric mucosa the mucosal damage induced by aspirin alone and aspirin combined with bile acids at pH values of both 1.5 and 6.5 and that the protective effect of sucralfate against mucosal injury was not dependent on an acid medium.
23. Eastwood GL: Effect of pH on bile salt injury to mouse gastric mucosa. *Gastroenterology* **68**:1457–1465, 1975. This publication demonstrates that the erosive activity of aspirin and bile acids is pH-dependent.
24. Morris GP, Williamson TE, Abonyi S: The effect of sucralfate and luminal stasis on recovery of the chambered rat gastric mucosa from taurocholate-induced damage. *Am J Med* **91**(suppl 2A):2S–14S, 1991. Sucralfate reduced taurocholate-induced damage of chambered rat gastric mucosa. Pretreatment with indomethacin reduced the acceleration of mucosal recovery induced by sucralfate.
25. Romano M, Razandi M, Ivey KJ: Effect of sucralfate and its components on taurocholate-induced damage to rat gastric mucosal cells in tissue culture. *Dig Dis Sci* **35**:467–476, 1990. It is concluded that sucralfate, but not its components, protected rat gastric mucosal cells against taurocholate-induced damage. Sucralfate stimulated prostaglandin production by cultured cells, but the protective effect of sucralfate did not depend on its stimulatory effect on endogenous prostaglandin synthesis.
26. Ligumsky M, Karmell F, Rachmilewitz D: Sucralfate protection against gastrointestinal damage: Possible role of prostanoids. *Isr J Med Sci* **22**:801–806, 1986. Sucralfate provided protection against taurocholate-induced gastric mucosal damage. Speculation: stimulation of endogenous gastric mucosal prostanoid formation may, at least in part, explain the protective properties of sucralfate.
27. Harrington SJ, Schlegel JF, Code CF: The protective effect of sucralfate on the gastric mucosa of rats. *J Clin Gastroenterol* **3**(suppl 2):129–134, 1981. Sucralfate decreased H^+ disappearance from rat stomach induced by taurocholate and significantly reduced the index of mucosal damage.
28. Buch KL, Weinstein WM, Hill TA, *et al*: Sucralfate therapy in patients with symptoms of alkaline

reflux gastritis. A randomized, double-blind study. *Am J Med* **79**(suppl 2C):49–54, 1985. Clinical trial comparing the therapeutic effect of sucralfate versus placebo in patients with alkaline reflux gastritis. Symptom score and endoscopic findings were not improved on sucralfate treatment, but the inflammatory cell score of the sucralfate-treated group was improved.

29. Meshkinpour H, Elashoff JD, Stewart H, *et al*: Effect of cholestyramine on the symptoms of reflux gastritis. A randomized double-blind crossover study. *Gastroenterology* **73**:441–443, 1977. Clinical trial showing that treatment of alkaline reflux gastritis with cholestyramine was not beneficial.
30. Nicolai JJ, Speelman P, Tytgat GNJ, *et al*: Comparison of the combination of cholestyramine/alginate with placebo in the treatment of postgastrectomy biliary reflux gastritis. Eur J Pharmacol **21**:189–194, 1981. This study did not show significant beneficial effects of cholestyramine in biliary reflux gastritis.
31. Petit D, Bonnefis M-T, Infante R: Fecal bile acid excretion and liver cholesterol synthesis after sucralfate and cholestyramine administration in the rat. *Pharmacol Res Commun* **187**:317–226, 1986. Cholestyramine induced greater fecal loss of bile acids than sucralfate.
32. Hunter JR, McCullagh L, Hoeg JM: Sucralfate ameliorates perirectal pain due to bile acid malabsorption. *Lancet* **1**:435, 1986. Anecdotal report on the beneficial effect of sucralfate in treatment of cholerrheic enteropathy.
33. Maas LC, Kikoler DJ: Sucralfate therapy for choleretic diarrhea. *South Med J* **76**:98, 1983. Anecdotal report on the beneficial effect of sucralfate in treatment of cholerrheic enteropathy.

IV

Mechanisms of Action of Sucralfate

7

Binding of Sucralfate to the Mucosal Surface

GERALD P. MORRIS

Introduction

Much of the appeal of sucralfate as a subject of study for the experimental biologist lies in the numerous unknowns that surround its mode of action. The concept of a non-systemically acting agent that is therapeutically useful for the treatment of peptic ulcer and that works independently of effects on gastric acid secretion has its own fascination. As will become apparent, even the initial event following administration of this agent—the binding of sucralfate to the mucosa of the upper gastrointestinal tract—is not as straightforward as it might seem.

Most of us—both physicians and laypersons—have grown up with the concept of "coating agents." Years of exposure to commercials for agents such as Pepto-Bismol and others have introduced into our subconscious a readiness to accept the idea that there are agents that form a creamy, white or pink barrier over the surfaces of our stomach or duodenum and, by so doing, protect the mucosa from whatever harsh and damaging substances lurk in those cavities. The concept has gained new life in the guise of the mucus–bicarbonate barrier that supposedly lines the stomach with a protective coat of viscous mucus within which luminal acid is neutralized and thus is kept from damaging the cells of the mucosal surface. From this, it is only a short step to the apparently obvious conclusion that at least part of sucralfate's antiulcer activity must result from its ability to complex with extracellular protein and mucus and thus form an adherent complex that excludes acid, pepsin, and bile salts. Certainly, when one looks at a mucosa to which sucralfate has been applied, it is apparent that this agent does adhere tenaciously and that adhesion to the mucosa may persist for many hours in humans and in animals. However, careful consideration reveals that such a simple explanation for the effects of sucralfate is

GERALD P. MORRIS • Department of Biology, Queen's University, Kingston, Ontario K7L 3N6, Canada.

Sucralfate: From Basic Science to the Bedside, edited by Daniel Hollander and G. N. J. Tytgat. Plenum Press, New York, 1995.

improbable. The coat of sucralfate is by no means continuous and is unlikely to form a permeability barrier, at least to acid. Nor is sucralfate an inert compound. Rather, the presence of bound sucralfate results in marked changes in cell function in the adjacent mucosa. The cytoprotective and ulcer-healing actions of sucralfate result from effects on mucosal functions such as local release of mediators of inflammation which, in turn, affect mucosal blood flow and secretion of fluid and/or mucus.

Sucralfate is the aluminum salt of sucrose octasulfate. It polymerizes under acid conditions to form a viscous, adherent mass. It also provides a source of aluminum and sulfate ions that can diffuse into the underlying mucosa. Thus, an immobilized, adherent mass of sucralfate can exert effects beyond the site of the visible mass, since diffusible components may be capable of acting on nearby mucosa, and of affecting both the surface epithelium and the cells of the lamina propria (such as endothelial cells and fibroblasts), and—in the case of damaged or inflamed tissues—of also affecting different populations of inflammatory cells such as neutrophils, eosinophils, macrophages, and mast cells. For instance, the presence of sucralfate in the gastric lumen decreases the levels of mucosal myeloperoxidase (indicating actions on mucosal neutrophils), elevates leukotriene synthesis,[1] and increases mucosal blood flow and secretion of both bicarbonate and fluid. These effects cannot be readily explained if sucralfate is considered to be a passive, mucus-bound barrier. This concept of bound sucralfate affecting different cell populations, at a distance from the bound mass, is developed in a subsequent section of this chapter.

Some studies suggest that although accelerated healing of chronic ulcers occurs in the presence of inhibition of acid secretion, sucralfate is only cytoprotective in an acid environment. We and others have found that this is not the case and equal protection against aspirin, bile acids, and ethanol is obtained when sucralfate is administered either in near-neutral or in acid solution.[2] Similarly, binding to the extracellular mucus coat occurs at both acid and neutral pH. There is evidence that the duration of the cytoprotective effects of sucralfate is longer in an acid environment and this may be related to the enhanced dissociation of aluminum ions from sucrose sulfate that occurs at low pH.

Bound Sucralfate Exerts Its Effects Locally

The effects of sucralfate are restricted to those regions of the mucosa to which sucralfate is bound. As is discussed below, sucralfate binds particularly tenaciously to ulcerated sites and this may produce persistent, local concentrations at ulcerated sites throughout the upper gastrointestinal tract. Cytoprotective effects of orally administered sucralfate are also limited to the stomach and duodenum, at sites where sucralfate is bound to the mucosa. In a simple experimental verification of the ability of sucralfate to produce local protection, we have shown that when sucralfate is placed on one-half of a chambered rat stomach, only the half that is covered is protected against the formation of hemorrhagic erosions when a barrier breaker such as 40% ethanol is placed on the entire stomach.[1] This local action is in contrast to agents such as prostaglandins, which can affect the entire GI tract if the dose is sufficiently large. There are obvious theoretical advantages to agents that act locally, at sites of injury. For instance, secretory diarrhea and effects on motility are major side effects of prostaglandin therapy, and may also be viewed as systemic manifestations of effects that are locally protective. The localization of action of sucralfate to the sites of mucosal binding minimizes the likelihood of deleterious side effects.

Mechanism of Binding of Sucralfate to the Gastrointestinal Mucosa

Binding of sucralfate occurs by electrostatic or ionic binding of the negatively charged molecule with positively charged proteins in the mucus or ulcer crater. Mucus glycoprotein is typically negatively charged and will bear numerous carboxyl groups and, in some sites, sulfate groups. The nature and extent of negatively charged components in mucus glycoprotein varies greatly from species to species and within regions of the GI tract and will also vary with changes in luminal pH. It must also be appreciated that the extracellular mucus is not composed only of mucus glycoprotein. In the GI tract, the extracellular mucus is a complex amalgam of mucus glycoprotein, phospholipids, and a great variety of proteins. What we see as mucus contains large quantities of nucleic acids, nucleoproteins, and membranes from shed cells (Fig. 1), as well as occasional bacteria and food particles. In the human stomach, for instance, a quantity of epithelial cells equivalent to a 5- × 5-mm square is shed by normal cell-loss processes every minute. It is the fragments of these disintegrated cells, their contained mucus, and the mucus that is released by exocytosis from the remaining cells that make up the "mucus" coat. When the stomach or intestine is damaged, the luminal mucus contains an even greater quantity of cellular debris plus fibrin, serum components, and additional mucus that was contained within the damaged cells. All of these components offer potential sites to which sucralfate can bind.

As a result, the mechanisms of binding and the consequences of binding of sucralfate to the mucosa will vary greatly in three different situations: (1) the intact or normal GI mucosa; (2) the acutely damaged mucosa, such as would be produced by recent exposure to aspirin, concentrated ethanol, or bile; (3) chronically inflamed tissue of an ulcer crater or of gastritis.

Binding of Sucralfate to Undamaged Mucosa

In an undamaged mucosa, binding of sucralfate to the extracellular mucus could influence the gastric or intestinal mucosal barriers in various ways: (1) A complex of sucralfate and extracellular mucus could form an impenetrable barrier—a true coat; (2) sucralfate could influence the physical or chemical properties of the mucus to which it binds; (3) sucralfate could bind to extracellular mucus but act by influencing the biochemical and physiological functioning of the underlying mucosa and, thus, produce its effects in an indirect manner.

Sucralfate as a Barrier to Acid Diffusion

There are studies suggesting that sucralfate can form a barrier to acid diffusion under certain circumstances. Some *in vitro* studies use diffusion chambers in which layers of

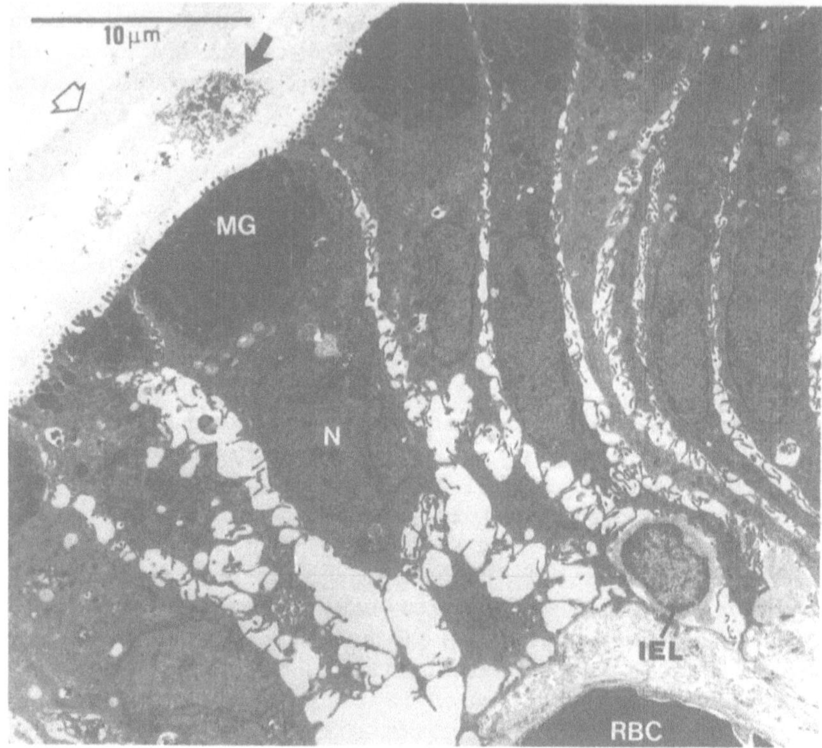

Figure 1. Transmission electron micrograph of surface epithelial cells from human antral mucosa. The edge of the mucus coat that covers this region is indicated by the open arrow. The solid arrow indicates a piece of cytoplasm from a shed cell. IEL, intraepithelial lymphocyte; MG, intracellular mucus granules; N, nucleus; RBC, red blood cells in subepithelial capillary.

sucralfate or sucralfate complexed with protein are tested for their ability to retard diffusion of acid from one side of the chamber to another. Experiments of this type do show impressive abilities of sucralfate to retard acid diffusion. It is still open to question whether a retardation of acid diffusion is a significant factor *in vivo*. Our experience, based on visualization of sucralfate that is bound to the mucosal surface, microscopical studies of tissues to which sucralfate is bound, and physiological studies where the effects of sucralfate on mucosal secretion are examined, suggest that the bound sucralfate does not form an impenetrable barrier. Rather, particles and patches of sucralfate are scattered over the surface of the mucosa (Figs. 2–5). Particles of sucralfate are only rarely seen associated with surface epithelial cells. Most particles of sucralfate are associated with the luminal surface of the extracellular mucus. It is evident that the particles do not form a continuous layer. Interpretation of fixed and sectioned material prepared for both light and electron microscopy is complicated by the inevitable loss of some material during the processes of fixation and embedding. However, the impression that is given by the accompanying micrographs—a sporadic cover of adherent, but discontinuous, particles—is borne out by our high-magnification examinations of chambered mucosae. When viewed with a dissecting microscope through an optically clear chamber, it is possible to see the particles on the mucus coat and, at some sites, to measure the distance between the particles and the mucosal surface.

Effects of Bound Sucralfate on Physical Characteristics of Mucus

There is a great deal yet to be learned about the structure, organization, and functions of GI mucus. The extent to which it forms a continuous or discontinuous coat, the depth of the mucus over normal and damaged sites, the question of its possible barrier roles are all subjects of vigorous debate. Sucralfate may affect the physical properties, such as viscosity, of mucus to which it binds. However, such studies are of necessity carried out on isolated mucus, and the consequences of such effects *in vivo* are difficult to assess.

Helicobacter pylori has been reported to negatively affeet the cation exchange (Na^+ for H^+) capabilities of gastric mucus. The ion exchange capability may be restored by sucralfate and could aid unidirectional flow of secreted acid into the lumen and prevent backdiffusion of acid into the mucosal epithelium. Similarly, sucralfate may decrease the rate at which pepsin digests gastric mucus, both by adsorbing pepsin and possibly by forming a barrier that limits diffusion of pepsin and access to mucus.

"Cytoprotection" by Indirect Effects of Bound Sucralfate

As is documented elsewhere in this volume, sucralfate has been shown in numerous experiments to be "cytoprotective" and it is argued that this could be beneficial in therapy. These studies on cytoprotection suggest an ability to protect an undamaged mucosa from damaging agents and this could be of importance in prevention of initial damage to the gastric or duodenal mucosa or, more likely in a clinical setting, could prevent relapse of healed ulcer.

It has been suggested that sucralfate could protect the mucosa against acute damage by stimulating the production of prostaglandins. Sucralfate is almost entirely associated with extracellular mucus and we do not find any significant damage to surface epithelium in the rat stomach after exposure to sucralfate. However, the epithelial cells do undergo certain characteristic changes that are associated with exposure to sucralfate and that are suggestive of active secretion (Fig. 2), and both sucralfate and prostaglandins may stimulate mucus release (Figs. 3 and 4).

The protective actions of sucralfate are likely related to the persistent binding of sucralfate to the mucosa. Effects on prostaglandin (PG) synthesis may not be central to sucralfate protection because although sucralfate produces a significant elevation in PG synthesis, this increase disappears after about 30 min. The protection afforded persists for at least 8 hr and is manifested even when animals are pretreated with indomethacin.

When sucralfate is applied to layers of cultured gastric surface epithelial cells, it reportedly adheres tightly to the surfaces of the cultured cells.[3] There are no published

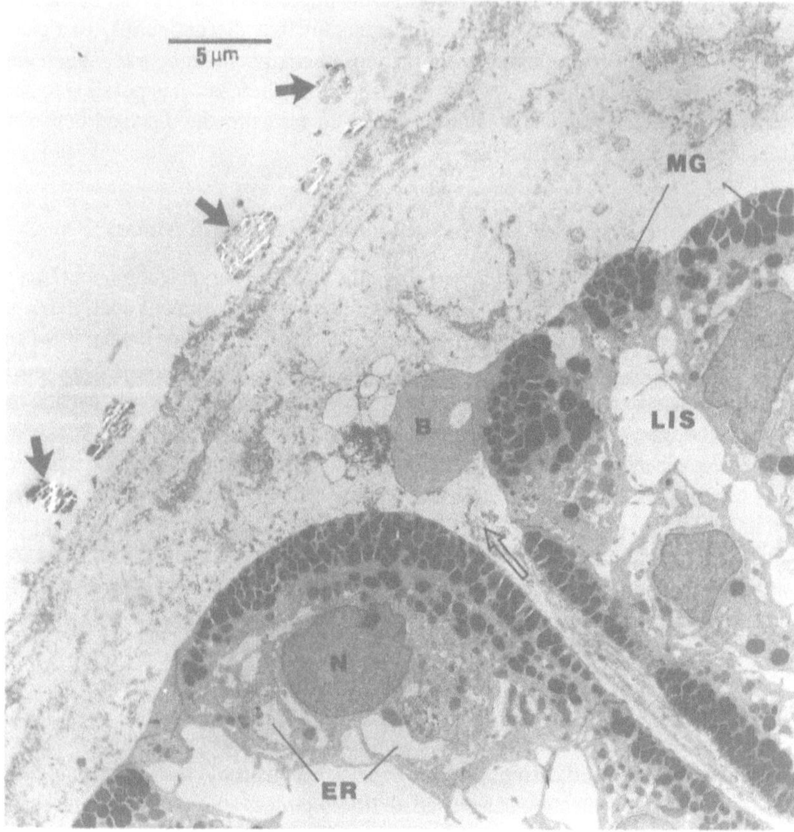

Figure 2. Transmission electron micrograph of surface epithelial cells from chambered rat gastric mucosa 10 min after exposure to 500 mg sucralfate in 10 ml normal saline. Solid arrows indicate particles of sucralfate adhering to the mucus coat. Note the presence of numerous membrane fragments and vesicles in the mucus. The swollen endoplasmic reticulum (ER) and lateral intracellular spaces (LIS) are often associated with nearby adherent sucralfate. The open arrow indicates the direction of flow of mucus from a gastric gland. B, bleb or protrusion of apical cytoplasm; MG, intracellular mucus granules.

electron micrographs of these preparations, so it is not possible to determine whether the attachment is directly to the cell surfaces or to mucus and proteins that have been released into the extracellular environment. There is no evidence that this adherent sucralfate damages the cultured cells; supporting our ultrastructural studies. The lack of damage is supported by direct observation of the cell cultures and by determination of ^{51}Cr release as an index of damage. It is also apparent that even though sucralfate effectively protects cultured cells against solutions containing up to 10 mM sodium taurocholate, it does not form a continuous barrier over the layer of cultured cells.

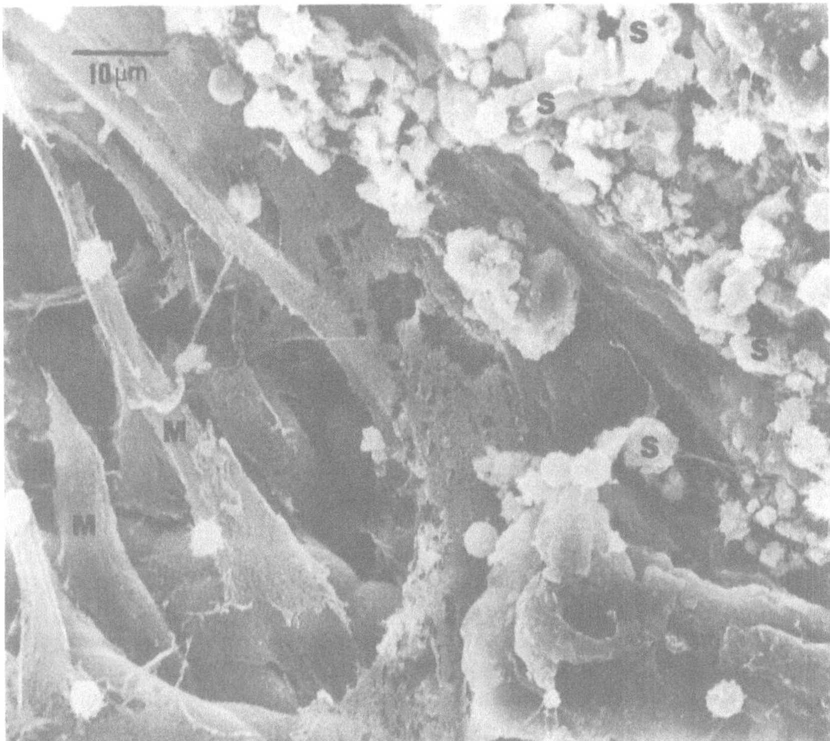

Figure 3. Scanning electron micrograph of rat gastric mucosa 10 min after exposure to 500 mg sucralfate in 10 ml normal saline. The extracellular mucus is covered with adherent, shed cells and with particles of sucralfate (S). Continuous sheets and ropes of mucus (M) issue from the gastric glands.

Binding of Sucralfate and Release of Mediators of Inflammation

As is described elsewhere in this volume, the presence of sucralfate is often associated with elevated levels of PG synthesis. This is not always the case and some studies do not detect increased PG synthesis subsequent to binding of sucralfate. We also find that sucralfate is protective in a rat model when gastric cyclooxygenase activity is nearly 90% inhibited by indomethacin. The same study shows that sucralfate elevates levels of leukotriene C_4 synthesis and causes a decrease in myeloperoxidase activity. Collectively, studies of this type show that when sucralfate is bound to an intact mucosa, it produces effects on the synthesis and release of various mediators of inflammation. This, once again, raises the question of how sucralfate exerts its protective effects. Szabo has pointed out that a single, definitive mechanism probably does not exist.[4] Rather, sucralfate produces multiple effects on mucosae that are normal or damaged in different ways.

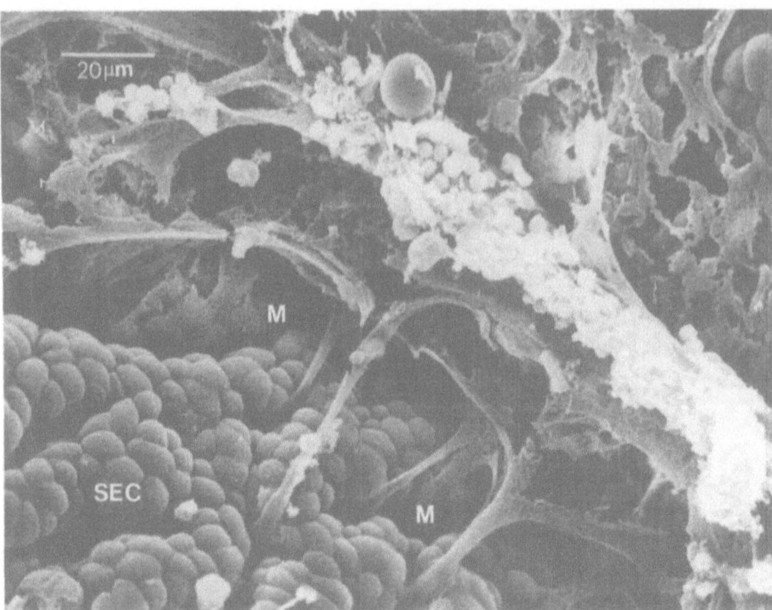

Figure 4. Scanning electron micrograph of rat gastric mucosa exposed for 10 min to a prostaglandin E_1 analogue (rioprostil). Mucus ropes and sheets (M) issue from the gastric glands and fuse with the overlying mucus network. This mucus network is the primary site of sucralfate binding. SEC, surface epithelial cells.

Sucralfate May Affect Local Mucosal Secretion

The mechanism behind cytoprotection produced by any agent remains elusive. Sucralfate is no exception. There is little doubt that the presence of bound sucralfate stimulates synthesis of mediators such as prostaglandins and leukotrienes, accelerated secretion of mucus and bicarbonate, and can produce elevated mucosal blood flow. We also find that sucralfate increases the thickness of a juxtamucosal pH gradient that we measure over the gastric mucosa with antimony microelectrodes.[5] We do not, however, see this gradient as a protective zone within which acid is neutralized. In fact, the magnitude of the gradient is typically less than one pH unit, and the juxtamucosal pH is often less than 3. The pH gradient that we measure is probably a manifestation of mucosal fluid secretion. It is in some ways similar to the unstirred water layer in thickness, but is more accurately visualized as a zone of secreted fluid that must be traversed by any necrotizing agent, before damage will occur to the epithelial surface and to the underlying cells of the lamina propria. A dynamic layer of secreted fluid could thus attenuate the damage produced by an acute exposure to a damaging agent. The ability to stimulate mucosal secretion is a feature of most agents that protect against topical damage and this

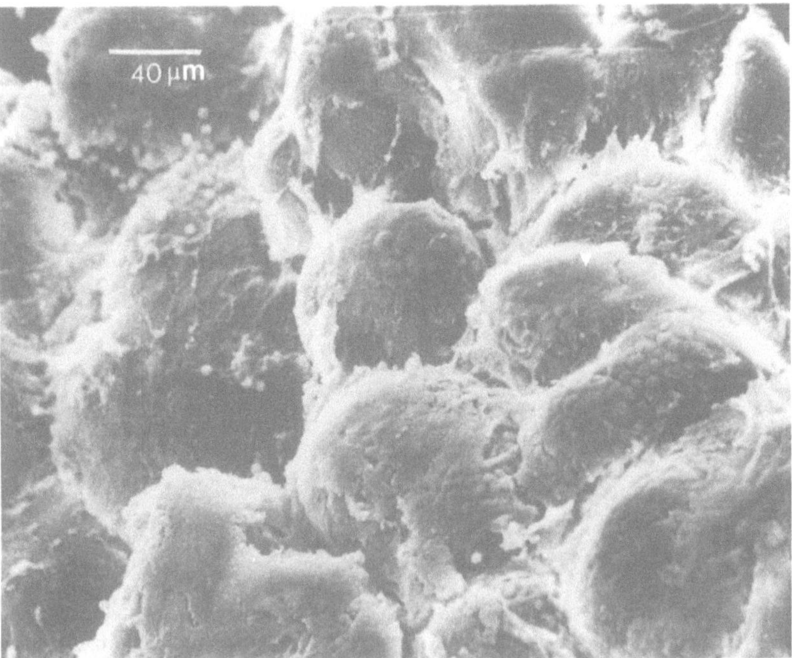

Figure 5. Scanning electron micrograph of human gastric mucosa 1 hr after administration of a 1-g sucralfate tablet. Much of the mucosa is covered with a coat of mucus, although there are also exposed surface epithelial cells. This dose of sucralfate is protective against ethanol-induced acute damage (see Cohen *et al*: *Gastroenterology* **96**:292–298, 1989, for details), but there is no continuous sucralfate coat. Scattered aggregates of sucralfate can be seen in sections of this tissue but cannot be distinguished from luminal debris in scanning electron micrographs.

may explain many examples of cytoprotection. Sucralfate similarly enhances mucosal secretion, but could do so for long periods of time and only at sites to which it is bound.

Binding of Sucralfate to Sites of Acute Damage

When used in therapy of existing peptic ulcer, one must also consider the ability of sucralfate to bind to ulcerated tissue. Acutely damaged sites present a very different substrate to sucralfate than does either a chronically inflamed or an intact mucosa. The chronically inflamed tissue does not usually secrete mucus and that which is secreted by surrounding tissues may be altered in composition. The acutely injured mucosa may be coated with a layer of shed cells and released mucus. In addition, there is typically an efflux of plasma proteins and the deposition of large quantities of fibrin (Fig. 6). Sucralfate appears to bind avidly to fibrin and our microscopical observations show that large aggregates of sucralfate are preferentially located at sites where the mucosal surface is

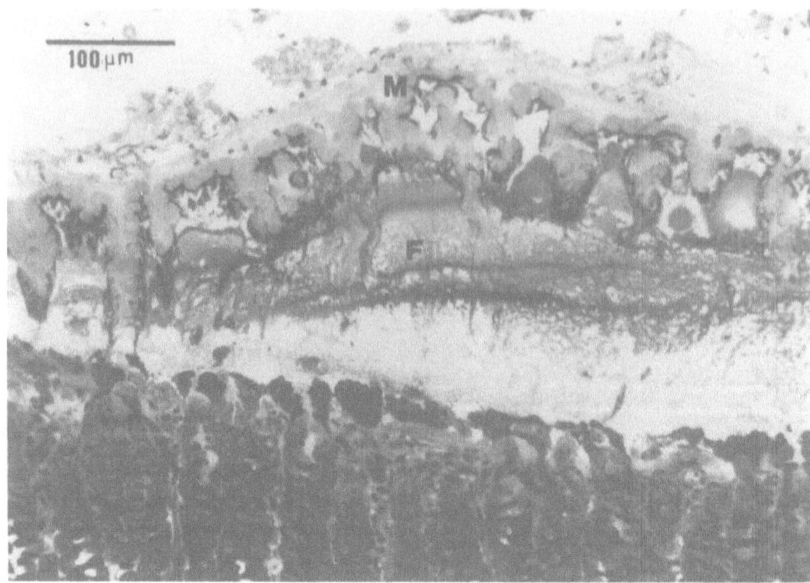

Figure 6. Toluidine blue-stained plastic section showing thick mucus cap (M) over region of damage produced by exposure of chambered rat gastric mucusa to acidified taurocholate. A layer of fibrin (F) often accumulates under the mucus cap as a result of the efflux of plasma from the damaged site during the time when repair by epithelial migration is taking place. Sucralfate enhances recovery from this damage; probably by effects on mucosal blood flow. See Ref. 5 for details.

coated with adherent fibrin, which is released during plasma efflux from sites of epithelial damage.

Most attention has been directed to the ability of sucralfate to prevent acute damage ("cytoprotective effects" which are manifested over undamaged mucosae) or to accelerate healing of chronic ulcer. We have also studied the ability of sucralfate to prevent acute damage caused by exposure of chambered rat gastric mucosae to bile salts from becoming converted into bleeding erosions. In this model system, the application of sucralfate *after* the production of bile damage, prevented the otherwise inevitable development of hemorrhagic erosions.[5] Within the limitations of a model based on animal experiments, this provides an example of another intermediate stage in the sequence of development of GI damage at which sucralfate administration could be useful. The mechanism behind this ability to prevent surface damage from being converted into hemorrhagic erosions probably relates to the ability of bound sucralfate to stimulate both mucosal fluid secretion and blood flow. Sucralfate thus provides the damaged gastric mucosal surface with time to repair itself by short-term healing involving rapid migration of cells from the glands. Unlike cytoprotection which is effective before exposure to damaging agents, protection of the acutely damaged mucosa by bound sucralfate is prevented by prior treatment with indomethacin.

Binding of Sucralfate to Chronic Ulcers

Several studies have examined the ability of sucralfate to bind to ulcerated tissue in animal models. Chronic-type gastric and duodenal ulcers are readily prepared in rats by a brief application to the serosal surface of the stomach or duodenum of a small quantity of concentrated acetic acid. This produces necrosis in the overlying mucosa and an ulcer crater of relatively constant size at a predetermined location. Sucralfate is capable of accelerating the healing of these ulcers, indicating that they have some relevance to human therapy despite the artificial means by which they are produced.

Sucralfate is widely distributed over normal and ulcerated mucosa for at least 6 hr, but is almost completely gone by 24 hr. Coverage on normal mucosa is sparse and irregular, but dense coats remain for at least 6 hr over the ulcers.[6] The specificity of attachment is probably related to the presence in the ulcer craters of exposed, basic proteins and, in humans, the ulcerated sites contain six to seven times more sucralfate than adjacent, nonulcerated mucosa following oral administration.[7] There is no way of knowing at this time whether such attachment is capable of producing a barrier to influxing acid or whether sucralfate accelerates healing by other mechanisms. The abilities of sucralfate to bind growth factors, to adsorb bile acids, and to inactivate pepsin could aid ulcer healing and are discussed elsewhere in this volume. It is also likely that the ability of sucralfate to stimulate mucosal blood flow would have a beneficial effect at sites of chronic ulcer.

The relative selectivity of binding of sucralfate to sites of mucosal ulceration can also be used for location of ulcer sites throughout the GI tract. When patients with Crohn's disease and with ulcerative colitis were given oral sucralfate complexed with technetium-99*m*, and isotope localization was carried out with a gamma camera, there was a high degree of accuracy in locating lesions in the small intestine and in the colon. Similar studies have shown localization of experimental gastric ulcers in rabbits and of gastric ulcer and duodenal ulcer in humans. Very little sucralfate is absorbed from the GI tract and these studies verify not only the preferential binding to ulcerated sites, but also the ability of sucralfate to bind to lesions throughout the GI tract.

References

1. Wallace JL, Morris GP, Beck PL, *et al*: Effects of sucralfate on gastric prostaglandin and leukotriene synthesis: Relationship to protective actions. *Can J Physiol Pharmacol* **66**:666–670, 1988. Demonstrates localization of protection to areas in contact with bound sucralfate and that protection is independent of prostaglandin synthesis. This study also shows that adherent sucralfate has local effects on other mediators (leukotriene C_4 and myeloperoxidase).
2. Morris GP, Keenan CM, MacNaughton WK, *et al*: Protection of rat gastric mucosa by sucralfate. Effects of luminal stasis and inhibition of prostaglandin synthesis. *Am J Med* **86**(suppl 6A):10–16, 1989. This paper describes the ability of sucralfate to maintain a pH gradient over the surface of the gastric mucosa at sites to which it is bound. The paper also describes the effects of sucralfate on gastric ultrastructure and shows that there is no significant damage produced by sucralfate.
3. Romano M, Razandi M, Ivey KJ: Effect of sucralfate and its components on taurocholate-induced damage to rat gastric mucosal cells in tissue culture. *Dig Dis Sci* **35**:467–476, 1990. The authors show that sucralfate adheres tightly to cultured gastric cells and protects them against sodium taurocholate-

induced damage. Protection is not produced by sucrose octasulfate or aluminum hydroxide and does not depend on elevated prostaglandin synthesis or sulfhydryl compounds.

4. Szabo S: The mode of action of sucralfate: The 1 × 1 × 1 mechanism of action. *Scand J Gastroenterol* **26**(suppl 185):7–12, 1990. A brief and readable review that emphasizes the dynamic actions of sucralfate on the mucosa, which lists some of the mechanisms that could be involved in protection against different stages of damage, and that deals realistically with the barrier or "Band-Aid" theories of action.
5. Morris GP, Williamson TE, Abonyi S: The effects of sucralfate and luminal stasis on recovery of the chambered rat gastric mucosa from taurocholate-induced damage. *Am J Med* **91**(suppl 2A):2S–14S, 1991. This paper establishes that, in an animal model, sucralfate can counteract the effects of indomethacin on the juxtamucosal pH gradient and can also accelerate repair mechanisms and thus prevent the development of otherwise inevitable damage in stomachs that have been damaged by bile salts.
6. Nagashima R: Mechanisms of action of sucralfate. *J Clin Gastroenterol* **31**(suppl 2):117–127, 1981. Comprehensive review of possible interactions of sucralfate with surfaces of both damaged and undamaged mucosae. Provides a good overview of the rationale behind various barrier hypotheses for actions of sucralfate.
7. Nakazawa S, Nagashima R, Samloff IM: Selective binding of sucralfate to gastric ulcer in man. *Dig Dis Sci* **26**:297–300, 1981. Demonstrates, in humans, preferential binding of sucralfate to ulcerated tissue.

8

Stimulation of Mucus Production

CLIFFORD TASMAN-JONES

Introduction

Mucus is a slippery hydrophilic, viscoelastic gel covering the surface epithelium of the stomach to form a lining superbly protecting the delicate columnar epithelial cells of the stomach from aggressive factors. Major luminal aggressors are ingested food, secreted hydrochloric acid, peptic enzymes, and free radicals generated in the lumen.[1]

Mucus

Mucus consists mainly of mucins, water, electrolytes, immunoglobulins, enzymes, and DNA. Its unique protective capacity is dependent on mucinous glycoproteins. Gastric mucins are synthesized and secreted by the continuous columnar epithelium as well as by specialized mucous neck cells distributed within the stomach as well as glands. Histochemical staining of gastric tissue shows mucins concentrated at the apex of epithelial cells and in the mucous neck cells of the gastric glands. The epithelial cells are joined tightly at their apical poles to present an occluding intercellular junction. The presence of mucus and a tight epithelium is an efficient combination protecting the stomach.

The complex processes of mucin formation and secretion are poorly understood. Mucin-containing cells release their mucins in a densely condensed form which on release by exocytosis are very rapidly hydrated with rapid massive swelling to form a viscoelastic gel layer.[2] The complex polymer structure of mucous glycoproteins are difficult to study because standard biochemical analysis destroys their macromolecular architecture.

Mucus once formed firmly adheres to the gastric epithelium and as newly formed mucins are released they constantly add to the underside of an existing insoluble mucous

CLIFFORD TASMAN-JONES • Department of Medicine, University of Auckland, Auckland, New Zealand.

Sucralfate: From Basic Science to the Bedside, edited by Daniel Hollander and G. N. J. Tytgat. Plenum Press, New York, 1995.

layer. In the stomach mucus contains some sloughed cells, bacteria, bacterial products, and some products of food digestion. Although some earlier studies suggested otherwise, recent scanning electron microscopy studies show the gel to be a continuous layer over the stomach. This is consistent with barrier functions shown to be important in protection of the delicate gastric epithelium.[3]

Release of Mucins

Cholinergic innervation has been implicated in the release of gastric mucins. Topically applied acetylcholine to the stomach of dogs produces a visible increase in the thickness of the mucous gel layer.[4] Infusion of acetylcholine results in a thick mucous gel secretion[4] and electron microscopy after the infusion shows a loss of mucus granules from the surface epithelial cells. On the other hand, adrenergic stimuli do not influence the release of granules from the gastric mucous cells.

Prostaglandins E and F if applied topically or given systemically increase the thickness of the mucous layer in the human stomach by stimulating release of gastric mucins.[5]

Protein-calorie malnutrition in rats decreases the concentration of small intestinal mucin.[6] Animals fed soluble nonstarch polysaccharide (dietary fiber) have increased amounts of mucin in samples of gastric luminal secretion and gastric tissue.[7]

In the small intestine, parasite infection is associated with a copious mucus discharge as well as a vigorous monocyte cell inflammatory response. Macrophages are pivotal in antigen processing producing a variety of molecules including the cytokine interleukin 1. Interleukin 1 is capable of promoting mucin release.[8] The place of cytokines in release of gastric mucus needs further study especially in *Helicobacter pylori* infection.

Composition and Physical Properties of Mucus

The capacity of mucins to protect epithelial surfaces depends on their rich and heterogeneous polysaccharide composition and their ability to form gels. Only five monosaccharides appear in mucin:

- *N*-Acetylglucosamine
- *N*-Acetylgalactosamine
- Fucose
- Galactose
- Sialic acid

Despite the heterogeneity of mucins they have a number of characteristic features. The protein content is low (20% by weight) and the individual protein constituents are present in two regions. Carbohydrate comprises 70–80% of the weight of mucins but with a wide variety of oligosaccharide chain lengths. The carbohydrate for linear or branched chain carbohydrate profile is not uniform. Carbohydrates are linked by *O*-glycosidic bonds to either serine or threonine of the peptide backbone. As sialic acid/glycosidic linkages are acid-labile, gastric acidity ensures that there is a paucity of sialic acid mucins in the stomach. However, discrete populations of highly sulfated mucins are present.

Chemical contaminants in mucus gel include DNA, polysaccharides, proteins, neutral lipids, fatty acids, and some drugs.

Mucus is an elastic layer maintaining a stability of structure without being rigid. It has enough fluidity to flow under mild shearing forces and yet it is porous enough to allow rapid diffusion of nutrients and secretions backward and forward between the lumen and the mucosal cells. The gel layer is continually changing in both thickness and quality with the changes governed by shearing forces, luminal enzyme digestion, and ongoing replacement of mucin by secretion from the cells below.

Although mucus is generally considered to be a porous layer, it is an ion exchanger aiding the maintenance of a pH gradient between gastric lumen and epithelial cell surface.[9] Epithelial cell secretion of bicarbonate is the other major factor in the generation and maintenance of the pH gradient.

While the pH gradient across the mucus layer is considered to have an important protective role against injury of tissue by acid in the lumen, the gradient can be dissipated by acid concentrations sometimes present in the stomach. Dissipation of the pH gradient across the mucus layer may not result in injury to the epithelium, possibly because of the local availability of bicarbonate ions in interstitial tissues.

Mucus and *Helicobacter pylori*

Mucus provides an ecological niche for some organisms. *Helicobacter pylori* distributes itself through the mucus in a distribution which can be clearly seen when the mucus has been antibody stabilized[10] (Figs. 1 and 2).

Protective Effects of Sucralfate

In the rat model, sucralfate has a protective effect against the formation of deep necrotic lesions when exposed to alcohol. Sucralfate showed no significant protection against surface epithelial damage, however.

The mechanisms of sucralfate protection of the stomach are unclear. It has been proposed that sucralfate may act by mediating prostaglandin synthesis with stimulation of mucin formation. In the human, sucralfate stimulates gastric bicarbonate secretion and prostaglandin E_2 output[11] and this may explain some protective effects of sucralfate. However, when indomethacin is given in doses that should completely block the synthesis of endogenous prostaglandins, there is still a protective effect of sucralfate. Pathways other than mucin formation stimulated by prostaglandin are therefore responsible for the protective activity.

Other protective mechanisms may be physicochemical, related to binding to the endogenous sulfhydryl groups of mucus. The donation of sulfate groups makes mucins less readily attacked by proteolytic enzymes, explaining reduced peptic digestion of gastric glycoprotein when sucralfate is present.[12]

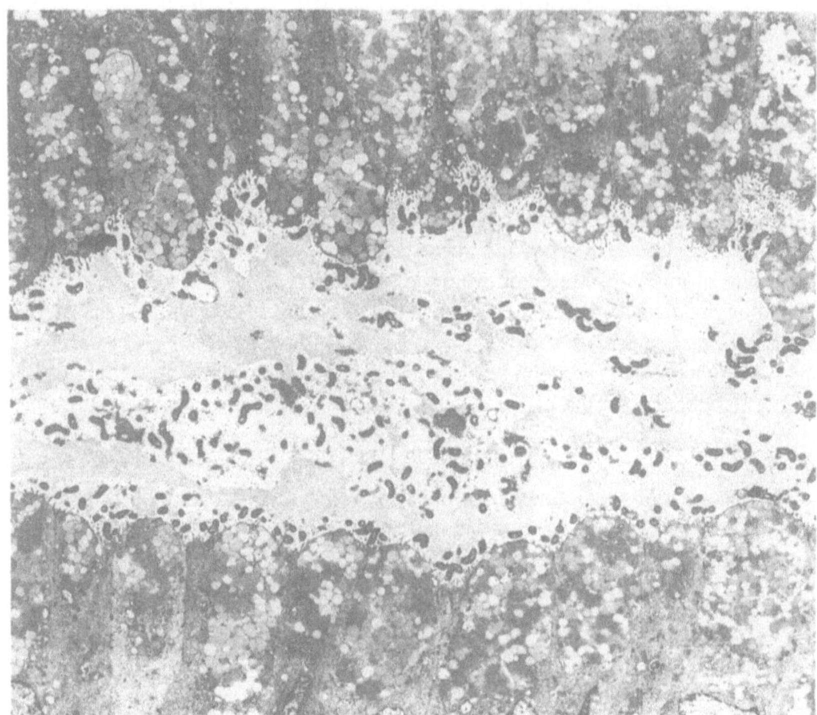

Figure 1. Distribution of *Helicobacter pylori* in antral glands. The mucus has been stabilized by incubation with antibody against human gastric mucus. × 1900.

Sucralfate will penetrate the mucus layer. Rat gastric mucosa incubated with sucralfate and analyzed for intramucus aluminum by Xrays generated by an electron beam on windows of mucus, shows a decreasing concentration gradient from lumen to epithelial surface. The concentration of aluminum is higher in the outer (luminal) layer of mucus than in the inner layer and significantly higher in both layers than in control tissue. Sucralfate is thus distributed through the full thickness of mucus.

In rats the addition of sucralfate causes only a small increase in mucus gel thickness but there is an associated increase in mucus gel viscosity, hydrophobicity, and mucin content.[13] Other studies in pigs have suggested that sucralfate acts by its physical barrier but with no increase in mucus secretion or identifiable changes in endogenous prostaglandin secretion.[14]

The Gel Layer

The gel layer in gastric ulceration has a reduced viscoelasticity suggesting a reduction in its ability to protect the gastric mucosa. The Na^+/K^+ ion exchange properties

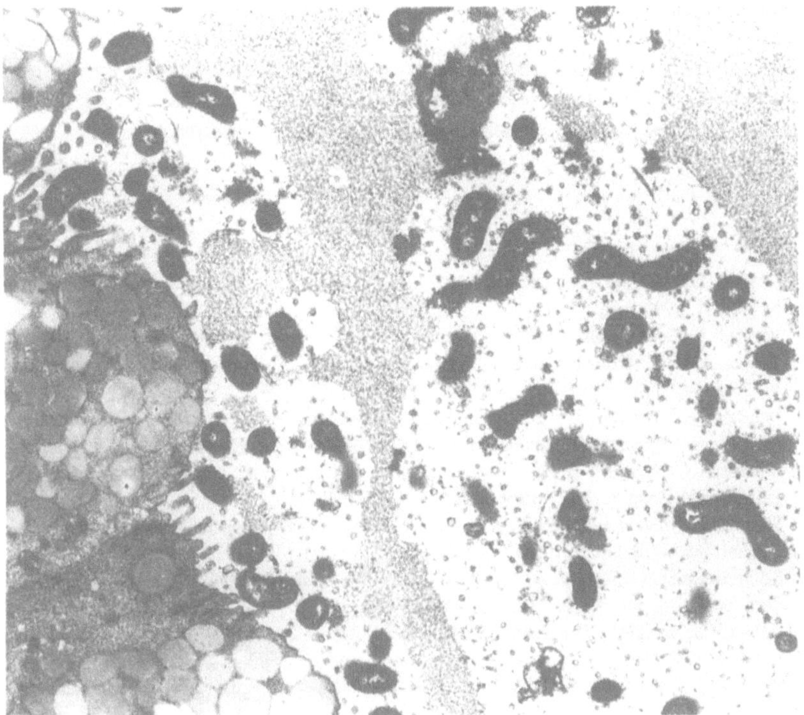

Figure 2. *Helicobacter pylori* in gastric mucus. × 8000.

of *H. pylori*-infected mucus are impaired.[15] It is speculated, but not proven, that this reduction is a result of the increased production of ammonia which modifies the physical characteristics of mucus. *In vitro* incubation of infected mucus with sucralfate returns the ion exchange to near normal suggesting that the gelling properties of mucus may have been restored.[16]

New Directions for Research

Basic information on the activity of sucralfate with mucus is incomplete. There is evidence that sucralfate binds throughout the mucus layer, but further work is necessary to determine the conditions under which this binding occurs.

Because of its binding with mucus, in addition to providing a physical barrier, sucralfate may have potential as a vehicle to ensure the transport of antibiotics which may be effective against *H. pylori*. Sucralfate itself does not have any specific antibacterial or inhibitory action and by itself is not an effective treatment against intramucus organisms.

A better understanding of the mechanisms whereby sucralfate may increase the production and/or release of mucins is desirable. Does sucralfate act through prostaglandins or are the effects of prostaglandins an index of other activities of sucralfate? As the spectrum of mechanisms involved in cytoprotection by epidermal growth factor, cytokines, etc. and as the importance of aggressors such as free radicals are defined, the interaction of surface protective agents such as sucralfate provides new directions for understanding and the development of exciting therapeutic derivatives.

References

1. Otamiri T, Sjodahl R: Oxygen radicals: Their role in selective gastrointestinal diseases. *Dig Dis* **9**:133–141, 1991.
2. Verdugo P: Goblet cells secretion and mucogenesis. *Annu Rev Physiol* **52**:157–176, 1990.
3. Tasman-Jones C: Gastric mucus—Physical properties in cytoprotection. *Med J Aust* **142**:55–56, 1985.
4. Neutra MR, Forster JF: Gastrointestinal mucus: Synthesis, secretion and function, in Johnson LR (ed): *Physiology of the Gastrointestinal Tract*, ed 2. New York, Raven Press, 1987, pp 975–1009.
5. Johansson C, Kollberg B: Stimulation by intragastrically administered E_2 prostaglandin human gastric mucus output. *Eur J Clin Invest* **9**:229–232, 1979.
6. Sherman P, Forstner J, Roomi N, *et al*: Mucin depletion in the intestine of malnourished rats. *Am J Physiol* **248**:G418–G423, 1985.
7. Satchithanandam S, Vargofcak-Apker M, Calvert RJ, *et al*: Alteration in gastrointestinal mucin by fiber feeding in rats. *J Nutr* **120**:1179–1184, 1990.
8. Cohan VL, Scott AL, Dinarello CA, *et al*: Interleukin-1 is a mucus secretagogue. *Cell Immunol* **136**:425–434, 1991.
9. Thomsen L, Tasman-Jones C, Maher K, *et al*: Na^+/H^+ ion exchange of postmortem gastric mucus. *Scand J Gastroenterol* **23**:701–704, 1988.
10. Thomsen LL, Gavin JB, Tasman-Jones C: Relation of Helicobacter pylori to the human gastric mucosa in chronic gastritis of the antrum. *Gut* **31**:1230–1236, 1990.
11. Shorrock CJ, Rees WDW: Effect of sucralfate on human gastric bicarbonate secretion and local prostaglandin E_2 metabolism. *Am J Med* **86**(suppl 6A):2–4, 1989.
12. Slomiany BL, Laszewicz W, Slomiany A: In vitro inhibition of peptic degradation of porcine gastric mucus glycoprotein by sucralfate. *Scand J Gastroenterol* **20**:857–860, 1985.
13. Slomiany BL, Slomiany A: The effect of intragastric sucralfate administration on the content, comparison and physical properties of the gastric mucosal barrier, Abstracts 6th International Sucralfate Symposium, August 19–21, 1990, Gold Coast, Australia.
14. Mall A, Fourie AJ, McLeod H, *et al*: Sucralfate protects the pig stomach from ulceration induced by bile duct ligation, Abstracts 6th International Sucralfate Symposium, August 19–21, 1990, Gold Coast, Australia.
15. Tasman-Jones C, Thomsen L, Vanderwee M, *et al*: Sucralfate enhances Na^+/H^+ exchange of uninfected and Campylobacter pylori infected mucus. *Gastroenterol Int* **1**(suppl):758, 1988 (Abstract).
16. Tasman-Jones C, Morrison G, Thomsen L, *et al*: Sucralfate interactions with gastric mucins. *Am J Med* **86**(suppl 6A):5–9, 1989.

9

Gastroduodenal Bicarbonate Secretion and Its Response to Sucralfate

W. D. W. REES

Bicarbonate Secretion by the Upper Gastrointestinal Tract

Reduction of gastric acidity by ingestion of alkali has been used for decades to alleviate the symptoms and heal mucosal damage in peptic ulcer disease. The possibility that intrinsic secretion of alkali into surface mucus gel could protect gastric epithelium from acid attack was raised by Heatley some 40 years ago. However, because of limitations in experimental techniques, the existence of such alkali secretion was not proven until 25 years later. The advent of potent inhibitors of acid secretion coupled with the development of techniques for measuring small amounts of bicarbonate *in vitro* and *in vivo* has confirmed the existence of bicarbonate secretion by esophageal, gastric, and duodenal mucosa. This alkali secretion is capable of sustaining a significant pH gradient across gastric and duodenal surface mucus gel thereby reducing exposure of underlying cells to a damaging acid environment (Fig. 1). However, the importance of bicarbonate secretion to mucosal integrity within the proximal gut remains uncertain. It is conceivable that alkali secretion by the esophagus and duodenum plays a far greater role in protection against the smaller quantities of luminal acid found in these organs than in the stomach where luminal acidity is consistently higher and capable of overwhelming the mucus pH gradient. Stimulation of alkali secretion may have important implications for the management of peptic ulcer disease and may enhance ulcer healing or prevent ulcer recurrence without altering luminal acidity.

W. D. W. REES • Hope Hospital, Salford, and University of Manchester School of Medicine, Manchester, England.

Sucralfate: From Basic Science to the Bedside, edited by Daniel Hollander and G. N. J. Tytgat. Plenum Press, New York, 1995.

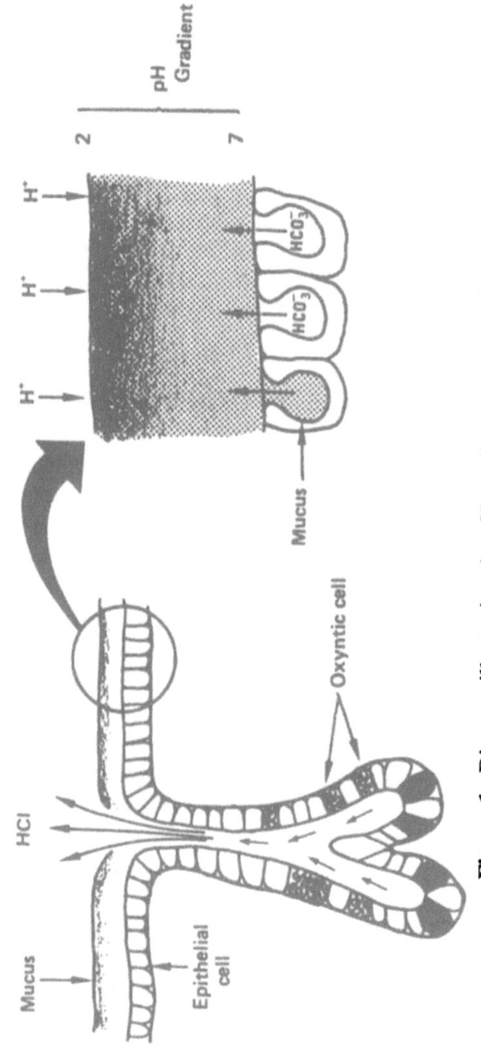

Figure 1. Diagram illustrating the pH gradient across gastric mucus gel.

Esophageal Bicarbonate Secretion

Traditionally, esophageal defense mechanisms were thought to rely on motor functions of the esophagus and gastroesophageal junction which either prevented acid entry from the stomach or enhanced its clearance from the esophageal lumen. In recent years it has been suggested that swallowed salivary bicarbonate may be important in the acid clearance.

The esophageal epithelium is largely squamous and therefore functionally quite different from that of the stomach and duodenum which has been shown to transport bicarbonate into the lumen. Studies in the rabbit have shown that the squamous epithelium does not transport bicarbonate unless damaged by acid. In the opossum, the esophageal submucosa contains glands connected by ducts to the lumen and this species has been shown to possess esophageal bicarbonate secretion. The clear inference is that esophageal bicarbonate output is derived from the submucosal glands. Since a network of such glands has been demonstrated in the human esophagus, it is not particularly surprising that similar bicarbonate secretion has recently been reported in man. Quantitatively, this delivery of bicarbonate into the esophagus is much smaller than that from saliva but may represent an important defense against acid at times when saliva is not being swallowed. The physiological regulation of this secretion and whether it is susceptible to pharmacological manipulation remain unknown. Sucralfate has been shown to protect the esophagus from acid but there is as yet no evidence that the effect is mediated through stimulation of bicarbonate secretion.

Gastric Bicarbonate Secretion

The existence of active bicarbonate transport by fundic and antral epithelium was first demonstrated in 1975 by Flemstrom and Sachs using isolated pieces of mucosa mounted in Ussing chambers. Since then a number of investigators have confirmed this observation using amphibian, mammalian, or human mucosa studied either *in vitro* or *in vivo*. Both fundic and antral epithelium transport bicarbonate with the basal rate amounting to between 2 and 10% of acid output. The rate of gastric bicarbonate secretion can be influenced by a variety of neurohormonal agents although the physiological significance of such observations remains unknown (Table I). The stimulant action of prostaglandins of the E and F series may be important in maintaining normal rates of gastric alkali secretion, and inhibition of cyclooxygenase activity by nonsteroidal anti-inflammatory drugs may cause mucosal damage, in part, by a reduction in bicarbonate secretion. Experimental proof for this hypothesis, however, remains unsatisfactory.[1]

Vagal activity and luminal acid have been shown to play an important role in regulating gastric alkali secretion. Such observations suggest a close relationship between acid and alkali secretion which in turn may help maintain a balance between aggressive luminal factors and mucosal defense mechanisms. An increase in luminal acidity is therefore accompanied by an increase in bicarbonate secretion, although at luminal pH less than 1.5 there is evidence that the alkali response is overwhelmed.

In comparison with acid secretion, bicarbonate output from gastric mucosa is small

Table I. Modulators of Gastric Bicarbonate Secretion[a]

Stimulants	
	Dibutyryl cyclic GMP, calcium, cholinergic agents, cholecystokinin, pancreatic glucagon, neurotensin, pancreatic polypeptide, E-type prostaglandins, prostaglandin $F_{2\alpha}$
Inhibitors	
	Acetazolamide, anoxia, atropine, cyanide, cyclooxygenase inhibitors, DIDS (4,4-diisothiocyano-2,2-disulfonate stilbene), 2,4-dinitrophenol, ethanol, noradrenaline, ouabain, parathyroid hormone, taurocholate
No effect	
	Dibutyryl cyclic AMP, ACTH, amiloride, carbenoxolone, enkephalins, gastrins, histamine, hydrocortisone, isoprenaline, morphine, motilin, prostacyclin, secretin, serotonin, somatostatin, substance P, urogastrone, vasoactive intestinal polypeptide

[a]After Flemstrom (1987).

and likely to be completely overwhelmed if delivered directly into the lumen. However, if such neutralization is confined to the epithelial surface by overlying mucus gel, then the magnitude of bicarbonate transport is capable of generating a significant pH gradient across the unstirred gel. In combination, bicarbonate secretion and gastric mucus gel therefore constitute the first-line defense against luminal acid. The importance of this "mucus–bicarbonate" barrier as a defense mechanism remains controversial. In the stomach it probably represents a weak defense which may even be overcome by physiological concentrations of gastric acid, while in the duodenum, which is exposed to lower and intermittent levels of acidity, it probably confers significant protection against acid-induced injury.

The potential importance of gastric bicarbonate secretion in mucosal defense has been studied in detail. As a component of the "mucus–bicarbonate" barrier it is only one of several "in series" defense mechanisms that protects the stomach from acid attack (Fig. 2). Damaging agents such as nonsteroidal anti-inflammatory drugs, bile salts, and ethanol inhibit bicarbonate secretion while "cytoprotective" prostaglandins are stimulants of secretion. Such observations would support the involvement of gastric bicarbonate secretion in mucosal defense and in the pathophysiology of mucosal damage but provide little information on its importance relative to the other defense mechanisms. Whether abnormal bicarbonate secretion into mucus gel plays a role in causing gastric ulcer or erosive gastritis remains uncertain. Studies of alkali secretion in gastric ulcer disease are limited and plagued by methodological difficulties. Initial observations suggest normal secretory activity in such patients although there is some evidence that the polymeric structure of mucus could be impaired in gastric ulcer leading to a less stable gel layer. As a result, the pH gradient sustained across gastric mucus gel may be impaired despite normal rates of bicarbonate transport across the surface epithelium. Such a generalized abnormality of mucosal defense is unable to explain the focal nature of gastric ulcer and may represent only one of several pathogenic mechanisms.

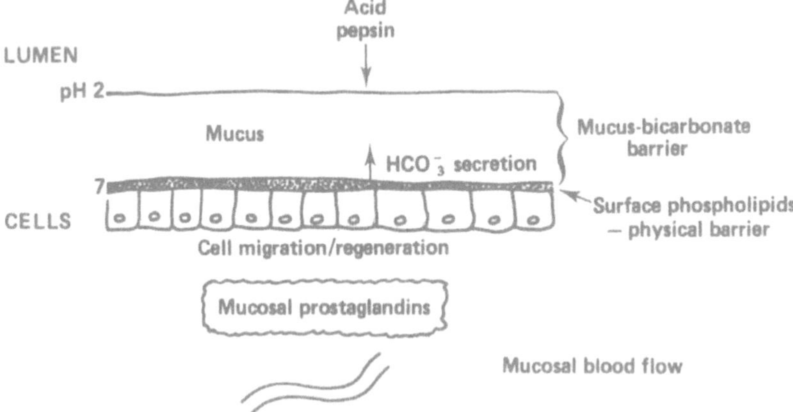

Figure 2. Some of the "in series" defense mechanisms protecting gastric mucosa.

Measurement of Gastric Bicarbonate Secretion

The presence of gastric acid precluded accurate measurement of alkali secretion from the stomach until the advent of H_2-receptor antagonists in the mid-1970s. Earlier studies had documented the existence of such alkali production in patients with pernicious anemia and canine antral pouches devoid of parietal cells. Gunner Flemstrom used isolated pieces of fundic and antral mucosa mounted in Ussing chambers to measure bicarbonate secretion in amphibian species. Alkali delivery into the lumen was recorded using a "pH stat" system (Fig. 3) and acid output from fundic epithelium was inhibited by an H_2-receptor antagonist. This pioneering work allowed the cellular mechanisms of bicarbonate transport to be explored and provided some insight into neurohormonal regulation of secretion. Bicarbonate transport is a metabolically dependent process although in the antrum, up to one-third of bicarbonate enters the lumen by a passive, intercellular route. Intracellular bicarbonate is derived from endogenous production, dependent on carbonic anhydrase activity, and transport across the basal epithelium by a sodium-dependent mechanism. The rate of bicarbonate secretion can therefore be influenced by the serosal supply of bicarbonate and is enhanced by the alkaline tide generated during acid secretion. Delivery of this alkaline tide to the surface epithelial cells is facilitated by capillaries that carry blood past the parietal cells toward the surface epithelium. Pharmacological studies have revealed a number of neurohormonal agents that either stimulate or inhibit bicarbonate transport (Table I). Apart from cholinergic stimuli, there is as yet little evidence that these responses have any physiological significance.

Similar bicarbonate secretion has been demonstrated using mammalian mucosa mounted in Ussing chambers and the characteristics of the transport process are remarkably similar to those seen in amphibian species. In intact animals, gastric bicarbonate secretion has been measured in a number of species and the results of such experiments are in general accord with those performed under *in vitro* conditions. In man, two different

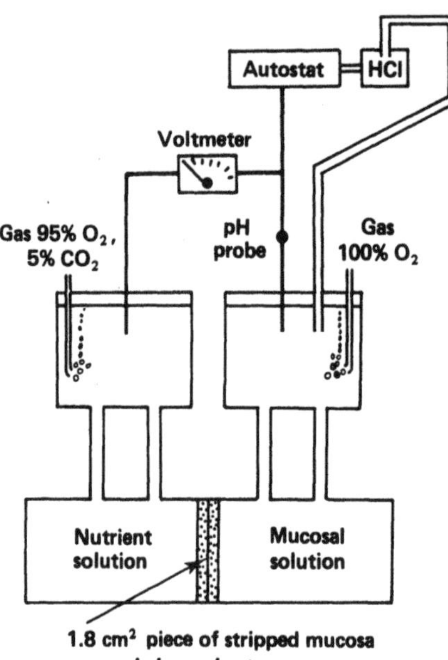

Figure 3. Diagram of a chamber acid pH stat system used to measure gastric or duodenal alkali secretion.

methods have been used to measure gastric alkali secretion. The earliest of these depends on gastroduodenal intubation, perfusion of the stomach with a nonabsorbable marker to determine gastric volume and measurement of the pH and pCO_2 of gastric aspirates to calculate bicarbonate concentration. The appearance of a second duodenal marker in the gastric aspirate is used to determine duodenogastric reflux and from amylase estimations contamination from swallowed saliva can be excluded. The second method also relies on gastric intubation but uses a two-compartment model of gastric secretion to calculate bicarbonate production from the hydrogen ion concentration and osmolality of gastric juice. Rates of bicarbonate secretion using this method are fivefold higher than by the other direct method and the validity of the calculations remains controversial. Studies of human gastric bicarbonate secretion have demonstrated the existence of a stimulatory vagal cholinergic pathway and autoregulation by luminal acid similar to those found in animal models. Human alkali secretion is also inhibited by damaging agents, such as nonsteroidal anti-inflammatory agents and bile salts.

Duodenal Bicarbonate Secretion

Acid delivered into the proximal duodenum is quickly neutralized resulting in a relatively stable, near-neutral pH. This was thought to depend mainly on intraluminal neutralization by pancreatico-biliary secretion. However, studies about 20 years ago suggested that the duodenal mucosa contributed to this process releasing carbon dioxide. Confirmation of bicarbonate transport across duodenal epithelium was provided by the work of Flemstrom and Silen using isolated pieces of amphibian mucosa devoid of Brunner glands. The rate of duodenal bicarbonate secretion was two to three times greater than gastric output but the cellular transport mechanisms were very similar. About a third of secretion occurred by passive diffusion while active cellular transport depended on either chloride/bicarbonate exchange or an electrogenic mechanism. Using mainly the *in vitro* preparation a number of stimulants and inhibitors of this bicarbonate secretion have been identified (Table II). As in the stomach, the physiological significance of these observations remains uncertain. Stimulants may activate either of the cellular transport mechanisms, with prostaglandins increasing output by an electrogenic pathway and the hormones GIP and VIP by chloride/bicarbonate exchange.

A variety of intact animal models have been developed to study duodenal alkali secretion and an intubation technique isolating a short segment of proximal duodenum has been used in man. Using these techniques luminal acid has been shown to be a potent stimulant of duodenal bicarbonate secretion, as in the stomach (Fig. 4). This response is likely to represent an important defense mechanism against acid injury and experiments have shown an inverse correlation between the extent of acid-induced villus damage and the magnitude of duodenal bicarbonate secretion. How this response is mediated remains speculative and at present prostaglandin E_2, VIP, and β-endorphin are potential candidates for producing the alkali response. Local nerves may also be important in regulating duodenal bicarbonate secretion. Activation of local neurons by field stimulation increases duodenal alkali output while capsaicin-sensitive afferent neurons may be involved in the acid response. Duodenal bicarbonate secretion is stimulated by cephalovagal activation and inhibited by splanchnic sympathetic nerves.

As in the stomach, duodenal bicarbonate enters surface mucus gel creating a significant pH gradient. Abnormality of duodenal alkali secretion and juxtamucosal pH has been described in duodenal ulcer. Basal bicarbonate transport and its response to luminal acidification is impaired in duodenal ulcer disease. This is probably responsible for the lower juxtamucosal pH in the duodenal cap of such patients compared with healthy subjects (Fig. 5). Impaired duodenal alkalinization may therefore be involved in the

Table II. Modulators of Duodenal Bicarbonate Secretion[a]

Stimulants
Dibutyryl cyclic AMP, arachidonic acid, β-endorphin, carbachol, cholecystokinin, diazepam, enkephalins, gastric inhibitory peptide, IMX (3-isobutyl-1-methyl xanthine), morphine, neurotensin, noradrenaline, pancreatic glucagon, pancreatic polypeptide, PHI, phenylephrine, theophylline, vasoactive intestinal polypeptide, E-type prostaglandins, prostaglandin $F_{2\alpha}$
Inhibitors
Acetazolamide, anoxia, clonidine, cyanide, cyclooxygenase inhibitors, dinitrophenol, ouabain, thiocyanate
No effect
Dibutyryl cyclic GMP, bombesin, carbenoxolone, cimetidine, gastrin, histamine, insulin, isoprenaline, omeprazole, propranolol, prostacyclin, serotonin, SITS (4-acetamido-4-isothiocyanostilbene-2,2-disulfonic acid), somatostatin, substance P, taurocholate, urogastrone

[a]After Flemstrom (1987).

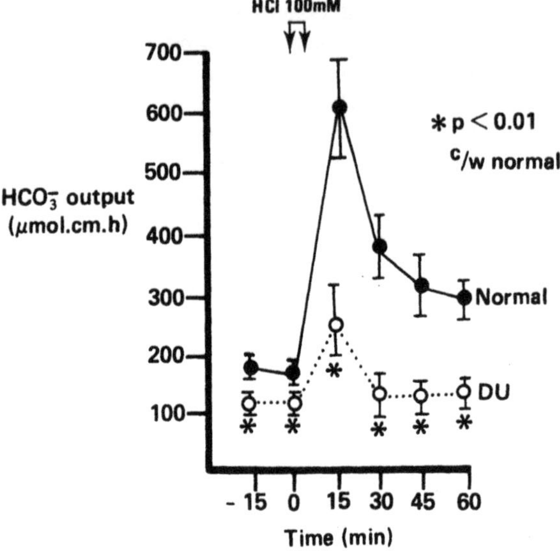

Figure 4. Stimulation of duodonel bicarbonate secretion by luminal acid in normal subjects and duodenal ulcer patients.

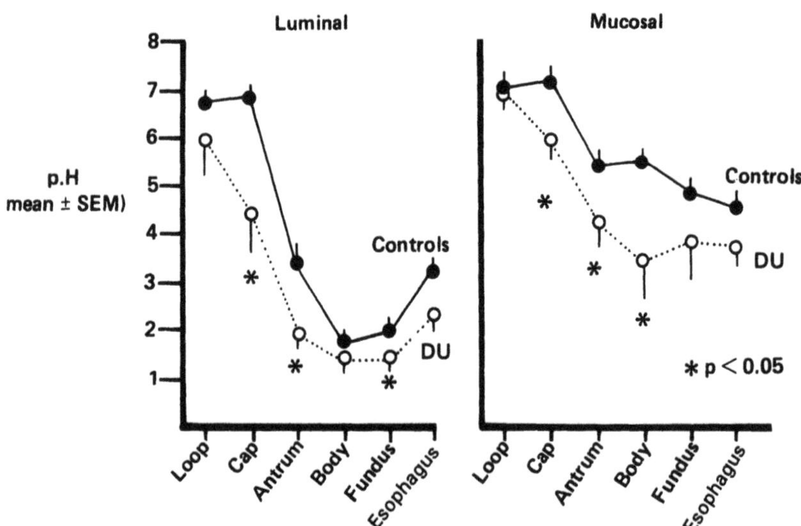

Figure 5. Luminal and mucosal pH in the stomach and duodenum of healthy subjects and duodenal ulcer patients.

pathogenesis of duodenal ulceration but its importance relative to other factors such as mucosal blood flow remains uncertain.

Effect of Sucralfate on Gastroduodenal Bicarbonate Secretion

Sucralfate has been shown to stimulate gastric and duodenal bicarbonate secretion both in isolated preparations and *in vivo*.[2] Using isolated amphibian gastric mucosa, luminal application of sucralfate produces a dose-dependent increase in bicarbonate transport from fundic and antral tissue without altering transmucosal potential difference (Fig. 6). An identical response can be observed in the duodenum, although compared with gastric studies, the dose–response curve was shifted to the right. Addition of the various components of sucralfate, sucrose, sucrose octasulfate, or potassium sulfate failed to alter bicarbonate secretion. However, luminal exposure to either aluminum potassium sulfate or

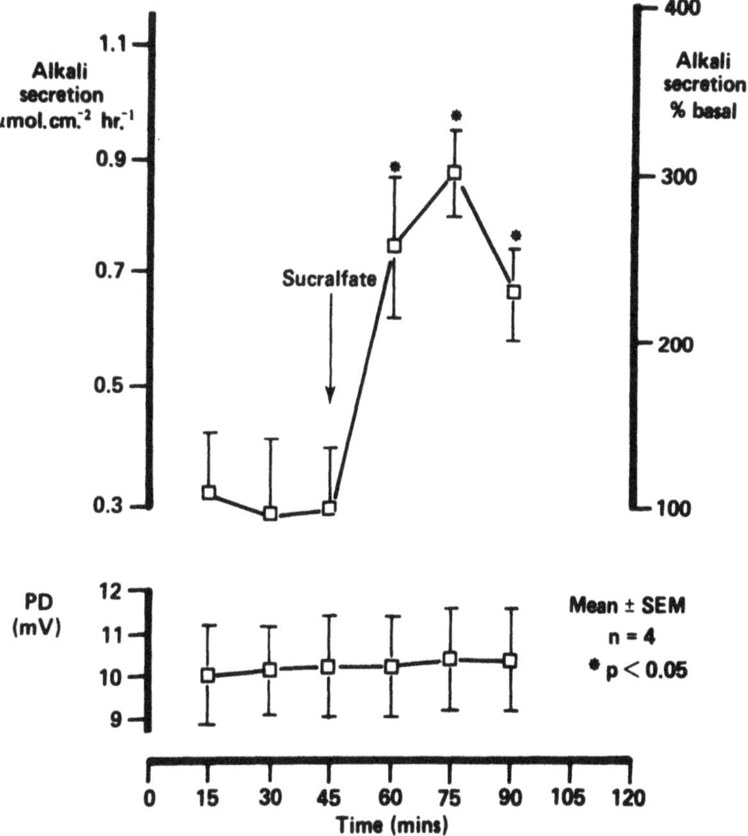

Figure 6. Stimulation of antral bicarbonate secretion by sucralfate, using amphibian mucosa.

aluminum acetate, equivalent to the total aluminum content of sucralfate, increased bicarbonate secretion by fundic, antral, and duodenal mucosa (Fig. 7). The magnitude of this secretory response was similar to that observed with sucralfate and it occurred without change in transmucosal potential difference.

These observations suggest that the aluminum component of sucralfate is responsible for the alkali response and that increased bicarbonate transport is probably mediated by enhanced chloride bicarbonate exchange. A number of studies have shown that sucralfate increases local formation of prostaglandins, such as PGE_2, and it is conceivable that the secretory response is mediated by enhanced PGE_2 formation (Fig. 8). *In vitro* experiments using indomethacin pretreatment to inhibit prostaglandin synthesis have shown that this has little effect on either the sucralfate or aluminium induced increase in gastric bicarbonate secretion. It therefore seems unlikely that the alkali response to sucralfate is mediated through increased synthesis of local prostaglandins.

Studies in man, using both the direct and indirect methods for calculating gastric bicarbonate output have demonstrated stimulation of alkali secretion by sucralfate (Fig. 9). This effect is accompanied by an increase in prostaglandin E_2 output from gastric mucosa but it remains controversial whether the alkali response is mediated by enhanced prostaglandin synthesis. In one study, the sucralfate-induced stimulation of gastric secretion was not affected by indomethacin pretreatment while in another the response was almost entirely prevented by aspirin. In view of the *in vitro* findings, it seems unlikely that local formation of prostaglandins plays a major role in mediating sucralfate stimulation of gastroduodenal bicarbonate transport.

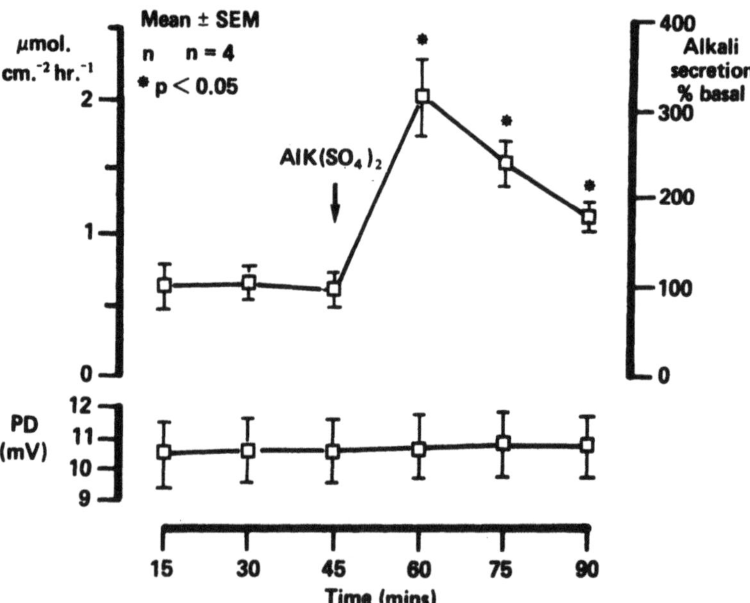

Figure 7. Stimulation of antral bicarbonate secretion by aluminum, using amphibian mucosa.

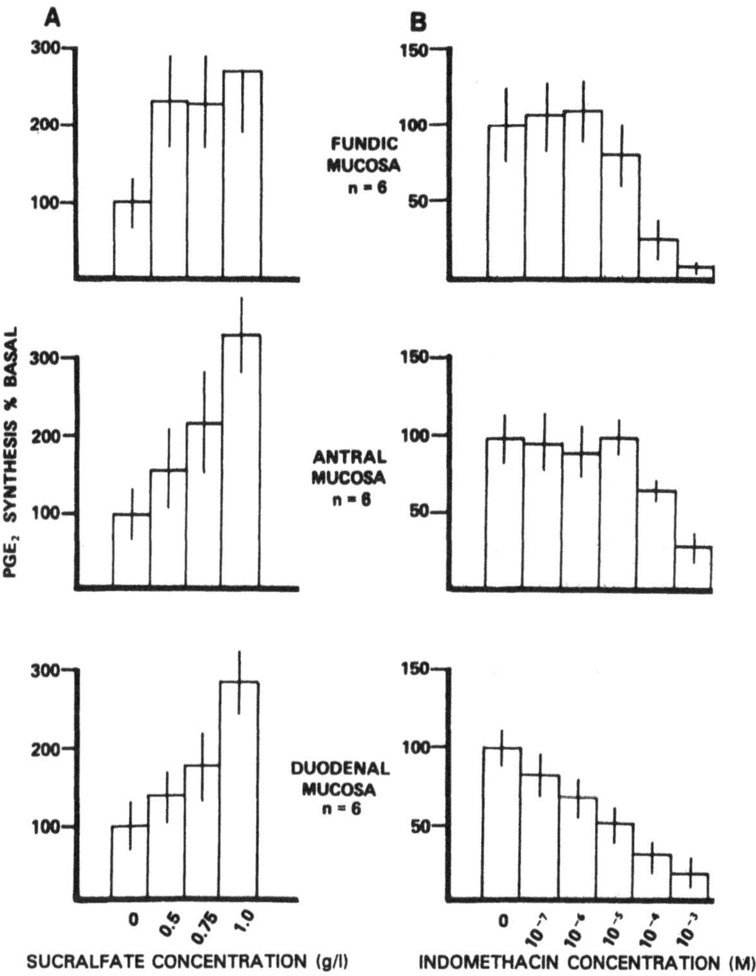

Figure 8. Effects of sucralfate (A) and indomethacin (B) on prostaglandin E_2 synthesis by isolated gastric and duodenal mucosa.

Relevance of Increased Bicarbonate Transport to Mucosal Protection and Ulcer Healing

As discussed elsewhere, sucralfate protects normal mucosa from damage and heals peptic ulcers.[3,4] It has a variety of site protective and cytoprotective actions mediated by its components aluminum, sulfate and sucrose octasulfate. The relative importance of stimulated bicarbonate secretion to its protective actions remains speculative. Increased delivery of bicarbonate into the unstirred mucus gel would in theory enhance the quality of the "mucus–bicarbonate" barrier overlying gastric and duodenal mucosa. This would be

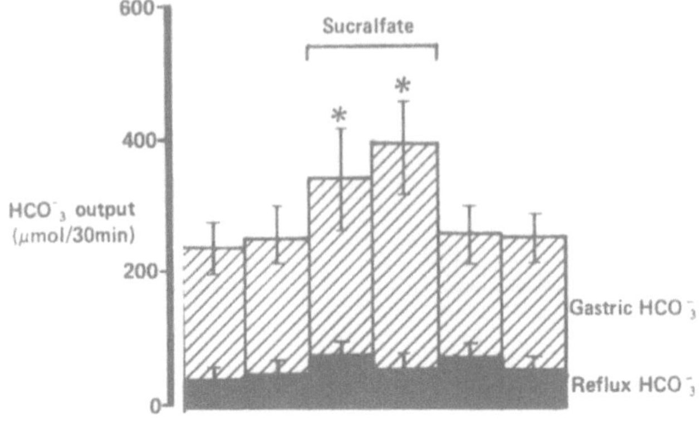

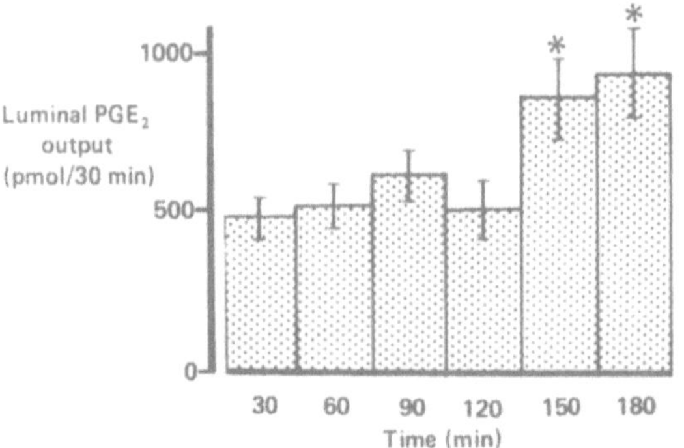

Figure 9. Stimulation of human gastric bicarbonate and prostaglandin E_2 output by sucralfate.

expected to reduce acid-induced injury to surface epithelial cells and would help preserve the integrity of normal mucosa.[5]

It seems very unlikely that stimulation of bicarbonate transport plays any role in the healing of damaged mucosa. Gastric mucosa exposed to high concentrations of ethanol shows severe damage to surface epithelial cells and the damaged mucosa may be covered by a thick layer of sloughed cells, fibrin, and mucus called the "mucoid cap." Passive delivery of bicarbonate from the interstitial space into this layer provides a neutral environment adjacent to the regenerative zones that is essential for reepithelialization. The actions of sucralfate on bicarbonate transport across normal gastric epithelial cells are clearly irrelevant to this healing process. Neither do these actions contribute to the healing of a focal ulcer, which is devoid of a surface epithelium.[6,7]

It seems highly likely that the action of sucralfate on bicarbonate secretion is most relevant to preserving normal epithelium following ulcer healing or as prophylaxis against an anticipated damaging agent.

ACKNOWLEDGMENTS. The author is grateful to Mrs. Julie Young for preparing the manuscript and the Department of Medical Illustration at Hope Hospital for providing the figures.

References

1. Shorrock CJ, Rees WDW: Gastroduodenal bicarbonate secretion, in Salmon PR (ed): *Key Developments in Gastroenterology*. New York, John Wiley & Sons Ltd, 1988, pp 171–187. Contains an up-to-date review of the physiology of gastroduodenal bicarbonate secretion. Written mainly for clinicians.
2. Rees WDW: Mechanisms of gastroduodenal protection by sucralfate. *Am J Med* **91**(2A):58S–63S, 1991. Up-to-date review of the mechanisms whereby sucralfate is thought to protect the stomach and duodenum.
3. Szabo S, Hollander D: Pathways of gastrointestinal protection and repair: Mechanisms of action of sucralfate. *Am J Med* **86**:23–31, 1989. Excellent review of the mechanisms of action of sucralfate.
4. Tarnawski A, Erickson RA: Sucralfate—24 years later: Current concepts of its protective and therapeutic actions. *Eur J Gastroenterol Hepatol* **3**:795–810, 1991. Recent review of the pharmacology and clinical actions of sucralfate.
5. Shorrock CJ, Rees WDW: Bicarbonate secretion and alkaline microclimate, in Hollander D, Tarnawski A (eds): *Gastric Cytoprotection*. New York, Plenum Press, 1989, pp 91–108. Review of the physiology of bicarbonate secretion and the "mucus–bicarbonate" barrier aimed at practicing clinicians.
6. Crampton JR, Gibbons LC, Rees WDW: Stimulation of amphibian gastroduodenal bicarbonate secretion by sucralfate and aluminum: Role of local prostaglandin metabolism. *Gut* **29**:903–908, 1988. Article documenting some of the original observations on sucralfate and gastroduodenal bicarbonate secretion *in vitro*.
7. Shorrock CJ, Rees WDW: Effect of sucralfate on human gastric bicarbonate secretion and local prostaglandin E_2 metabolism. *Am J Med* **86**:2–4, 1989. Article documenting original observations on the effect of sucralfate on human gastric bicarbonate secretion and local prostaglandin E_2 output.

10

Effect of Sucrose Octasulfate on Isolated Gastric Cells

MICHAEL R. LUCEY and TADATAKA YAMADA

Introduction

Sucralfate, which is an aluminum salt of the sulfated disaccharide sucrose octasulfate, has been shown to promote healing of experimental gastric ulcers in rats and duodenal ulcers in humans.[1] Sucralfate has been approved by the Food and Drug Administration as therapy for duodenal ulcers, both for healing and as prophylaxis against recurrence. The mechanisms whereby sucralfate exerts its salutary effects on gastric and duodenal mucosa are insufficiently understood. In 1991, McCarthy listed the possible actions of sucralfate to include antipeptic effects, cytoprotective effects, actions on arachidonic acid metabolites, mucus, and bicarbonate, and finally effects on tissue growth, regeneration, and repair.[1] However, he did not consider whether sucralfate or sucrose octasulfate, its presumed active constituent, could either promote ulcer healing or prevent ulcer recurrence by influencing the secretion by the stomach of either acid or regulatory peptides.

Somatostatin is a naturally occurring small peptide secreted by endocrine D cells located in the gastric and duodenal mucosa and in the endocrine pancreas is a major local regulator of gastric physiology, modulating acid secretion, endocrine function, and probably blood flow.[2] Animal studies suggest that somatostatin plays an important role in regulation of ulcer healing.[3] We decided therefore to examine whether sucralfate may exert its ulcer healing effects in part via release of endogenous gastric somatostatin. The data have been reported in greater detail elsewhere.[4]

MICHAEL R. LUCEY and TADATAKA YAMADA • Department of Internal Medicine, University of Michigan Medical Center, Ann Arbor, Michigan 48109.

Sucralfate: From Basic Science to the Bedside, edited by Daniel Hollander and G. N. J. Tytgat. Plenum Press, New York, 1995.

Investigations

We utilized two experimental models which have been studied extensively in our laboratory. First, the interaction of sucrose octasulfate with isolated canine gastric mucosal cells maintained in short-term culture was examined. Cells were dispersed from freshly obtained adult canine gastric mucosa as reported previously.[5] The cell fractions utilized for study consisted of roughly 70% somatostatin-containing D cells on the basis of immunocytochemistry. After 40 hr stabilization, the cells were incubated with various test substances for a 2-hr test period and the somatostatin-like immunoreactivity released into the medium was measured by radioimmunoassay.

Fractions enriched in parietal cells were isolated to a purity of 60–70% in a similar fashion. Viability of the parietal cells exceeded 95% as judged by trypan blue exclusion. [^{14}C]-Aminopyrine and various test materials were added to a 4×10^6 cell suspension and incubated for 20 min at 37°C. Thereafter, cells were pelleted by centrifugation and accumulation of radiolabeled aminopyrine within the pellet, an indirect measure of hydrogen ion production, was measured by scintigraphy.

In our initial experiments we examined the effects of sucrose octasulfate on basal secretion of somatostatin-like activity as well as somatostatin secretion induced by epinephrine or gastrin-17. We chose these secretagogues because they activate different intracellular signal transduction pathways in canine fundic D cells. Epinephrine stimulates canine fundic D cells via cyclic AMP generation whereas gastrin's effects are mediated by induction of membrane inositol phospholipid and activation of protein kinase C. As shown in Fig. 1, sucrose octasulfate dose-dependently stimulated somatostatin secretion in all three circumstances. Of particular interest was the observation that the combined stimulatory action of sucrose octasulfate at the two highest doses (10 and 20 mg/ml) against a background of epinephrine exceeded the sum of the somatostatin responses to each secretagogue administered alone. In contrast, a similar potentiating phenomenon was not observed when sucrose octasulfate and gastrin-17 were combined. From these data we inferred that sucrose octasulfate and epinephrine may interact via separate signal transduction mechanisms. To examine further the potential interactions of sucrose octasulfate with these intracellular signal transduction mechanisms, we investigated the somatostatin-like

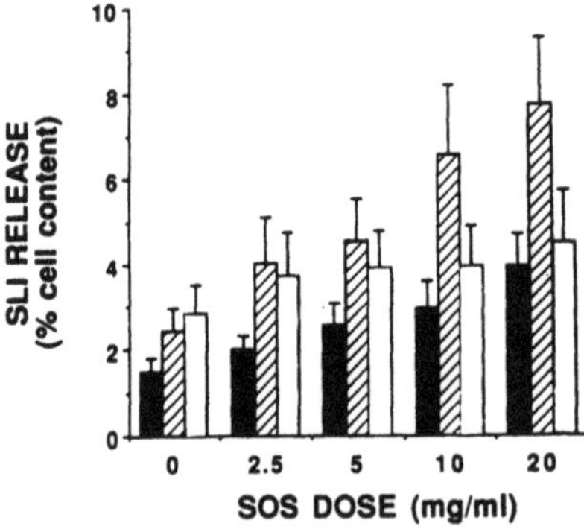

Figure 1. The effect of sucrose octasulfate either alone or in combination with epinephrine (▨, 10^{-6} M) or gastrin heptadecapeptide (□, 10^{-8} M) on somatostatinlike immunoreactivity release by fundic D cells. The data represent means ± SEM from four separate cell preparations (■, control). (Reproduced from Ref. 4, with permission).

immunoreactivity response to combined administration of sucrose octasulfate and either dibutyryl cAMP or TPA (12-*O*-tetradecanoylphorbol 13-acetate), a direct stimulant of protein kinase C. As shown in Fig. 2, sucrose octasulfate potentiated the somatostatin-stimulatory action of dibutyryl cAMP but not that of TPA.

To determine whether the effect of sucrose octasulfate represented nonspecific irreversible stimulation of, or possibly even damage to, D cells, we investigated whether the stimulation of somatostatin release by sucrose octasulfate could be inhibited. As shown in Fig. 3, octreotide, a functional analogue of somatostatin which is not immunoreactive in our somatostatin radioimmunoassay, inhibited at least partially the somatostatin-stimulating effect of sucrose octasulfate alone and sucrose octasulfate in combination with either epinephrine, gastrin-17, dibutyryl cAMP, or TPA. We also explored whether the stimulatory effect of sucrose octasulfate was selective for D cells by examining its action on gastric parietal cells. As shown in Fig. 4, sucrose octasulfate in a dose which was effective in stimulating somatostatin secretion did not affect aminopyrine uptake by isolated enriched parietal cells, either basally or when coadministered with acid secretagogues.

In our second experimental model, we used perfusion of vascularly intact isolated rat stomachs to investigate the influence of sucrose octasulfate on gastric somatostatin release into the portal venous flow. In all experiments, the responsiveness of the preparation was established by administration of isoproterenol, a known secretagogue of somatostatin, before and after the test periods.

As shown in Fig. 5, sucrose octasulfate produced a modest but significant increase in basal somatostatin release. When sucrose octasulfate was administered with a background infusion of low-dose isoproterenol, a similar modest increment in somatostatin concentration was observed in the portal venous effluent (Fig. 6).

Discussion

Although sucralfate has become a widely used agent to prevent or treat gastric and intestinal mucosal injury, the cellular basis of its action is uncertain. Much of the effort to

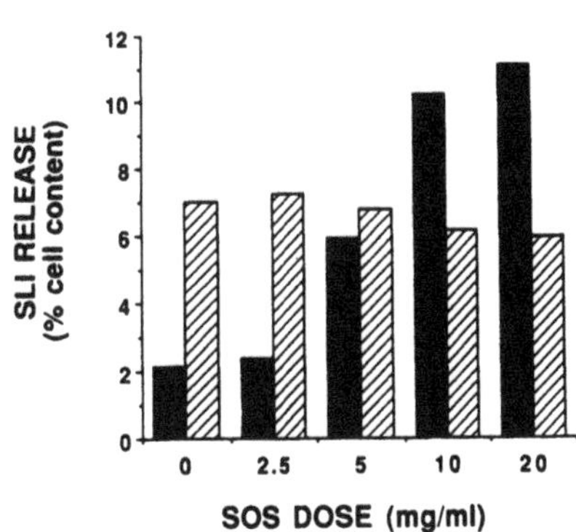

Figure 2. The effect of sucrose octasulfate either alone or in combination with dibutyryl cyclic AMP (■, 10^{-3} M) or 12-*O*-tetradecanoylphorbol 13-acetate (TPA) (▨, 10^{-6} M) on somatostatin release by fundic D cells. The data are from a single cell preparation and are representative of data obtained from two other preparations. (Reproduced from Ref. 4, with permission).

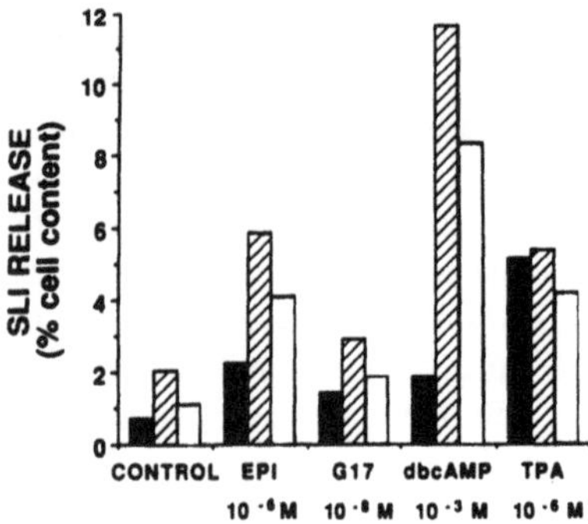

Figure 3. The effect of octreotide on somatostatin release in response to sucrose octasulfate (SOS) either alone (■) or in combination with other secretagogues (▨, plus 10 mg/ml SOS; □, plus 10 mg/ml SOS plus 10^{-6} M sandostatin). The data are from a single cell preparation and are representative of data obtained from two other preparations. (Reproduced from Ref. 4, with permission).

determine the mechanism of sucralfate's efficacy has been focused on its ability to enhance mucosal defense. The cells that function as targets for sucralfate or sucrose octasulfate have not been identified and the possibility that the gastric D cell could be a target for sucralfate has received little attention heretofore. D cells produce somatostatin. Somatostatin has been shown previously to prevent experimentally induced gastric ulcers, and in contrast to its usual inhibitory actions, has been found to enhance gastric mucus production. Our present studies showing that sucrose octasulfate stimulates somatostatin release from the stomach via direct action on D cells in the gastric mucosa support the hypothesis that sucralfate may mediate its effect through somatostatin.

The action of sucrose octasulfate on isolated fundic D cells resembles that of other neurohormonal stimuli of somatostatin release in that it is dose-dependent and potentiates the somatostatin response to agents that activate the cyclic AMP messenger pathway, but influences only in additive fashion agents that act via the Ca^{2+}/protein kinase C pathway. This would imply a direct receptor-mediated action of sucrose octasulfate linked to a calcium-dependent intracellular second messenger mechanism. Further studies are necessary to define the nature of this receptor and to confirm this intracellular mode of action. Nonetheless, the action of sucrose octasulfate is clearly not a nonspecific phenomenon

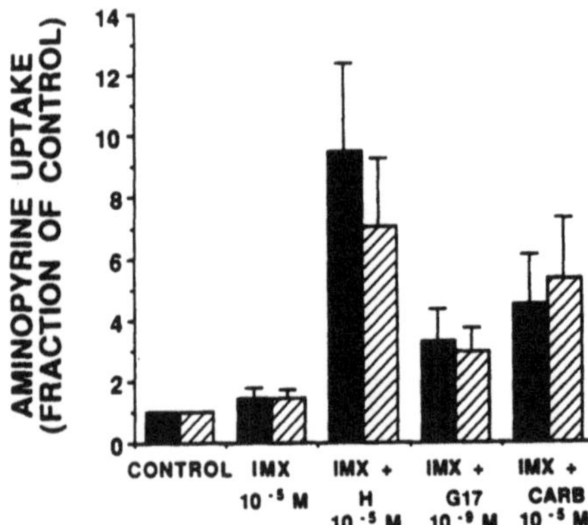

Figure 4. The effect of sucrose octasulfate (SOS) on uptake of radiolabeled aminopyrine by enriched canine parietal cells either alone or with coadministration of isomethylxanthine (IMX); histamine plus IMX, gastrin-17 plus IMX, and carbachol plus IMX. The data represent means ± SEM from three receptor cell preparations (■, no SOS; ▨, 10 mg/ml SOS). (Reproduced from Ref. 4, with permission.)

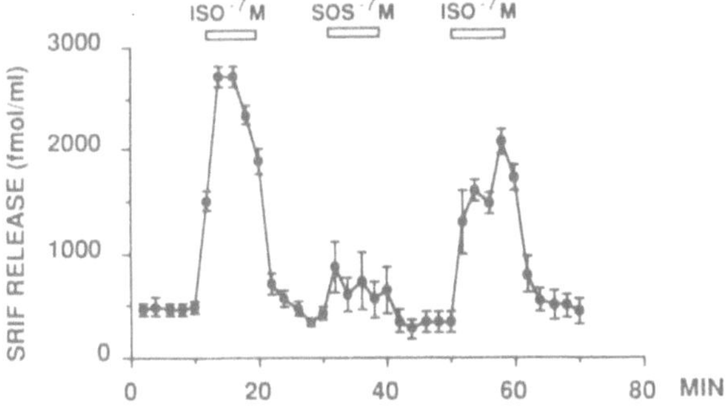

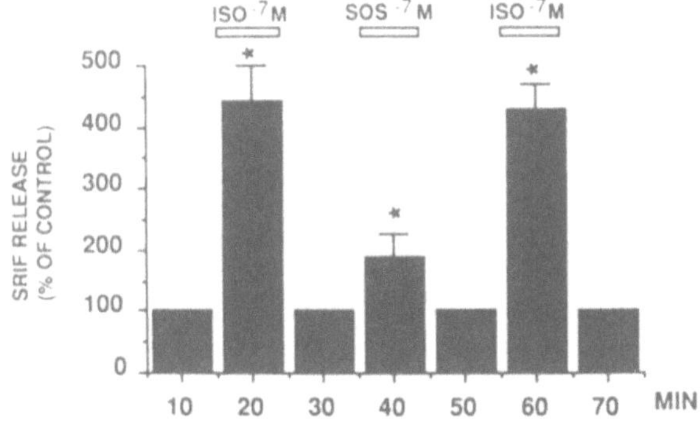

Figure 5. The effect of sucrose octasulfate on somatostatin release by the isolated perfused rat stomach. Data are represented as means ± SEM ($n = 5$) of absolute somatostatin concentration (upper panel) or % of control (lower panel). *$p < 0.05$, compared with basal (Student's *t* test for paired data). (Reproduced from Ref. 4, with permission.)

since it is reversible and D cell selective. Moreover, it is not likely to be an artifact of the culture D-cell system since it could be reproduced in the intact perfused stomach. However, because our D-cell preparations are not entirely pure, we cannot exclude the possibility that an intermediary target cell for sucrose octasulfate other than the D cell sequentially stimulates somatostatin release.

What is the relevance of our studies to the pharmacological action of sucralfate? Our use of sucrose octasulfate seems appropriate since sucralfate dissociates into its components Al^{3+} and sucrose octasulfate when present in an acid environment such as the stomach. The usual therapeutic doses of sucralfate are capable of producing local concentrations of sucrose octasulfate in the ranges described in our studies (2.5–20 mg/ml). Furthermore, D cells in the gastric antrum and possibly also in the fundus are configured with apical membranes that extend to the lumen of the stomach and are thus presumed capable of responding to stimuli present in the intragastric contents. This

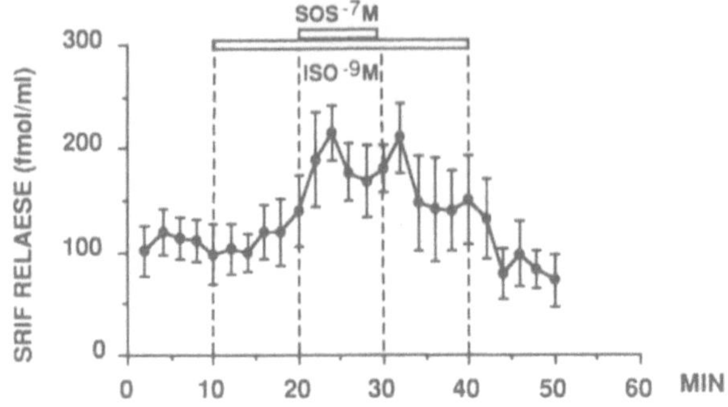

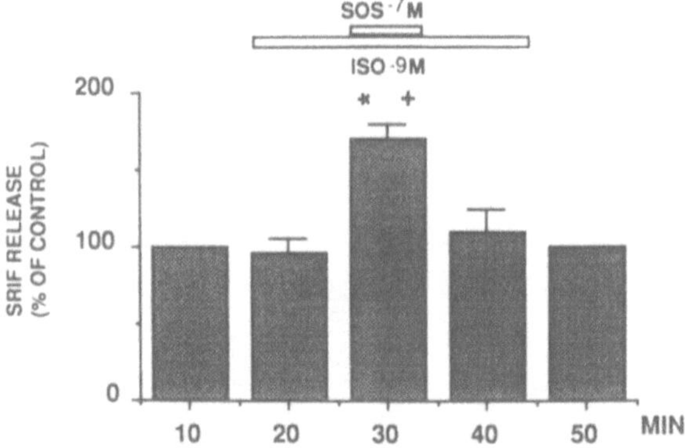

Figure 6. The effect of sucrose octasulfate in combination with low-dose isoproterenol (10^{-9} M) on somatostatin secretion from the isolated perfused stomach. The data, provided in the same format as in Fig. 5, represent means ± SEM from five separate perfusions. Sucrose octasulfate produced a response that was significantly greater than control on somatostatin secretion in response to low-dose isoproterenol $*p < 0.05$, compared with basal. $+ p < 0.05$, compared to isoproterenol alone. (Student's *t* test for paired data). (Reproduced from Ref. 4, with permission).

mechanism is thought to account for release of gastric somatostatin in response to intraluminal acidification.[6] Thus, it does not seem unreasonable to postulate that when sucralfate enters the gastric lumen it dissociates into its constituents including sucrose octasulfate, and that sucrose octasulfate then interacts with fundic D cells with consequential release of somatostatin.

Our perfused stomach studies were performed primarily to confirm the observations made in isolated gastric D cells. In these preparations, sucrose octasulfate was administered arterially rather than luminally and so may not have been physiological. However, despite the notion that sucralfate is poorly absorbed, there is evidence that some Al^{3+} and possibly sucrose octasulfate also can enter the circulation when standard doses of sucralfate are administered by mouth. The low doses used in the perfusion studies (10^{-7} M), therefore, may be a reflection of the amounts that circulate in plasma.

Conclusion

Our studies provide novel insight into the cellular mechanisms by which sucralfate works as a therapeutic or cytoprotective agent in the stomach. They are consistent with the hypothesis that sucralfate, acting through its constituent moiety sucrose octasulfate, stimulates release of somatostatin which, in turn, promotes ulcer healing via a variety of mechanisms. Sucrose octasulfate had no direct effect on acid secretion by gastric parietal cells, and appeared to act via specific receptor-mediated events to initiate somatostatin release from D cells.

ACKNOWLEDGMENTS. These studies were supported by NIH Grant RO1DK33500 and funds from the University of Michigan Gastrointestinal Peptide Research Center (NIH Grant P30DK34933).

References

1. McCarthy DM: Sucralfate. *N Engl J Med* **325**:1017–1025, 1991. An excellent overview of sucralfate, its potential mechanisms of action, and uses in gastrointestinal disorders.
2. Lucey MR, Yamada T: Biochemistry and physiology of gastrointestinal somatostatin. *Dig Dis Sci* **34**(3):5S–13S, 1989. A review of the role of somatostatin in the gastrointestinal tract.
3. Zierend H, Hengst K, Wagner H, *et al*: Inhibition of stress ulcer formation with somatostatin in rats. *Res Exp Med* **168**:199–204, 1976. *In vivo* study showing that somatostatin may modulate the formation of experimentally induced gastric ulcers.
4. Lucey MR, Park J, DelValle J, *et al*: Sucrose octasulphate stimulates gastric somatostatin release. *Am J Med* **91**(suppl 2A):52S–58S, 1991.
5. Yamada T, Soll AH, Park J, *et al*: Autonomic regulation of somatostatin release: Studies with primary cultures of canine fundic mucosal cells. *Am J Physiol* **247**:G567–G573, 1984. One of a number of papers in which the cell separation and culture methods used herein are described. Reference 4 includes a more comprehensive list of references.
6. Lucey MR, Wass JAH, Rees LH, *et al*: Relationship between gastric acid and elevated plasma somatostatin-like immunoreactivity after a mixed meal. *Gastroenterology* **97**:867–872, 1989. A study in humans showing that luminal factors such as gastric acid influence release of somatostatin.

11

Effect on Gastric Surfactant

BRIAN A. HILLS

Gastric Surfactant

Sucralfate is unique among pharmaceutical approaches to peptic ulceration in that it binds to the ulcer site as described in more detail in Chapter 10. However, the binding of a protective agent to the surface it protects has been exploited in the protection of nonbiological surfaces since ancient man first put bear grease on his spears to stop them from rusting. The same principle is retained in modern-day corrosion inhibitors which are surfactants that function by coating the surfaces they protect by a process known in the physical sciences as adsorption,[1] the deposited lining often rendering the surface hydrophobic. This aspect has led to the realization[2] that many corrosion inhibitors closely resemble the highly surface-active disaturated phosphatidylcholine (DSPC) found in the lung where there is increasing evidence[3] for its binding to the alveolar mucosa in addition to its more traditional role of reducing surface tension. In this chapter we pursue the mounting body of evidence supporting the concept of endogenous gastric surfactant providing the gastric mucosal barrier and review the capability of sucralfate to compensate for any deficiency.

Gastric Mucosal Barrier

For centuries there has been the concept of an "inside lining" to the stomach, to use lay terms. However, it was not until the 1950s and 1960s that Davenport[4] performed numerous experiments elegantly designed to elucidate the fundamental physiology of the stomach wall, concluding that there is a "gastric mucosal barrier" to the backdiffusion of hydrogen ions.[5] However, failure to demonstrate this barrier morphologically, despite the advent of the electron microscope, has led to this term being regarded more as a physiological concept than a physical reality. Many theories of gastric mucosal protection

BRIAN A. HILLS • Department of Physiology, University of New England, Armidale, NSW 2351, Australia; *present address*: Pediatric Respiratory Research Centre, Mater Children's Hospital, South Brisbane, Queensland, Australia.

Sucralfate: From Basic Science to the Bedside, edited by Daniel Hollander and G. N. J. Tytgat. Plenum Press, New York, 1995.

have arisen,[6] often based on physiological parameters, e.g., Na^+ or Cl^-, which change on failure of the barrier; but one is confronted with the perennial problem of differentiating between cause and effect. However, after critical review of these theories in the light of more recent evidence, the consensus of opinion[6] would still seem to favor a gastric mucosal barrier as a *physical* entity.

Gastric Mucus

Until recently,[7] the only physical structure seen lining the epithelial surfaces of stomach wall has been the mucous layer and this has long been implicated as providing mucosal protection. This view is still supported by many[8] and the reader is advised to consult Chapter 4 for a more comprehensive treatment of the subject and the action of sucralfate.

The problem with the mucus theory is that the mucous lining would only appear to provide about 25% of the resistance to hydrogen ions required for protection, while it does not address the problem of the protection of the epithelial surface of oxyntic ducts. In these, the environment is particularly corrosive as hydrochloric acid from parietal cells mixes with pepsinogen from chief cells to form pepsin, all at a pH of 1, and yet there is *no mucous lining* to these surfaces.

Corrosion Inhibitors

Considerations such as those expressed above have led to the search for an alternative physical barrier against acid and one that might not have been conducive to visualization by conventional electron microscopy. For instance, it is particularly difficult to visualize a monomolecular layer—the form in which corrosion inhibitors are claimed[1,3] to function in protecting metals, for instance. Corrosion inhibitors are surfactants that bind to the metal surface by adsorption.[1] Surfactants are amphipathic substances, meaning that they possess a "dual personality" in which one end is polar, seeking aqueous environments or bonding by electrostatic forces to the surface, while the other is nonpolar—often hydrocarbon in nature—and is oriented outwards. If these outwardly oriented "tails" pack together with those of surfactant molecules adsorbed to neighboring sites—as depicted in Fig. 1a,c—then the adsorbed monolayer often forms an effective barrier to all manner of corrosive substances, including acids. Thus, strong cohesion between adsorbed molecules is as important as strong adsorption in determining the efficacy of a surfactant as a corrosion inhibitor.[1]

Often a binding agent is added to improve cohesion, a classical example being the addition of multivalent cations to phosphate "primers" as depicted in Fig. 1b, intimating a comparable role for Al^{3+} in sucralfate.

One of the incidental findings in the use of many corrosion inhibitors is the tendency to render the protected surface hydrophobic as manifest by water "beading up" when placed on the surface rather than wetting it. In fact, when working as an engineer several decades ago, this writer would use the hydrophobicity of the surface as an indication of the retention of the corrosion inhibitor.

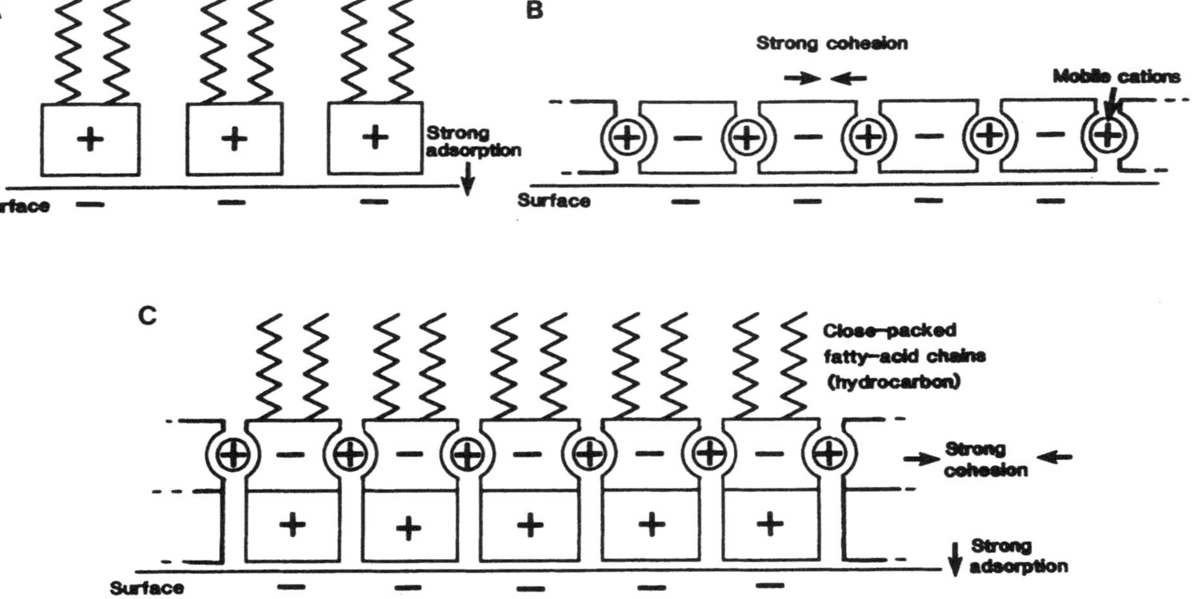

Figure 1. Three types of adsorption. (A) A cationic surfactant, typical of most corrosion inhibitors, can be strongly adsorbed to a negatively charged surface through ionic (electrostatic) bonding of the positive charges at the polar ends of the molecules. However, there is no force promoting cohesion of the adsorbed monolayer. (B) "Phosphating," in which the interspersion of mobile cations between phosphate ions pulls those ions into a most cohesive layer with no gaps for penetration of corrosive solutes. However, adsorption and general binding to the surface is ofter poor in "phosphating." (C) The situation envisaged *in vivo*[12] where mobile cations pull together not only the phosphate ions but also the attached fatty-acids chains to form a close-packed hydrocarbon barrier to hydrated hydrogen ions as shown in Fig. 6. Note also how neutralization of the negative phosphate ions by the intercalated mobile cations now leaves the terminal positive charges of the phospholipid zwitterions free to form a strong ionic bond with the surface—as applies to the simple cationic surfactant depicted in panel a.

Mucosal Hydrophobicity

In view of the above experience it was very interesting to find evidence for direct adsorption to tracheal mucosa[9] of the particularly surface-active disaturated phospholipid (DSPC) which comprises the major component (67%) of pulmonary surfactant. A simple and very convenient index of surface hydrophobicity is provided by the contact angle (θ). This is the angle between the tissue surface and the tangent to the surface of a droplet of saline placed on it as it "beads up" rather than wetting the surface. For a spontaneously wettable surface, θ is zero, whereas it reached 70° for tracheal epithelium exposed to DSPC.[9]

In view of the similarity of surface-active phospholipid (SAPL) to many surfactants used as corrosion inhibitors,[2] it was particularly interesting to find that the canine gastric mucosa was so hydrophobic, giving a mean contact angle of 86 ± 5.4°.[10] This compares with a value of 95° for polyethylene,[1] which is similar in its hydrocarbon composition to the outwardly oriented nonpolar "tails" of adsorbed SAPL molecules as they pack together with their adsorbed neighbors—see Fig. 1a. A loose analogy can be made with a very thin polythene liner which is often used commercially to protect against acid attack, the best example being the modern polythene battery case.

Perhaps the most interesting aspect of this analogy is the loss of hydrophobicity with the common barrier breakers,[10] notably bile salts, aspirin, and alcohol, each of which is either a solvent for SAPL or reacts with it to form chemical complexes. The contact angle has now been adopted by some groups as a quantitative index of active gastritis, the measurement being performed routinely on biopsy samples of gastric mucosa procured during diagnostic endoscopy.

Hydrophobicity can be increased by protective agents such as prostaglandins, PGE_2 not only increasing the contact angle but also the quantity of gastric surfactant present in the stomach.[11] Hence, it has been tempting to speculate that DSPC—or SAPL, at least—is a mediator in the protective action of prostaglandins upon the gastric mucosa.

Although the experimental evidence leaves no doubt that the normal gastric mucosa is hydrophobic, it is difficult to explain on thermodynamic grounds. A lining of surfactant adsorbed to alveolar epithelium to render that surface hydrophobic[2,3] makes good sense because it will have low surface energy when in contact with air. On replacing the air by an aqueous fluid, however, the surface energy is greatly increased, raising the question of why the adsorbed layer would be stable. Such theoretical objections can be allayed by the fact that the hydrophobic surface would be in contact with gastric mucus which is an effective wetting agent,[12] thus reducing interfacial energy. Other aspects of the association of gastric mucus with surface hydrophobicity are discussed later (section The Mucous Lining) in connection with the ultrastructure of mucus. However, it should be mentioned at this point that sucralfate, being surface active, is also a mild wetting agent.

Morphology

If there really is a gastric mucosal barrier of gastric surfactant, then it should be capable of visualization by electron microscopy using fixatives designed to preserve any SAPL. One reason that a barrier of SAPL may have been missed in many morphological studies of the stomach wall is the almost universal use of glutaraldehyde as the primary fixative since its introduction in 1963 for its ability to fix protein. However, aldehydes are well known to destroy hydrophobic surfaces. Hence, in more recent studies the glutaraldehyde has been largely replaced by tannic acid which preserves not only the highly osmiophilic DSPC but is ideal for enabling any multilaminated structure to be resolved.[13] Other modifications include the use of extremely thin (<60 nm) sections to help to resolve any lamellar bodies and other lamellated structures and a long (72 hr) primary fixation time. This is needed to enable water-soluble fixatives to penetrate what is, after all, a gastric mucosal barrier to water-soluble solutes.

The results of this major deviation from conventional fixation procedures are quite spectacular. Aware of the implications of surfactant to the stomach,[10] Ueda *et al.*[14] have demonstrated a few lamellations of surfactant over some parts of the luminal lining of the stomach to which lamellar bodies could be seen to be attached. They have also shown many lamellar bodies in parietal cells and surface mucus cells and a few in chief cells. This was particularly interesting since lamellar bodies are unequivocally the form in which surfactant is produced in the alveolar Type II cell of the lung; although many pathologists dismiss such structures as simply the "membranous remains of dead cells"—even when found within nonphagocytic cells.

Our studies[7] confirmed the presence of many multilamellar bodies, i.e., multifocal LBs, in parietal cells (Fig. 2) and some in surface mucus cells. The former is particularly

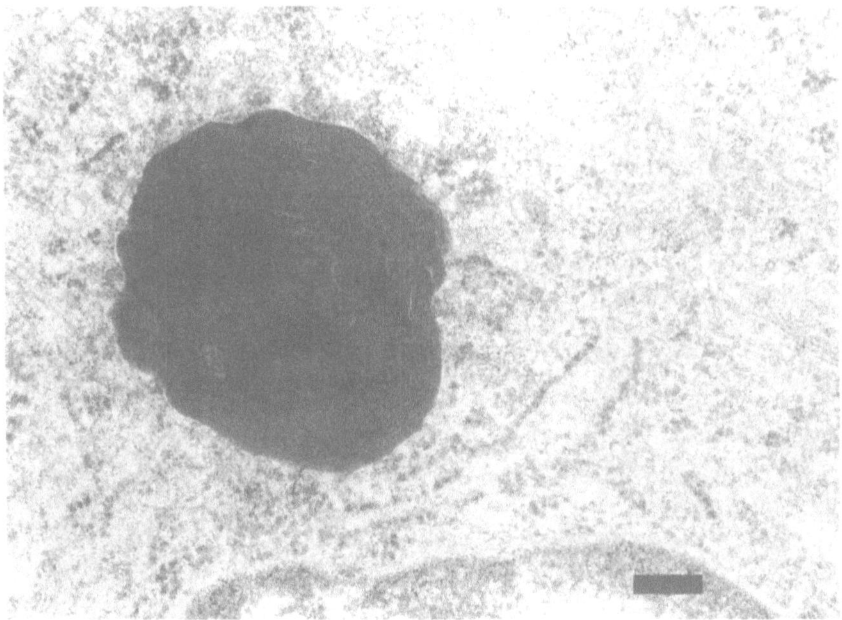

Figure 2. Electron micrograph of a lamellar body typical of those found in secreted gastric mucus and in the necks of oxyntic ducts. Bar = 200 nm.

interesting since it implies that, by co-secretion of acid and gastric surfactant, the stomach would be able to gear the release of protectant to that of the potential insult to the mucosal barrier. It was also possible to confirm Ueda's finding of an oligolamellar luminal lining to the stomach.[7]

A particularly exciting finding was the thicker oligolamellar lining coating oxyntic ducts (see Fig. 3) since these are known to be mucus-free and yet in contact with an environment even more corrosive than gastric juice, as described above. The number of lamellations ranged from 10 to 16. A similar oligolamellar lining of gastric surfactant was found[7] on the epithelial surfaces of the canaliculi of the parietal cells, i.e., on another surface of channels through which acid is transmitted. This finding has been subsequently confirmed[15] in human tissue (see Fig. 4).

Thus, there would indeed appear to be a physical structure of phospholipid lining the epithelial surfaces in contact with the most corrosive fluids in the stomach wall. This is almost certain to be predominantly DSPC, or phospholipid in some form, for several reasons. First, it is densely osmiophilic and is really only demonstrated effectively using fixatives known to preserve such structures.[13] Second, the interlamellar spacing of 45–55 Å is highly characteristic of lamellated SAPL either as the gastric mucosal barrier or as other examples of what is probably a "ubiquitous barrier." Third, where such barriers are accessible for extraction with lipid solvents, e.g., on pleural mesothelium,[3] the material recovered is predominantly DSPC and is recovered in quantities agreeing well (± 1) with

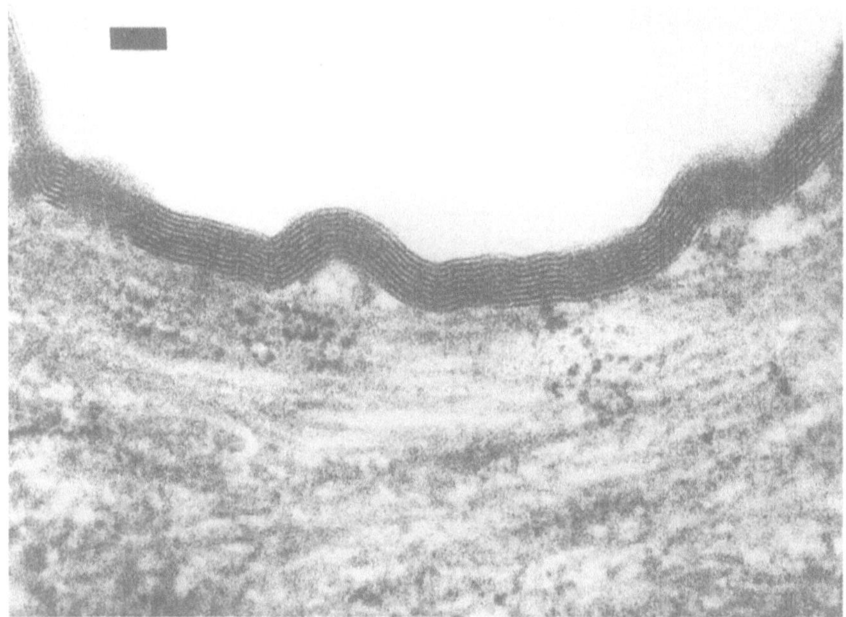

Figure 3. Electron micrograph of the luminal surface of a rat oxyntic duct visualizing an oligolamellar lining to the epithelium.[7] Bar = 50 nm.

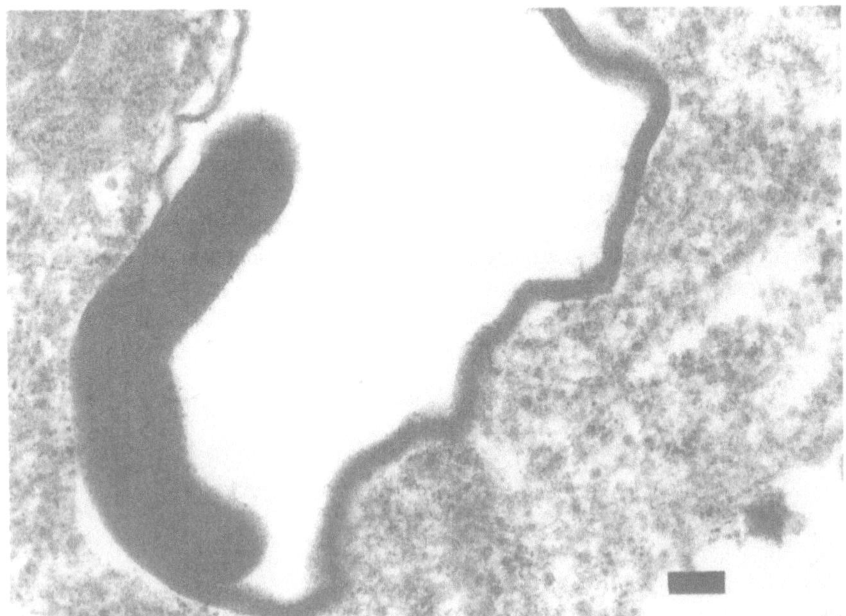

Figure 4. Electron micrograph of the luminal surface of a canaliculus in a human parietal cell demonstrating an oligolamellar lining to the epithelium.[15] Bar = 100 nm.

the number of monolayers visualized by electron microscopy. Fourth, synthetic DSPC dispersed by ultrasound forms lamellated structures in aqueous media[13] which appear identical to those seen in Fig. 2. Finally, there are many lamellar bodies in the vicinity of the oligolamellar lining and in adjacent secretory cells which are the obvious source.

Before turning to the evidence that these oligolamellar structures really are barriers to acid, it is necessary to reconsider the mucous lining of the stomach.

The Mucous Lining

Although the oligolamellar linings of epithelial surfaces *within* the stomach wall may explain one of the shortcomings of theories of mucosal protection based on gastric mucus, many aggressive and protective agents act by way of the luminal lining. Here the barrier protecting the vital organelles of surface mucous cells from gastric juice is not simply secreted mucus but includes highly granulated mucus *within* surface mucous cells which has been estimated from pH gradients to provide about 70% of the total barrier to acid backdiffusion.

Lipids have been implicated in the mucous barrier for some years and studied for the enhancement in resistance to acid transmission which they impart.[16] There are, however, widely differing opinions concerning the means by which lipids participate in mucosal defense. One view[16] has been their incorporation into mucin, i.e., into the mucosal proteins and glycoproteins as they are synthesized, while the other view is based on essentially the same phospholipid barrier already discussed in relation to the protection of epithelial surfaces deeper in the stomach wall. Reverting to traditional physical chemistry, it has been proposed that SAPL could migrate as micelles to the luminal surface to impart the characteristic hydrophobicity. However, this would seem unlikely if gastric surfactant is already present in surface mucous cells as multilamellar bodies and many lamellar bodies have been visualized in secreted mucus.[17]

At lower magnification, mucus in the surface mucous cells is highly granular. However, the intergranular matrix material is lamellated phospholipid as seen under higher magnification in Fig. 5. Thus, it has been proposed[17] that the luminal surface employs essentially the same basic barrier system as deeper epithelial surfaces, employing

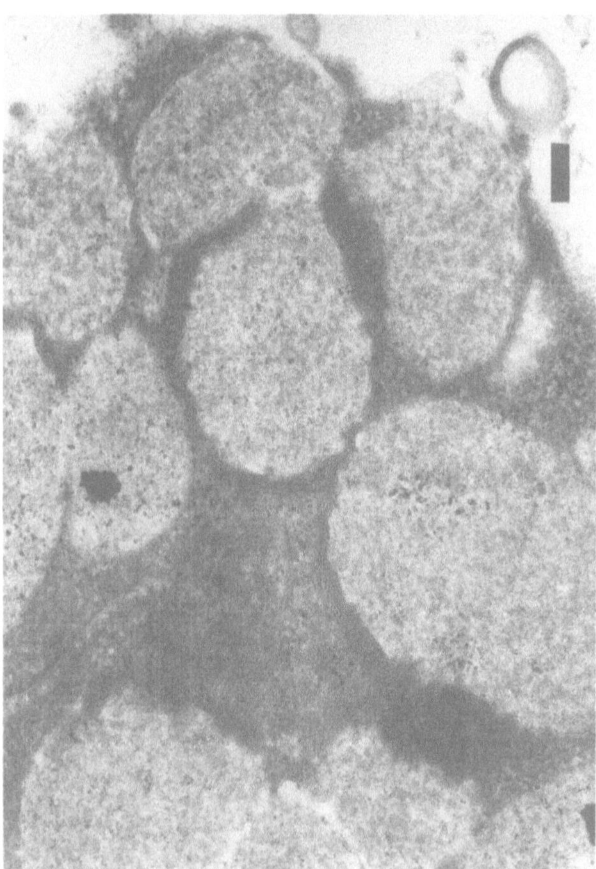

Figure 5. Electron micrograph of gastric mucus in a mucus-neck cell, visualizing the intergranular matrix material as oligolamellar SAPL. Bar = 100 nm.

minibarriers of only three to five lamellations each but arranged in series with respect to the backdiffusion of acid. Thus, an electrode gradually advanced across the mucosal lining would register a more or less continuous pH gradient as it penetrates successive minibarriers as envisaged in Fig. 5.

This model can also explain the drop in both resistance to acid transmission and viscosity as the mucin is "refined,"[8] refinement removing the intergranular matrix material of SAPL.

Secreted Mucus

After secretion from the surface mucous cells, mucus tends to lose its granular structure but the SAPL seems capable of re-forming as a continuous oligolamellar coating of SAPL at the interface with the gastric juice. It seems to be capable of re-forming as more mucin is eroded, probably aided by the many monolamellar bodies found in the vicinity. This could explain why the hydrophobicity is almost the same however much of the adhering mucous layer is rinsed away with saline and yet falls appreciably on ulceration.

Helicobacter pylori

Another facet of the mucus story is the role of *H. pylori* in causing peptic ulcer. These bacteria, when present, are located at the interface between secreted and nonsecreted mucus where they were first reported by Marshall and collaborators in Perth. It is now well established that they produce phospholipase A_2[18] which would explain their aggressive role in compromising the gastric mucosal barrier whether the digested phospholipid were in chemical association with mucin or present as oligolamellar SAPL.

Recently we have found evidence of densely osmiophilic granules within *H. pylori* which appear to be lamellated phospholipid.[19] This has led us to speculate that these bacteria act as an aggressive agent by ingesting a gastric mucosal barrier of oligolamellar SAPL. In this laboratory we refer to these bacteria jokingly as "*Helicopacman.*" Ingestion of the barrier would explain why acid is still needed to cause an ulcer and, hence, why acid suppression is successful in treating peptic ulcer even when they are left to proliferate at the higher pH.

A question seldom asked is why *H. pylori* are not themselves digested in the highly corrosive conditions of the stomach. Hence, it was most interesting to find that the densely osmiophilic outermost coating of these bacteria is oligolamellar and probably SAPL, the additional lamellae being most pronounced toward the pole of the organism. Hence, *H. pylori* could be deriving their protection from the host. It is also interesting to find evidence of an adsorbed lining on another parasite which thrives in the acidic conditions of the sheep abomasum—the barber's pole worm which is the scourge of the Australian sheep farmer.

If *H. pylori* adopt essentially the same mode of protection as the gastric mucosa itself, they should be subject to the same barrier breakers, including bile. Hence, this might be one of the reasons why so few of these bacteria, if any, are found in the duodenum.

The Barrier per se

Having outlined the morphological evidence for rekindling interest in the concept of a gastric mucosal barrier as a *physical* reality and having reviewed the evidence for the underlying structure to be essentially phospholipid in nature, it is now necessary to consider how such molecules can form an effective barrier to acid. The long fatty-acid chains of the DSPC molecules have an enormous repulsion for the aqueous environment from which they can escape in one of three ways. In the lung they can escape into the air as the polar end of the molecule "sits" in the aqueous hypophase while, in the absence of air, they can group together as micelles with the polar groups outwards. However, the fact that the cross-sectional areas of the polar and nonpolar moieties are equal means that these cylindrical molecules are ideal for packing as lipid bilayers.

In this configuration the long fatty-acid chains can exclude all water as they close-pack with those of similar DSPC molecules in the same monolayer while, by two monolayers coming together tails to tails, they can also exclude all water from the ends of the chains. This configuration is illustrated in Fig. 6 which depicts the central hydrophobic domain of hydrocarbon chains. Such structures, of course, provide the structural basis of all biological membranes in which most of the physiology is confined to the intercalated protein.

The various oligolamellar structures seen in gastric mucus and within the stomach wall closely resemble those on other epithelial surfaces which are more accessible, representing what has been termed a "ubiquitous barrier." In those cases, the underlying membrane displayed the same spacing as the additional lipid layers of the whole oligolamellar structure. However, on rinsing away those layers with a lipid solvent, they appear to contain little protein, if any (<1.5%). Thus, the outermost layers of predomi-

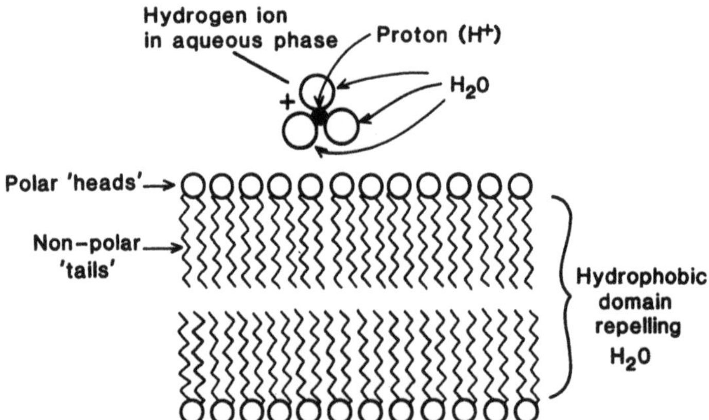

Figure 6. Depiction of the principle by which the fatty-acid chains of the nonpolar moieties of the DSPC molecules escape the aqueous environment by forming a lipid bilayer devoid of the intercalated protein found in regular membranes. The strongly hydrophobic central domain will repel the water of hydration without which a proton cannot exist alone in an aqueous environment.[20] Hence, it will act as a physical barrier to acid.

nantly DSPC would appear to protect the underlying membrane and, in particular, sealing the areas of intercalated protein which would be the most vulnerable to acid attack.[12] In any case these are the areas through which water and water-soluble solutes would be transmitted across the membrane.

Hydrogen Ions

The vital question remaining is why the close-packed bilayer of predominantly DSPC should be such an effective barrier to acid. This has been proven *in vitro* by placing pH electrodes on either side of a filter paper separating saline from saline + HCl at a pH of 2, when a very thin layer of DSPC decreased the rate of transmission of acid by about two orders of magnitude.[20]

In seeking an explanation at the molecular level it must be remembered that a hydrogen ion, as commonly depicted as H^+, is a physical impossibility in any aqueous environment. As a proton, it is so highly polarizing that it will instantly attach itself to water molecules and exists in solution as $H(H_2O)_3^+$.[20] Thus, the hydrophobic domain of the low-protein lipid bilayer will strongly repel molecules in the form of water of hydration and, hence, the proton attached to them (see Fig. 6). The same will apply to other hydrated ions which are also excluded by the gastric mucosal barrier, while it is permeable to lipophilic molecules.

Barrier Enhancement

If the barrier depicted in Fig. 6 represents the basic unit of resistance to acid transmission on the gastric mucosa, then it indicates several avenues to pursue in promoting mucosal protection. The most obvious approach is one of supplementing the indigenous DSPC barrier. This has been partially successful by administering drugs such as ambroxol to promote surfactant secretion,[21] or administering exogenous surfactant as DSPC[21] alone or in liposomal form, or as milk. However, whereas the extreme repulsion for water may impart ideal barrier properties, it has proven a major problem in administering DSPC on account of its low solubility in aqueous fluids where the critical micelle concentration is as low as 10^{-10} M.[3] This problem has been largely overcome by seeking natural sources of lamellar bodies, a delightfully simple and inexpensive source being the ripe banana.[22]

The second approach to fortifying a gastric mucosal barrier of lamellated DSPC is to promote tighter bonding of indigenous molecules, even if there is a quantitative deficiency. This returns us to the basic physical chemistry of corrosion inhibitors which must satisfy two basic criteria to be successful:

1. They must be strongly adsorbed (bound) to the surfaces they protect (see Fig. 1a). In this regard cationic surfactants are ideal since there is a strong electrostatic force of attraction of the positive charge on the polar ends of the molecules for the negative charges which abound on most surfaces, including mucosal surfaces.
2. There must be strong cohesion between the protectant molecules so as to avoid gaps which might permit passage of potentially corrosive ions (see Fig. 1b). A good example is "phosphating,"[3] i.e., the use of multivalent cations to pull

phosphate ions together into impermeable sheets—a principle exploited in "Pink Primer" and other phosphate primers widely sold in paint shops as a first coat for raw surfaces.

The problem with these two approaches is that the layers of simple cationic surfactants tend to lack cohesion while the cohesive phosphate layers tend to lack adhesion to the surfaces they protect. In monolayers of DSPC, nature may have solved this dilemma in a particularly ingenious way,[3] by separating the polar and nonpolar moieties of the standard cationic surfactant/corrosive inhibitor and placing a phosphate group in the center of the molecule, covalently bound to the two ends.

This achieves the best of both worlds because the positively charged polar groups are still ideally oriented for strong adsorption to the surface to be protected, while the location of mobile cations between the phosphate groups imparts strong cohesion between molecules adsorbed to neighboring sites. The mobile cations also effectively neutralize the phosphate ions electrostatically so that they do not compromise adsorption. The strong cohesive forces between the phosphate groups will also pull together the long straight fatty-acid chains to which they are covalently bound, thus producing a particularly tightly packed domain of hydrocarbon chains with very high repulsion for water in any form (see Fig. 1c). This includes water of hydration of hydrogen ions as discussed above. In some ways the outer layer of fatty-acid chains resembles paraffin wax or even polyethylene which is used to fabricate acid containers, notably the modern car battery.

If the above discussion represents the basic chemistry of the gastric mucosal barrier, we can now address the question of how sucralfate can interact with such a structure or attempt to substitute for gastric surfactant.

Sucralfate

We became particularly interested in sucralfate when we found that it was much more surface active than any other synthetic pharmaceutical agents currently prescribed to treat peptic ulcers. This can be observed simply by shaking a suspension in water when it foams—rather like gastric juice. Surfactants that bind to solid surfaces by adsorption almost invariably reduce the surface energy of other interfaces, including liquid–air. This was demonstrated by placing a suspension of sucralfate on the Langmuir trough—the standard instrument for studying surface activity—and compressing the monolayer that gradually forms on the surface. When the sucralfate is well dispersed in water by ultrasonication, the surface tension (γ) is reduced from 72 to 52 dyn/cm (mN/m). On compression of the monolayer γ is further reduced to a value of 35 dyn/cm at 20% of the initial area (A). On reversal of the barrier there is hysteresis in surface tension *vs.* area, the γ:A loops resembling those for most surfactants.

Effect of Cations

When different cations are present in the aqueous solution in which sucralfate is dispersed, it can be seen in Fig. 7 that cations with a higher ionic charge are more effective in promoting the reduction in γ on initial compression of the monolayer. This is consistent

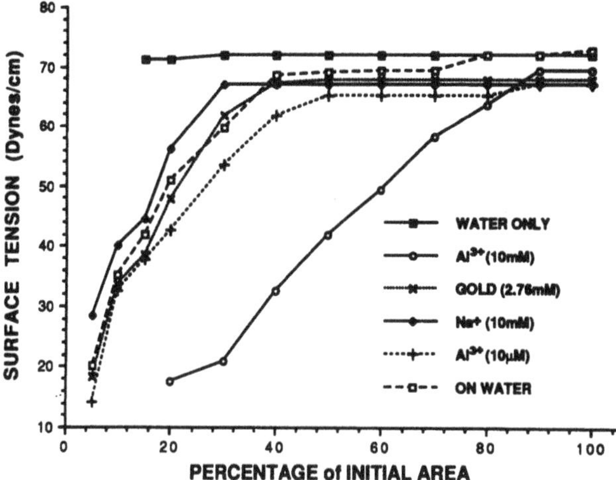

Figure 7. Demonstration of the surface activity of sucralfate in reducing the surface tension of water on compression of the monolayer recruited to the surface of the pool of a Langmuir trough. Note how the activity (reduction in surface tension) is so much greater when the cation is the aluminum ion.

with comparable changes observed with other surfactants, including SAPL.[17] However, the enhancement found in the presence of Al^{3+} appears to exceed that anticipated by comparison with other surfactants and would help to explain why sucralfate is so effective as its aluminum salt.

Ulcer Trials

Cations can also influence the packing of SAPL molecules as described above and, hence, they can influence the efficacy of indigenous gastric surfactant. In trials of SAPL administered as egg lecithin (200 mg/ml) dispersed in water, the ulcerated area of the non-pylorus-ligated rat model was reduced significantly on adding 10 mM aluminum chloride to the aqueous phase. Relative to saline controls, the protection rate imparted by SAPL was increased from 65% to 78% by coadministering aluminum ions, compared with 50% by sucralfate alone.

Compatibility with Surface-Active Phospholipid

Despite the enhancement of surface activity by Al^{3+}, SAPL would still appear more surface active than sucralfate. Hence, it could be argued that the sucralfate anion might have an adverse effect if it could complete more effectively than the indigenous SAPL for the sites on the ulcer. At the air–liquid interface, however, this reservation does not seem to be substantiated with mixtures of sucralfate and SAPL displaying $\gamma{:}A$ loops intermediate between those for the two systems standing alone.[17] This indicates that a more surface-active SAPL molecule will occupy a site at the interface in preference to a sucralfate molecule but the latter will occupy any remaining sites and thus make up any deficiency in SAPL.

Adsorption

Substances which are surface-active at liquid–air interfaces, where surface tension is easy to measure, are almost invariably surface-active at solid surfaces, but not necessarily to the same extent. At the beginning of this chapter it was described how the contact angle provides a good index of surface hydrophobicity and, hence, the degree of adsorption of a surfactant to a hydrophilic surface.

A convenient flat hydrophilic surface is provided by quartz. Deposition of SAPL by slowly withdrawing the quartz plate through a monolayer on the Langmuir trough renders it moderately hydrophobic as manifest by a contact angle of about 55°. However, if Al^{3+} ions are substituted for Na^{+} in the aqueous hypophase from which the monolayer is being transferred, then the contact angle is 71°, i.e., the surface is significantly more hydrophobic. Thus, the aluminum ions would appear to be promoting the adsorption of SAPL as indicated by the higher protection rate against acid-induced ulcers described above.

The Sucralfate Anion

The anions represent an interesting comparison between sucrose sulfate and the SAPL molecule reduced to a cation by suppression of ionization of the central phosphate ion at a normal gastric pH of 2. When an SAPL molecule is adsorbed, the increase in hydrophobicity increases the surface energy and, at first sight, would therefore appear to decrease stability of the adsorbed layer. However, the actual interface on the luminal surface is between the hydrophobic adsorbed layer and mucus which, as an excellent wetting agent,[12] reduces surface energy to stabilize the coating. When the sucrose sulfate anion is adsorbed, however, it does not render the surface hydrophobic, somehow orienting the sucrose moiety toward the aqueous environment. Although it may not impart the same surface activity as the SAPL anion, it could be just as effective because it plays the dual roles of corrosion inhibitor and mucous stabilizer.

The nature of bonding of the sucralfate anion to the ulcer site is described elsewhere in this book, chelate binding of the anion to negative charges on the mucosal surface requiring Al^{3+} "bridges." Similar "bridging" *between* sucralfate anions adsorbed to neighboring sites by Al^{3+} ions would improve the cohesion of the adsorbed layer vital to protection as described above. Research is continuing to determine whether the aluminum ions which act on each anionic species alone can also act to promote cohesion of a layer composed of both anions. This would seem highly relevant to the practical case of sucralfate binding to the site of an ulcer caused by depletion of the indigenous SAPL providing the gastric mucosal barrier.

Effect on SAPL Secretion

While the foregoing discussion would indicate that sucralfate and the indigenous SAPL are mutually supportive in providing the gastric mucosal barrier at the molecular level, there would need to be no suppression of the indigenous gastric surfactant by this drug. It has been reported* that sucralfate might actually increase the rate of secretion of phospholipid by cells in the stomach wall. In our studies using the novel fixation procedure described earlier, much of this phospholipid would appear to take the form of lamellar bodies represented at the lower magnification by the many densely osmiophilic "granules" which can be visualized. At higher magnification these "granules" are no different from the lamellar bodies found in the absence of sucralfate, but the increase in numbers did not reach statistical significance.

Conclusions

If one accepts the model of a physical gastric mucosal barrier provided by gastric surfactant, then sucralfate could enhance that barrier in any of four ways or in any combination of the following:

1. The aluminum ions promote cohesion of the indigenous phospholipid to enhance the natural barrier.
2. The sucralfate anions can be adsorbed to the ulcer at sites left vacant by the deficiency of SAPL which allowed the ulcer to form in the first place.
3. The sucralfate anions can supplement the barrier without rendering the surface hydrophobic, assuming something of the role of mucin in stabilizing the natural barrier.
4. Sucralfate might also be promoting the secretion of SAPL as lamellar bodies to fortify the natural gastric mucosal barrier.

Thus, a good scientific basis for prescribing sucralfate for peptic ulcer disease would appear to be emerging based on the application to gastrointestinal physiology of principles of corrosion protection well established in the physical sciences.

References

1. Adamson AW: *Physical Chemistry of Surfaces*, ed 2. New York, John Wiley & Sons, 1967.
2. Hills BA: What is the true role of surfactant in the lung? *Thorax* **36**:1–4, 1981.
3. Hills BA: *The Biology of Surfactant*. London, Cambridge University Press, 1988. References 1–3 provide a general background in surfactants in general (No. 1) and pulmonary surfactant (Nos. 2 and 3), including an outline of its possible roles in many organs (No. 3).
4. Davenport HW: *The Gastric Mucosal Barrier—A Swan Song*. Ann Arbor, University of Michigan, 1983.
5. Davenport HW: Destruction of the gastric mucosal barrier by detergents and urea. *Gastroenterology* **54**:175–181, 1968. References 4 and 5 refer to the classical *physiological* studies of Davenport which led him to propose the "gastric mucosal barrier" as a *physical* barrier.
6. Fromm D: Gastric mucosal barrier, in Johnson LR (ed): *Physiology of the Gastrointestinal Tract*. New York, Raven Press, 1981, pp 733–748.
7. Hills BA: A physical identity for the gastric mucosal barrier. *Med J Aus* **153**:76–81, 1990.

*Comment by T. Yamada at the 1990 Sucralfate Symposium.

8. Allen A: Gastrointestinal mucus, in Schultz SG, Forte JG, Rauner BB (eds): *Handbook of Physiology*. Washington, DC, American Physiological Society, 1989, sect 6, vol III, pp 359–382. Reference 6 is one of the best reviews of the various theories of gastric mucosal protection while No. 8 is selected as a good recent review of gastric mucus and its role in cytoprotection.
9. Hills BA, Barrow RE: The contact angle induced by DPL at pulmonary epithelial surfaces. *Respir Physiol* **38**:173–183, 1979. The first evidence for the adsorption (direct bonding) of surfactant to any epithelial surface is given in No. 9, while specific ultrastructural evidence for a surfactant lining within gastric mucosa is presented in No. 7.
10. Hills BA, Butler BD, Lichtenberger LM: Gastric mucosal barrier: Hydrophobic lining to the lumen of the stomach. *Am J Physiol* **7**:G651–G658, 1983.
11. Lichtenberger LM, Richards JE, Hills BA: Effects of prostaglandin PGE_2 on the surface hydrophobicity of aspirin-treated canine gastric mucosa. *Gastroenterology* **88**:308–314, 1985.
12. Hills BA: Gastric mucosal barrier: Stabilization of hydrophobic lining to the stomach by mucus. *Am J Physiol* **244**:G561–G568, 1985. The physiological evidence for a mucosal barrier of gastric surfactant is presented in Nos. 10–12, including the telltale hydrophobicity which led to its discovery (No. 10).
13. Kalina M, Pease DC: The preservation of ultrastructure saturated in phosphatidyl cholines by tannic acid in model systems and type II pneumocytes. *J Cell Biol* **74**:726–741, 1977.
14. Ueda S, Kawamura K, Ishii N, *et al*: Morphological studies on surface lining layer of the lungs. Part VI. Surfactant-like substance in other organs (pleural cavity, vascular lumen and gastric lumen) than lungs. *Jpn Med Soc Biol Interface* **17**:132–156, 1986. References 13 and 14 refer to the special fixation procedures which are needed in order to visualize oligolamellar layers of surfactant by electron microscopy, indicating why this barrier was not discovered in earlier ultrastructural studies.
15. Hills BA: A mucosal barrier of gastric surfactant identified on the human stomach. *Aus NZ Med J* **22**:441–444, 1992. This paper describes morphological evidence for a mucosal barrier of gastric surfactant in *human* tissue.
16. Slomiany A, Slomiany BL, Horowitz MI: Studies in changes in lipid profiles of the rat gastric mucosa with stress ulcers. *Clin Chim Acta* **59**:215–216, 1975. This paper acknowledges earlier work demonstrating an effect of phospholipids in enhancing the resistance of mucus to the transmission of acid.
17. Hills BA: A common physical basis for the gastric mucosal barrier and the action of sucralfate. *Am J Med* **91**(2A):43S–51S, 1991. This paper demonstrates how the mucus barrier would appear to be provided by the intergranular matrix of gastric surfactant. It also demonstrates the surface activity of sucralfate and how it is more surface active as the aluminum salt.
18. Raedsch R, Stiehl A, Phol S, *et al*: Quantification of phospholipase A_2 activity of *Campylobacter pylori*. *Gastroenterology* **89**:A478, 1989.
19. Hills BA: Gastric mucosal barrier: Evidence for *Helicobacter pylori* ingesting gastric surfactant and deriving protection from it. *Gut* **34**:588–593, 1993. References 18 and 19 are included to demonstrate how the *Helicobacter* story fits in with the model of the gastric surfactant barrier as *H. pylori* ingest surfactant (No. 19) and produce the enzymes to digest it (No. 18).
20. Hills BA, Kirwood CA: Gastric mucosal barrier: Barrier to hydrogen ions imparted by gastric surfactant *in vitro*. *Gut* **33**:1039–1041, 1992. This paper describes direct *in vitro* evidence for surface-active phospholipid acting as a barrier to acid.
21. Szelenyi I, Engler H: Cytoprotective role of gastric surfactant in the ethanol-produced gastric mucosal injury in the rat. *Pharmacology* **33**:199–205, 1986.
22. Hills BA, Kirwood CA: Surfactant approach to the gastric mucosal barrier: Protection of rats by banana even when acidified. *Gastroenterology* **97**:294–303, 1989. References 21 and 22 refer to the prophylactic use of gastric surfactant in preventing gastric ulcer.

12

Stimulation of Mucosal Prostaglandins by Sucralfate

DANIEL RACHMILEWITZ

Introduction

Sucralfate enhances ulcer healing and protects the mucosa of the stomach against damage induced by various irritants in human subjects as well as in experimental animals. Since sucralfate does not affect gastric acid secretion, other mechanisms are responsible for its protective and healing effects. Sucralfate's efficacy in the prevention of gastric mucosal injury induced by various irritants mimics to some extent the protection afforded by prostaglandins. The hypothesis that sucralfate enhances mucosal defense and induces ulcer healing via stimulation of endogenous gastric prostaglandin synthesis was therefore thoroughly investigated in experimental models and also in human subjects. Whereas in many studies the direct effect of sucralfate on gastric generation and release of prostaglandins was evaluated, another approach elucidated the effect of cyclooxygenase inhibitors such as indomethacin on the protection afforded by sucralfate.

Prostaglandins and Their Effects on Gastric Mucosa

Prostaglandins, 20-carbon fatty acid derivatives, are synthesized from arachidonic acid by most tissues. Gastric mucosa synthesizes and secretes several prostanoids, prostaglandin E_2 (PGE_2), prostacyclin (PGI_2), and thromboxane A_2 (TxA_2) being the major ones. Prostacyclin and thromboxane A_2 are not stable and are immediately metabolized to stable compounds, namely 6-keto-$PGF_{1\alpha}$ and thromboxane B_2 (TxB_2). PGE_2 inhibits gastric acid secretion and exerts protective mucosal properties. Prostaglandins prevent gastric ulceration induced by extreme challenges such as 100% ethanol, 0.6

DANIEL RACHMILEWITZ • Department of Medicine, Hadassah University Hospital, Mount Scopus, Hebrew University Hadassah Medical School, Jerusalem, Israel.

Sucralfate: From Basic Science to the Bedside, edited by Daniel Hollander and G. N. J. Tytgat. Plenum Press, New York, 1995.

M HCl, 0.2 M NaOH, 25% NaCl, and even boiling water. The term *cytoprotection* was employed to describe this property. However, the term is somewhat misleading since careful histological evaluations of the mucosa subjected to such insults reveal almost complete destruction of the surface epithelial cells even in the presence of prostaglandins. Prostaglandins reduce the degree and extent of the deep mucosal necrosis induced by these noxious agents. Prostaglandins seem to affect the vascular rather than the epithelial level and to prevent hemorrhage lesions.

Several mechanisms were suggested to be responsible for prostaglandin enhancement of mucosal defense[1]: stimulation of bicarbonate and mucus secretion, enhancement of mucosal blood flow, stimulation of cellular transport processes, stabilization of tissue lysosomes, and maintenance of gastric sulfhydryl compounds. It seems that enhancement of mucosal blood flow supplying buffer capacity and volume to dilute luminal agents is one of the most important mechanisms of action. With respect to all prostaglandins, the dose that provides mucosal protection is small and does not affect gastric acid secretion. It is therefore beyond any doubt that inhibition of gastric secretion is not the mechanism to explain their protective effects.

Gastric mucosal damage induced by aspirin and NSAIDs is ascribed to their inhibition of mucosal cyclooxygenase activity, the enzyme responsible for prostanoid generation from arachidonic acid. In addition, in patients with peptic ulcer disease gastric mucosal prostaglandin generation was found to be decreased, suggesting that mucosal prostaglandin deficiency may contribute to the pathogenesis of peptic ulcer disease. In view of the antisecretory properties of prostaglandins and in view of their enhancement of mucosal defense, synthetic prostaglandins were tested for their efficacy in the treatment of peptic ulcer disease. Several synthetic prostaglandin analogues, i.e., arbacet, enprostil, and misoprostol, were found to be more potent than placebo in the healing of GU and DU but only when administered in antisecretory doses. None of the synthetic prostaglandins was found to be effective when administered in small doses that presumably only enhance mucosal defense but have no effect on gastric acid secretion. Healing rates of both DU and GU with any of the synthetic prostaglandins are lower than those achieved in comparative studies with H_2 RAs or with sucralfate. Because of this and because of potential side effects and especially of diarrhea, synthetic prostaglandins are usually not accepted as a treatment of choice for peptic ulcer disease.

In contrast, prostaglandins could theoretically be very useful for the treatment of NSAID-induced damage and ulceration of the gastroduodenal mucosa and also could be useful in the prevention of such damage. However, despite efforts and clinical trials at present only a few studies indicate their efficacy in preventing NSAID-induced damage. Misoprostol, a synthetic PGE_1 analogue, was found to be more effective than placebo in the prevention of gastric and duodenal ulceration during 3-month treatment of chronic rheumatic patients on NSAID therapy. It is disappointing that only an antisecretory dose was found to be effective, thus casting doubt on enhanced protection as the main mechanism responsible for its efficacy.

In spite of all of the reservations it is clear that prostaglandins are important agents in the upper gastrointestinal tract contributing to maintaining its integrity both by decreasing gastric acid secretion and by enhancing protective mucosal mechanisms.

Effect of Sucralfate on Gastric Prostanoids in Experimental Animals

Most of the studies in experimental animals were conducted in rats. In the majority, the effect of sucralfate was evaluated on gastric prostanoids.[2] Investigations on sucralfate's effect on prostanoid generation by cultures of gastric epithelial cells and by small intestinal mucosa were also conducted. Prostanoids generated by the mucosa are secreted into the lumen and sucralfate's effects on both mucosal prostanoid generation and secretion were evaluated.[3] In almost all of the studies the protection afforded by sucralfate against gastric damage induced by irritants was correlated with its effect on gastric mucosal prostanoid generation and release.

The protection afforded by sucralfate against gastric damage induced by irritants was found to be accompanied by increase in gastric mucosal cyclooxygenase activity.[4] The stimulation of cyclooxygenase activity was evident irrespective of the irritant used. Sucralfate 125 mg, administered intragastrically 30 min prior to induction of mucosal damage with irritants such as ethanol, 0.6 N HCl, 0.2 N NaOH, and 30 mM sodium taurocholate provided significant reduction in the lesion score. Gastric mucosal PGE_2 and TxB_2 generation were significantly higher in sucralfate-treated rats when compared with their respective generation in control rats.[5] Sucralfate pretreatment was also found to reduce the inhibitory effect of indomethacin on cyclooxygenase activity. At 15 min, 1 hr, and 3 hr after intragastric instillations of sucralfate, there was a significant drop in gastric mucosal potential difference and a significant increase in luminal release of PGE_2 to the rat stomach. Sucralfate's effect on gastric mucosal prostaglandin generation is not correlated in all instances with its effect on luminal prostaglandin levels. Ethanol-induced gastric ulceration is effectively prevented by sucralfate 200–800 mg/kg. This protection is accompanied by increased luminal PGE_2 levels but with no effect on prostaglandin synthesis in gastric mucosal biopsy specimens.[6]

Sucralfate 2 and 5 mg/ml significantly decrease taurocholate-induced damage to cultured rat gastric mucosal cells by 29 and 56%, respectively. This protection is not afforded by its components, aluminum hydroxide and sucrose octasulfate. Sucralfate but not its components significantly and dose dependently stimulate PGE_2 and 6-keto-$PGF_{1\alpha}$ production by cultured gastric mucosal cells. Stimulation of PGE_2 formation by mucosal homogenates of isolated amphibian mucosa was also documented.

One study evaluated the influence of sucralfate treatment on gastric prostanoid levels and damage induced by gastric surgery. Sucralfate 100 mg/kg per day was administered to rats for 1 year following performance of Billroth I, Billroth II, or vagotomy and pyloroplasty. In sucralfate-treated rats, gastric mucosal PGE_2 and 6-keto-$PGF_{1\alpha}$ levels were increased as well as the ratio 6-keto-$PGF_{1\alpha}$: TxB_2. It therefore seems that sucralfate protection against gastritis induced by gastric surgery is also accompanied by changes in mucosal prostanoid generation.

There is only one study in which oral administration of sucralfate at a dose causing a significant reduction of ethanol-induced gastric damage (500 mg/kg) did not significantly alter gastric 6-keto-$PGF_{1\alpha}$ synthesis. In this study, using an *ex vivo* gastric chamber model, application of sucralfate to one side of the mucosa did not affect gastric prostaglandin synthesis but did cause a significant increase in leukotriene C_4 synthesis together with a fall in transmucosal potential difference. It was concluded that prostaglandins do not mediate the protection afforded by the exposure to sucralfate. Whereas the negative effect of sucralfate on gastric mucosal prostaglandin generation in the *ex vivo* model may be related to the model, it is difficult to explain the negative effect in the intact stomach.

Few studies explored the effect of sucralfate on small intestinal lesions induced by indomethacin and on small intestinal prostaglandin generation. Sucralfate 450 mg/12 hr did not affect PGE_2 generation in the small intestine of normal rats. Indomethacin-induced intestinal lesions in the refed rat model were significantly inhibited by pretreatment with sucralfate which had no significant effect on intestinal PGE_2 generation. In another study, sucralfate was found to possess a marked protective effect on the intestinal mucosa against indomethacin-induced ulceration. However, in contrast to the previous study, this protection was accompanied by significant elevation of basal mucosal PGE_2 generation and by partial reversal of the indomethacin-induced inhibition of PGE_2 synthesis.

The cumulative data therefore indicate that in experimental animals sucralfate stimulates gastric prostaglandin release in the lumen and most probably also increases gastric mucosal prostaglandin generation. It is also suggested that there is some kind of correlation between the stimulation of prostanoid generation and the provision of mucosal protection. Fewer studies were conducted in the small intestine and sucralfate effects on intestinal prostanoid generation deserve further clarification.

Effect of Sucralfate on Gastric Prostanoids in the Human

In the human, sucralfate increases gastric mucosal generation and release of prostaglandins. Perfusion of the human stomach with 1 g sucralfate stimulates bicarbonate output by 50% and PGE_2 output by 64%. Enhancement of gastric bicarbonate secretion which may play a role in the protective action of sucralfate may be related to its effect on gastric prostanoids since the latter are potent stimulators of bicarbonate secretion. Sucralfate 1.0 g qid significantly reduced spontaneous gastric damage manifested as spontaneous gastric microbleeding and DNA loss accompanied by increased mucosal biosynthesis and mucosal luminal release of PGE_2 and 6-keto-$PGF_{1\alpha}$ with reduction in the release of TxB_2. Sucralfate also protected against gastric damage induced by a single dose of 2.5 g aspirin but did not affect the suppressed mucosal generation and luminal release of PGE_2 and TxB_2. Is was therefore difficult to ascribe the protection against aspirin-induced damage to enhancement of mucosal prostanoid generation. The effect of sucralfate on human gastric prostanoid generation was assessed also prior to and following induction of acute injury with ethanol. Sucralfate was found to protect the stomach and to induce significant increase in antral and fundic 6-keto-$PGF_{1\alpha}$ synthesis.

Another insight into the possible effect of sucralfate on human gastric mucosal prostaglandin generation can be gained by its determination in patients before and after prolonged sucralfate administration. Gastric mucosal PGE_2 and 6-keto-$PGF_{1\alpha}$ generation were decreased in patients with duodenal ulcer prior to initiation of treatment. Ulcer healing induced by 6 weeks' treatment with H_2RAs was accompanied by significant increase in mucosal prostanoid generation. In contrast, both antral and corporal PGE_2 and 6-keto-$PGF_{1\alpha}$ generation were not affected following 6 weeks of treatment with sucralfate

1 g qid. However, in rheumatic arthritic patients with gastric and duodenal lesions while on continuous stable dosage of NSAIDs, 6 weeks' treatment with sucralfate 1 g qid was accompanied by significantly increased PGE_2 synthesis in the antrum and corpus but not in the duodenum. TxB_2 and 6-keto-$PGF_{1\alpha}$ synthesis were not affected by sucralfate.

It therefore seems that sucralfate stimulates the generation of mucosal prostanoids and their secretion in healthy human subjects. In pathological conditions, its stimulating effect on gastric prostanoids is less pronounced despite effective mucosal protection. It is also apparent that sucralfate's effects on mucosal prostanoids are more potent in experimental animals than in the human. This may relate to the different doses used. In the human, the regular dose is about 55–50 mg/kg per day whereas in rats a significant effect is noted at a dose of 100 mg/kg or more but not when administered in lower doses.

Effect of Cyclooxygenase Inhibitors on Sucralfate Stimulation of Gastric Prostanoids

The tendency of sucralfate to stimulate mucosal prostaglandin generation does not necessarily mean that this is the only or one of the mechanisms responsible for its protective and healing effects. Modulation of the protective effects of sucralfate and/or its stimulation of mucosal prostaglandin generation by pretreatment with cyclooxygenase inhibitors such as indomethacin should resolve the issue. However, both in experimental animals and in the human results are not conclusive and to some extent even controversial.

In one study the protection provided by sucralfate against injury induced in the rat stomach by ethanol, acidified aspirin, water immersion, and restraint stress was reversible by pretreatment with indomethacin to suppress the generation of endogenous prostaglandins. However, in another study conducted by the investigators who did not observe stimulation of 6-keto-$PGF_{1\alpha}$ generation by sucralfate, pretreatment of rats with indomethacin at a dose that inhibits gastric cyclooxygenase activity by about 88% did not affect the protective effect of sucralfate against ethanol-induced gastric damage. Pretreatment with indomethacin also did not prevent the protective effect of sucralfate against damage induced by sodium taurocholate to rat cultured gastric mucosal cells nor did it abolish the stimulating effect of sucralfate on bicarbonate secretion by amphibian gastric mucosa. In the small intestine, sucralfate was found to partially overcome the inhibition of PGE_2 synthesis induced by indomethacin, thus suggesting that its protection of small intestinal ulceration induced by indomethacin is related at least in part to its effect on mucosal prostaglandins.

In the human, the possibility to modulate the effect of sucralfate with indomethacin is limited because of technical and ethical problems. Results of the few studies designed to modulate the effects of sucralfate with indomethacin in the human are also controversial. Pretreatment with indomethacin abolished the protective effect of sucralfate against damage induced by a single aspirin dose of 1200 mg. On the other hand, 50% stimulation of bicarbonate output induced by perfusion of the human stomach with 1 g sucralfate was unaffected by pretreatment with indomethacin.

The cumulative data from experimental animals and from human subjects definitively suggest that inhibition of cyclooxygenase activity with indomethacin to some extent decreases the protective effects of sucralfate. However, in most instances it is not an all-or-none phenomenon, thus suggesting that stimulation of prostaglandin generation cannot be the sole mechanism to explain the protective effects of sucralfate.

Summary

Both in experimental animals and in the human, sucralfate tends to stimulate gastric mucosal prostaglandin generation and release into the lumen. These effects seem to be dose dependent and to be clearly apparent above a dose of 100 mg/kg per day, a dose that is smaller than the one commonly used in human subjects. The mechanism whereby sucralfate affects gastric prostaglandin synthesis and release were never elucidated. Stimulation of endogenous prostaglandin generation may contribute to the protective and healing effects of sucralfate. Yet, stimulation of prostaglandin generation may be only one of the mechanisms and not the sole mechanism responsible for the beneficial effects of sucralfate.

References

1. Miller TA: Protective effects of prostaglandins against gastric mucosal damage: Current knowledge and proposed mechanisms. *Am J Physiol* **245**:G601–G623, 1983. A comprehensive review outlining the various effects of prostaglandins on the gastric mucosa with discussion of the mechanisms responsible for their provision of protection against injury.
2. Guth PH: Mucosal coating agents and other non anti-secretory agents. Are they cytoprotective? *Dig Dis Sci* **32**:647–659, 1987. Review of the various agents that provide protection to gastric mucosa and of the possible mechanisms to explain the protective effects of each of the agents.
3. Tarnawski A, Hollander D, Krause WJ, *et al*: Does sucralfate affect the normal gastric mucosa? Histologic, ultrastructural and functional assessment in the rat. *Gastroenterology* **90**:893–903, 1986. Correlation between the histological and ultrastructural effects of sucralfate on the gastric mucosa with its functional effects as well as on luminal release of PGE_2.
4. Hollander D, Tarnawski A: The protective and therapeutic mechanisms of sucralfate. *Scand J Gastroenterol* **S173**:1–5, 1990. Review article on the protective effects of sucralfate and on the possible mechanisms responsible for this unique property.
5. Ligumsky M, Karmeli F, Rachmilewitz D: Sucralfate protection against gastrointestinal damage: Possible role of prostanoids. *Isr J Med Sci* **22**:801–806, 1986. The protective effect of sucralfate against gastric injury induced by several irritants is correlated with its effect on gastric prostanoid generation.
6. Szabo S, Hollander D: Pathways of gastrointestinal protection and repair: Mechanism of action of sucralfate. *Am J Med* **86**:23–31, 1989. A detailed discussion of mucosal damage and the various mechanisms responsible for its repair. The various mechanisms responsible for the effects of sucralfate are discussed in detail.

13

Sucralfate and *Helicobacter pylori*

J. A. LOUW, G. O. YOUNG, T. A. WINTER, and I. N. MARKS

Introduction

The reason for the lower relapse rates following duodenal ulcer healing with the mucosal protective agents, as opposed to the H_2-receptor antagonists (H_2RAs), is unclear. The quality of ulcer healing has been shown to be better following healing with colloidal bismuth and sucralfate[1,2] and the tendency to "acid rebound" following withdrawal of the H_2RAs may have some relevance. A further consideration relates to the antimicrobial effect of the mucosal protective agents on *H. pylori*, at least as far as colloidal bismuth preparations are concerned.

This chapter will consider the available evidence regarding the possible effects of sucralfate on *H. pylori*.

In Vitro Observations

Central to the pathogenetic potential of *H. pylori* (Fig. 1) is its ability to colonize the gastric mucosa, to survive and in fact flourish in the hostile gastric milieu (Fig. 2), and finally to induce mucosal injury. There is evidence that sucralfate may influence at least some of these factors when studied *in vitro*.

J. A. LOUW, G. O. YOUNG, T. A. WINTER, and I. N. MARKS • Gastrointestinal Clinic and Department of Medicine, University of Cape Town and Groote Schuur Hospital, Observatory, South Africa.

Sucralfate: From Basic Science to the Bedside, edited by Daniel Hollander and G. N. J. Tytgat. Plenum Press, New York, 1995.

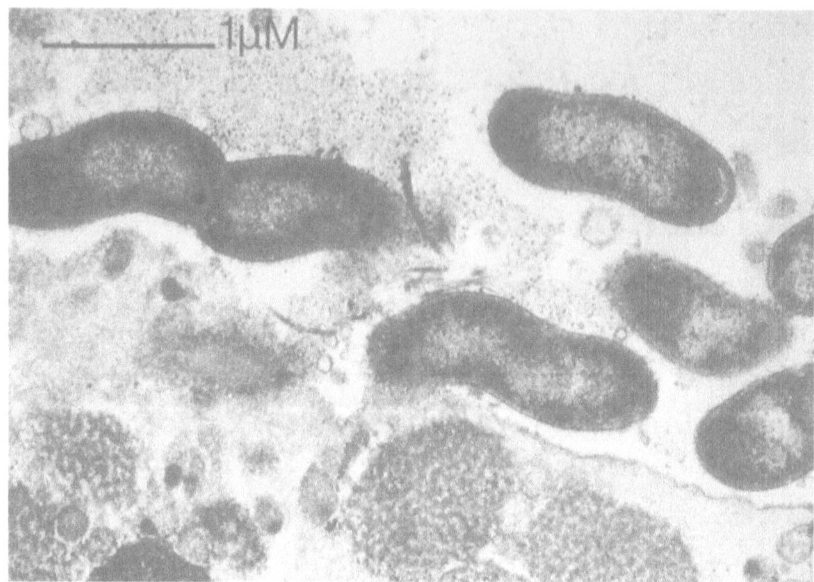

Figure 1. *Helicobacter pylori* ultrastructure. (A color version of this figure can be found in the color insert following p. 6.)

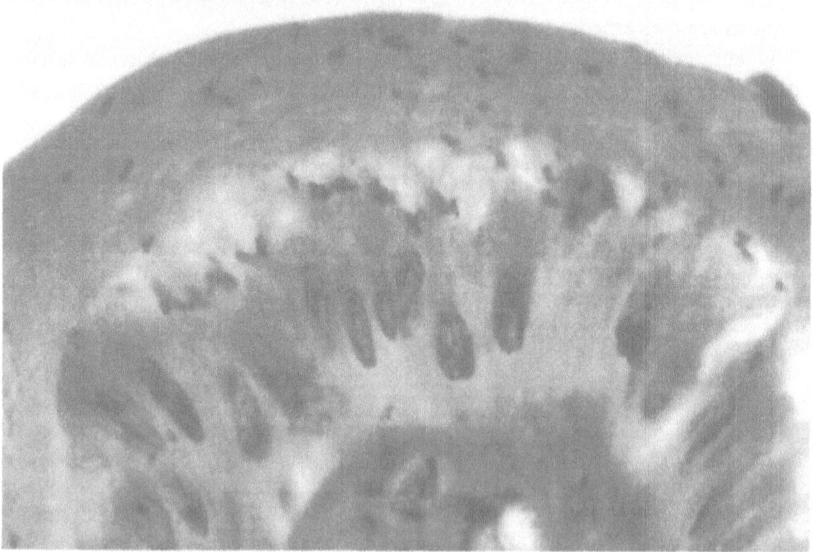

Figure 2. *H. pylori* in the mucus layer covering the epithelial cells. (A color version of this figure can be found in the color insert following p. 6.)

Colonization

H. pylori is a remarkable organism, adapted to specifically colonize gastric mucosa. This specificity of colonization appears to be mediated by the affinity of *H. pylori* colonization factors, thought to be associated with its fibrillar hemagglutinin activity,[3] for gastric glycolipid (sulfatides and GM_3 ganglioside) receptors.[4,5]

In their study evaluating the inhibitory effect of various sulfated and sialic acid-containing glycolipids on *H. pylori*-mediated hemagglutination, Slomiany *et al.* have demonstrated that sucralfate has a hemagglutinin inhibitory capacity surpassed only by GM_3 ganglioside and lactosylceramide sulfate.[6] Nakajima *et al.* also reported on a decrease in bacterial adhesion to gastric mucin in the presence of the components of sucralfate.[7] These data suggest that sucralfate has the potential, by competing with gastric glycolipid receptors, to interfere with *H. pylori* mucosal attachment.

Growth and Survival

It has been demonstrated that aluminum-containing antacids inhibit *H. pylori* growth *in vitro*, an observation apparently confirmed by *in vivo* observations.[8,9] Nakajima, studying the effect of the components of sucralfate on *H. pylori* viability, demonstrated an inhibition of *H. pylori* growth by the aluminum component of sucralfate.

Mucosal Injury

A host of the bacterium's enzymes, metabolic products, and toxins have the potential to damage the mucosa.[10] Ammonia, generated by the catalytic action of *H. pylori* urease on the substrate urea, is considered to be a toxin per sé and has the potential to generate cytotoxic products during the inflammatory cascade. There is some *in vitro* evidence, from the work of Tsuji *et al.*, that sucralfate may act as an ammonia scavenger, a factor that may protect the mucosa from ammonia-induced injury.[11]

Piotrowski *et al.*[12] have produced some evidence that sucralfate is capable of preventing the *H. pylori* lipopolysaccharide-mediated disruption of epithelial laminin/integrin interaction, thereby having the potential to prevent the disruption of (gastric) mucosal integrity by the organism. *In vitro* evidence from the same group suggests that sucralfate can counteract the mucolytic activity of *H. pylori*, by inhibiting the activity of the organism's proteinases and lipases.[13]

In Vitro Susceptibility

Despite these *in vitro* findings, the limited data published to date on *in vitro* susceptibility, using the recognized methodology for determining the minimum inhibitory capacity (MIC), indicate that *H. pylori* is resistant to sucralfate. It should be noted, however, that the methodology used to determine the MIC of sucralfate on *H. pylori* may only determine a direct antibacterial effect of the drug on the organism, and will not be able to assess the effect of the drug on the dynamics of the infection, such as its effect on bacterial adhesion, ammonia "scavenging," and inhibition of lipopolysaccharide-mediated disruption of mucosal integrity.

In Vivo Observations

A limited number of clinical studies have evaluated the effect of sucralfate treatment on *H. pylori* status—either as monotherapy or as a component of combination therapy. No monotherapy study has sought to demonstrate eradication as currently defined.

Monotherapy

Two early reports suggested that sucralfate has a suppressive effect on *H. pylori* and that antral clearance of the organism is not uncommonly achieved. De Korwin *et al.*[14] showed that sucralfate cleared the organism of 7 of 16 (44%) patients compared to only 1 of 12 (8%) of cimetidine-treated patients, when assessed by scanning electron microscopy. Kjoller *et al.*[15] compared the effect of sucralfate and colloidal bismuth in a group of 97 patients and noted clearance rates of 47% and 56%, respectively. This difference was not significantly different.

Subsequent reports focused on semiquantitative changes in antral *H. pylori* density. Hui *et al.*[16] in their study on 54 patients treated with sucralfate 1 g qid for 4 weeks, demonstrated a significant decrease in the *H. pylori* colonization density following treatment, when assessed histologically (Warthin–Starry stain). A similar suppressive effect on *H. pylori* density was noted by Winter *et al.*[17] in 43 duodenal ulcer patients following 6 weeks' treatment with sucralfate 1 g qid and by Banerjee *et al.*[18] in 11 duodenal ulcer patients treated with sucralfate 2 g bd for 4 weeks. Despite the significant decrease in antral *H. pylori* density in these studies, however, clearance of the organism was seldom achieved.

Combination Therapy

Five studies have investigated the efficacy of sucralfate-containing triple therapy in *H. pylori* eradication (Table I). Eradication rates in these studies vary from 60% to 89%. In all, eradication was noted in 130 of the total number of 163 patients studied. The sucralfate dosage regimen was 1 g (tablet form) qid in all but the study by Stupnicki *et al.*,[21] who used sucralfate suspension, 2 g bd. Antibiotics were started with the sucralfate as a rule, except in the Stupnicki study in which antibiotic therapy was begun 2 weeks after initiation of sucralfate treatment. The duration of the sucralfate and antibiotic cotreatment varied from 1 to 4 weeks, with 2 weeks the most common. The study by Sung *et al.*[23] is of particular interest since cotherapy was given for 1 week only, albeit in relatively high doses. This short course achieved an eradication efficacy of 84%.

Discussion

Evidence from *in vitro* studies would suggest that the mucosal protective agent, sucralfate, has the potential to influence *H. pylori*'s ability to colonize gastric mucosa, to inhibit the organism's growth, and to prevent mucosal injury through its effect on mucus stability, epithelial cell interaction, and ammonia scavenging. Both the aluminum and

Table I. Sucralfate Used in Antibiotic Combination Therapy

Study	*n*	Therapy	Eradication (%)
Dorval *et al.*[19]	9	Sucralfate 1 g qid, 7 wk Amoxicillin 1 g/day, 4 wk Metronidazole 0.75 g/day, 2 wk	8 (89)
Louw *et al.*[20]	20	Sucralfate 1 g qid, 2 wk Tetracycline 250 or 500 mg qid, 1 or 2 wk Metronidazole 400 mg tid, 1 or 2 wk	12 (60)
Stupnicki *et al.*[21]	56	Sucralfate 2 g bd, 8 wk Amoxicillin 750 mg tid, 2 wk Metronidazole 500 mg tid, 2 wk	44 (79)
Hui *et al.*[22]	33	Sucralfate 1 g qid, 4 wk Clarithromycin 250 mg qid, 2 wk Metronidazole 300 mg qid, 2 wk	28 (86)
Sung *et al.*[23]	45	Sucralfate 1 g qid, 4 wk Tetracycline 500 mg qid, 1 wk Metronidazole 400 mg qid, 1 wk	38 (84)

sucrose octasulfate components may be important in determining various aspects of this activity. These *in vitro* observations appear to be supported by the reports of clinically significant suppression of the organism with sucralfate therapy. They are, however, in conflict with the findings, both *in vitro* and *in vivo*, that sucralfate does not possess any antimicrobial activity against *H. pylori*. As pointed out, this should perhaps not be surprising in the case of standard MIC testing, as the test cannot evaluate the interaction between drug, host, and organism. Certainly, MICs appear to be poorly predictive of the *in vivo* efficacy of antibiotics against *H. pylori*, where *in vitro* efficacy is often not predictive of *in vivo* success.

It is of interest to note the disparities in suppressive effect shown by the *in vivo* studies. This justifiably raises questions with regard to the reproducibility of these findings. It is of course possible that these discrepancies reflect the inadequacies of current methodology used to detect *H. pylori*. Further studies, using methodology not subject to biopsy bias, such as the [^{14}C]urea breath test, are needed to confirm or refute the findings of a suppressive effect of sucralfate on *H. pylori*. Other factors may also be important in causing this discrepancy; these include the dose of sucralfate (high in the de Korwin study), the frequency of dosage (thought to be important in determining the efficacy of bismuth), and the relationship of medication to meals.

While there should still be some doubt with regard to the magnitude of the suppressive effect of sucralfate monotherapy on *H. pylori*, there is clear evidence, from the limited studies available, that it has an efficacy comparable to that of bismuth-containing triple therapy when used in combination therapy. This should be interpreted with caution, however, as it does not prove that sucralfate has an additive direct antimicrobial effect on *H. pylori*. It should be noted that combination therapy with sucralfate does not appear to have any advantage over conventional triple therapy. The regimen remains complicated and is associated with a significant incidence of side effects. The question arises whether dual therapy with a suitable antibiotic will not give equally acceptable eradication rates with a lower incidence of side effects, much as dual therapy with omeprazole has been reported to be effective.[24]

In conclusion, there is some evidence that sucralfate has activity *in vitro* against *H. pylori*. While this has not been shown to represent a bactericidal effect, a growing body of clinical evidence suggests that these *in vitro* observations may be translated into real clinical benefit. These observations may explain, at least partially, the clinically observed delaying effect of sucralfate healing on duodenal ulcer relapse. Finally, while sucralfate-containing combination therapy is clearly effective in eradicating *H. pylori*, the strategy of eradicating the organism with complicated treatment regimens, prone to cause side effects, needs to be reviewed and a simpler, more effective, and user-friendly treatment sought.

References

1. Moshal MG, Gregory MA, Pillay C, *et al*: Does the duodenal cell ever return to normal? A comparison between treatment with cimetidine and DeNol. *Scand J Gastroenterol* **54**(suppl):48–51, 1979. The ultrastructure of the duodenal cell was found to be normal in most cases following 6 weeks of De Nol therapy, whereas it remained abnormal after cimetidine therapy of similar duration.
2. Tovey FI, Husband EM, Yiu YC, *et al*: Comparison of relapse rates and mucosal abnormalities after healing of duodenal ulceration and after one year's maintenance with cimetidine or sucralfate: A light and electron microscopy study. *Gut* **30**:586–593, 1989. Duodenal mucosal biopsies abnormal after healing; on maintenance therapy, sucralfate-treated duodenal mucosa approached control mucosa characteristics, whereas cimetidine-treated mucosa did not (sucralfate group = 24, cimetidine group = 22).
3. Evans DG, Evans DJ, Houlds JJ, *et al*: N-Acetylneuraminyl-lactose-binding fibrillar hemagglutinin of *Campylobacter pylori*: A putative colonization factor antigen. *Infect Immun* **56**:2896–2906, 1988. Clinical isolates of *H. pylori* possess a cell-bound hemagglutinin with fibrillar morphology, which preferentially binds to isomers of *N*-acetylneuraminyl-lactose.
4. Saitoh T, Sugano K, Natomi H, *et al*: Glyco-sphingolipid receptors in human gastric mucosa for *Helicobacter pylori*. *Eur J Gastroenterol Hepatol* **4**(suppl 1):S49–S53, 1992. Demonstrates, by thin-layer chromatography immunostaining, that *H. pylori* binds specifically to sulfatide and GM_3 ganglioside in human gastric mucosa.
5. Lingwood CA, Lau H, Pellizzari A, *et al*: Gastric glycolipid as a receptor for *Campylobacter pylori*. *Lancet* **2**:238–241, 1989. Reports differential gastric distribution of glycerolipid substance, which is specifically recognized by *H. pylori*.
6. Slomiany BL, Piotrowski J, Samanta A, *et al*: *Campylobacter pylori* colonization factor shows specificity for lactosylceramide sulfate and GM_3 ganglioside. *Biochem Int* **19**(4):929–936, 1989. *Helicobacter pylori* hemagglutinin activity inhibited by lactosylceramide GM_3-ganglioside, as well as by sucralfate.
7. Nakajima M, Sunairi M, Tanaka N, *et al*: Effects of sucralfate, an anti-ulcer agent, on *Helicobacter pylori*. *Gastroenterology* **102**(4):A131, 1992. Sucralfate components inhibit the adhesion of *H. pylori* to mucosal surfaces, *in vitro*.
8. Berstad A, Alexander B, Weberg R, *et al*: Antacids reduce *Campylobacter pylori* colonization without healing the gastritis in patients with non-ulcer dyspepsia and erosive prepyloric changes. *Gastroenterology* **95**:619–624, 1988. Aluminum–magnesium-containing antacid decreases density of *H. pylori* colonization. No improvement in inflammatory reaction noted.

9. Berstad K, Weberg R, Berstad A: Suppression of gastric urease activity by antacids. *Scand J Gastroenterol* **25**:496–500, 1990. Employs [^{14}C]urea breath test to demonstrate a short-lived reduction in ^{14}C recovery following treatment with aluminum–magnesium antacid.
10. Tytgat GNJ, Noach LA, Rauws EAJ: *Helicobacter pylori*. *Eur J Gastroenterol* **4**(suppl 1):S7–S15, 1992. Review of the general state of knowledge regarding the pathogenesis of *H. pylori* infection, potential treatment strategies, and implications of eradication.
11. Tsuji S, Kawano S, Tsuzu M, *et al*: Sucralfate is an ammonia scavenger and protects gastric mucosa from ammonia-induced injury. *Gastroenterology* **102**(4):A706, 1992. Cotreatment of rats with sucralfate or ranitidine prevents ammonia-induced gastric mucosal injury; sucralfate claimed to be ammonia scavenger *in vitro*.
12. Piotrowski J, Yamaki K, Slomiany A, *et al*: Inhibition of gastric mucosal laminin receptor by *Helicobacter pylori* lipopolysaccharide: Effect of sucralfate. *Am J Gastroenterol* **86**(2):1756–1760, 1991. *In vitro* evidence that lipopolysaccharide from *H. pylori* interferes with laminin/integrin binding; this inhibition of binding prevented by sucralfate.
13. Slomiany BL, Piotrowski J, Slomiany A: Effect of sucralfate on the degradation of human gastric mucus by *Helicobacter pylori* protease and lipases. *Am J Gastroenterol* **87**(5):595–599, 1992. *In vitro* evidence that sucralfate is capable of counteracting the mucolytic activity of *H. pylori*-derived enzymes to human gastric mucus proteins and lipids.
14. de Korwin JD, Vicari FI, Chambre V, *et al*: Follow-up of *Campylobacter pylori* gastric infection after treatment of gastroduodenal ulcers with sucralfate or H_2-antagonists, in Mégraud F, Lamouliatte H (eds): *Gastroduodenal Pathology and Campylobacter pylori*. Amsterdam, Elsevier Science Publishers, 1989, pp 619–623. Retrospective study on 28 *H. pylori*-positive gastric and duodenal ulcer patients, treated with H_2-receptor antagonists or sucralfate for a period of 6 weeks. Clearance noted in 7 of 16 sucralfate-treated patients and 1 cimetidine-treated patient. *H. pylori* detection by scanning electron microscopy.
15. Kjoller M, Nielsen L, Kristensen E, *et al*: DeNol versus Antepsin in the treatment of gastric ulcer. World Congresses of Gastroenterology, Sydney, Australia, August 26–31, 1990, PD307. Gastric ulcer patients ($n = 97$) treated with either De Nol or Antepsin for a maximum of 60 days. Clearance rate of 56% in the De Nol group and 47% in the sucralfate-treated group. Method of *H. pylori* detection not specified.
16. Hui WM, Lam SK, Ho J, *et al*: Effect of sucralfate and cimetidine on duodenal ulcer associated antral gastritis and *Campylobacter pylori*. *Am J Med* **86**(suppl 6A):60–65, 1989. Antral colonization density of *H. pylori* decreased significantly after sucralfate 1 g qid for 4 weeks, but not after cimetidine 200 mg tid and 400 mg nocte.
17. Winter TA, Louw JA, Marks IN, *et al*: The effect of sucralfate on *Helicobacter pylori* status and gastritis in duodenal ulcer patients. *S Afr Med J* **83**:784, 1993. Decreased histologically assessed density of *H. pylori* colonization in the antrum following 6 weeks of sucralfate therapy.
18. Banerjee S, El Omar E, Mowat A, *et al*: Sucralfate suppresses *H. pylori* infection and reduces gastric acid secretion by 50% in DU patients. *Gut* (suppl 2):S35, 1994. Decreased histologically assessed antral *H. pylori* colonization density and urea breath test levels in 11 sucralfate-treated subjects.
19. Dorval ED, Barbieux JP, De Muret A, *et al*: Long term results of a triple therapy using sucralfate on *Helicobacter pylori* eradication and healing of duodenal ulcers (DU). *Gastroenterology* **100**:A55, 1991. Preliminary report evaluating nine patients.
20. Louw JA, Zak J, Lucke W, *et al*: Triple therapy with sucralfate is as effective as triple therapy containing bismuth in eradicating *Helicobacter pylori* and reducing duodenal ulcer relapse rates. *Scand J Gastroenterol* **27**(suppl 191):28—31, 1992. Comparable eradication rates found in 20 sucralfate- and 20 bismuth-treated patients.
21. Stupnicki TH, Taufer M, Denk H, *et al*: Triple therapy of duodenal ulcer with sucralfate and amoxycillin plus metronidazole. Abstract, 7th International Sucralfate Symposium, Santa Barbara, 1994. Forty-four of fifty-six patients treated with sucralfate based triple therapy successfully eradicated.

22. Hui WC, Lam SK, Ching CK, *et al*: Omeprazole or sucralfate combined with clarithromycin and metronidazole in *Helicobacter pylori* eradication and ulcer healing. *J Gastroent Hepatol* **9**:A11, 1994. Eradication achieved in 86% of patients treated with a sucralfate-based triple therapy compared with 87% in an omeprazole-based group.
23. Sung JY, Ling TKW, Suen R, Chung SCS: Can sucralfate replace bismuth in triple therapy for the treatment of *Helicobacter pylori* associated duodenal ulcers? Abstract, 7th International Sucralfate Symposium, Santa Barbara, 1994. 84% eradication with sucralfate-containing triple therapy, followed by sucralfate-healing therapy, versus 100% eradication in patients treated with bismuth-containing triple therapy and omeprazole cotreatment for healing.
24. Bayerdörrfer E, Mannes GA, Sommer A, *et al*: High dose omeprazole treatment combined with amoxicillin eradicates *Helicobacter pylori*. *Eur J Gastroenterol Hepatol* **4**(9):697–702, 1992. Eighty-two percent eradication reported in 27 patients treated with high-dose omeprazole (80 mg/day × 10 days, 20 mg/day for rest of 6-week period) in combination with amoxicillin, 1 g bid for the first 10 days. No side effects reported.

14
Sucralfate and Cell Proliferation

HAJIME KUWAYAMA

Introduction

The gastroduodenal epithelium is one of the most rapidly proliferating tissues in the body. The surface epithelial cells of the gastroduodenum are renewed every 2–3 days in rodents and 4–5 days in humans.[1] Why is there such rapid renewal? Possibly because mucosae of the stomach and duodenum are always exposed to irritants, including not only exogenous agents such as seasonings/spicy food, alcohol, nonsteroidal anti-inflammatory drugs (NSAIDs) but also physiological substances such as hydrochloric acid, pepsin, and bile acids. In addition, motor activity facilitates exfoliation of epithelial cells. Exfoliated cells are then promptly replaced with new cells. It seems to be the physiological destiny of epithelium of the gastroduodenum to be constantly damaged, exfoliated, and renewed.

Methods to Study Cell Renewal and Cell Renewal in the Normal Gastroduodenum

In the gastroduodenum, not only epithelial cells but also nonepithelial cells such as fibroblasts undergo renewal. However, because of their rapid renewal, most studies of cell renewal have focused on epithelial cells. The epithelium of the gastroduodenum is composed of heterogeneous cell populations. In the stomach, five major cell types are well characterized: surface mucus cells, mucous neck cells, chief cells (zymogenic cells), parietal cells (oxyntic cells), and endocrine cells (enteroendocrine cells). In the duodenum, absorptive cells, mucus cells, Paneth cells, and enteroendocrine cells are major cell types. Although a few of these differentiated cells undergo slow self-replication, the majority of these differentiated cells do not have this ability. Exfoliated cells are replaced with migrating cells which originate from proliferating cells.

HAJIME KUWAYAMA • Department of Medicine, Nihon University School of Medicine, Tokyo, and University of Texas Southwestern Medical School, Dallas, Texas 75216.

Sucralfate: From Basic Science to the Bedside, edited by Daniel Hollander and G. N. J. Tytgat. Plenum Press, New York, 1995.

Epithelial renewal is a dynamic process of cell proliferation, migration, senescence, and eventual cell loss by exfoliation (Fig. 1). The proliferating cells are located between the base of the pit and the upper portion of the glands (the proliferative zone) and are in various phases of the cell cycle. The cell cycle consists of four phases: mitotic (M), postmitotic gap 1 (G_1), DNA synthetic (S), and post DNA synthetic gap 2 (G_2). There are also some cells with proliferative capacity which are not actually cycling, and are said to be in G_0. These cells in G_0 are likely to reenter the cell cycle under certain conditions (see below).

The fact that gastroduodenal epithelium undergoes rapid proliferation was well recognized nearly 150 years ago by Bizzozero, a German pathologist who recognized the proliferating cells in M phase as mitotic cells by light microscopy. Today, additional techniques are available to visualize proliferating cells. Before mitosis, proliferating cells must double their DNA. Because radiolabeled thymidine or its analogue, bromodeoxyuridine (BrdU), is rapidly incorporated into newly synthesized DNA, visualization of radiolabeled thymidine or antibody staining of BrdU allows the identification of proliferating cells that are in S phase. Furthermore, because cells whose nuclei have incorporated labeled thymidine or BrdU retain these signals until cells are exfoliated, such DNA labeling techniques will also provide information about how cells migrate after mitosis if the histologic sections were obtained at adequate time intervals after thymidine or BrdU administration (usually after 24–72 hr). Immunohistochemical detection of proliferating cell nuclear antigen (PCNA), another proliferation marker, permits visualization of proliferating cells in all phases of the cell cycle. Although PCNA levels are maximal in S phase, the half-life of the protein is about 20 hr; thus, PCNA continues to be detectable for 20 or more hours, even as cells progress through G_2 and M phases into the subsequent G_1 phase. Because the average cell cycle time of proliferating gastroduodenal epithelial cells is about 25–50 hr, it is likely that PCNA would be detected in cycling cells throughout most of the cell cycle. From a clinical point of view, one advantage of PCNA as a marker of proliferating cells is the fact that this method does not require any specimen pretreatment

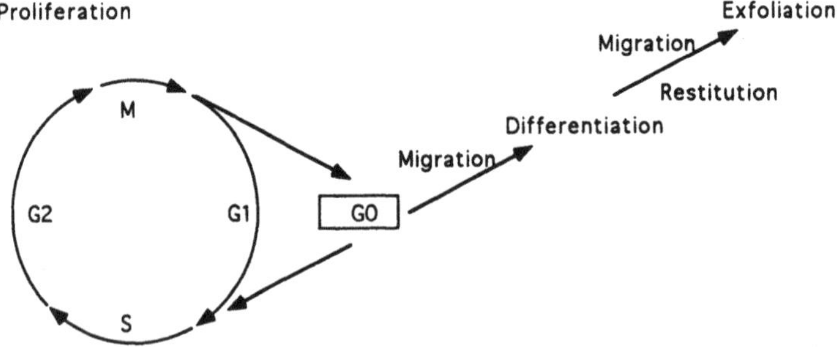

Figure 1. Cell cycle and cell renewal.

or labeling at the time of biopsy. Thus, this method can be applied to sections from routinely prepared tissue blocks from pathology archives. Other techniques that have been used for proliferation studies include scintillation counting, DNA flow cytometry, and biochemical markers such as ornithine decarboxylase.

After the mitosis, the majority of new cells migrate upward toward the lumen and only very few cells migrate downward. This reflects the fact that surface mucus cells have a much shorter turnover time compared with gastric glandular cells such as parietal and chief cells (life spans of these cells are estimated to be more than 200 days). As cells migrate, they differentiate and perform their specific function until exfoliated into the lumen. In addition to normal cell migration, rapid cell migration (also termed cell restitution) is an important element in replenishing lost cells.[2] When excessive cell loss is caused by noxious agents such as ethanol, viable cells located just beneath the lost cells rapidly migrate up and cover the eroded epithelium within minutes. This occurs only when damage is limited to the superficial epithelium and dose not extend into the proliferative zone. Possibly, this process of cell restitution requires an intact extracellular matrix.

Mechanisms that Control Cell Renewal of the Gastroduodenal Epithelium

The mechanisms that control epithelial renewal are not well understood. There are at least three mechanisms that exert some control over epithelial renewal: negative feedback, luminal factors, and peptides and polyamines.

Negative Feedback

Negative feedback is a local mechanism whereby nonproliferating mature cells may signal to the proliferating cells to decrease cell proliferation. Loss of negative feedback is illustrated by the fact that gastric mucosa adapts to repeated administration of NSAIDs. NSAIDs, including aspirin and indomethacin, are known to increase epithelial cell loss. Repeated aspirin and indomethacin administration, however, results in stimulated epithelial proliferation of the gastric mucosa.[3] Although the details of the mechanism of adaptive response have not been definitively elucidated, this enhanced proliferation may contribute to mucosal adaptation after repeated administration of NSAIDs.

Luminal Factors

The presence of food in the gastrointestinal lumen is one of the most potent stimuli of proliferation. When the amount of feeding and hence luminal food is increased, as in pregnancy or lactation, the mucosa undergoes hyperplasia. Conversely, when an animal is fasted, fed parenterally, or undergoes gut diversion surgery, those segments of the mucosa not exposed to luminal contents become atrophic. The mechanisms by which luminal contents stimulate proliferation may be modulated by associated hormonal and neural effects. Nevertheless, luminal factors including microbial flora, dietary amines, and fiber are important in the control of cell renewal.

Peptides and Polyamines

Growth-related peptides and polyamines play important roles in cell renewal.[4] These peptides include gastrin, epidermal growth factor (EGF), transforming growth factors (TGF) α and β, platelet-derived growth factor (PDGF), fibroblast growth factor (FGF), and insulinlike growth factor (IGF-I). In addition, classic hormones such as growth hormone and insulin also play important roles. The action of peptides is mediated by separate pathways: endocrine, paracrine, and autocrine. Also, from the cell proliferation point of view, these growth-related peptides can be divided into two classes: competence factors, which induce G_0 cells to enter G_1 phase, and progression factors, which induce G_1 cells to enter S phase. For example, PDGF and FGF are competence factors and EGF and IGF-I are progression factors. Recent evidence has indicated that EGF/TGFα, a pair of structurally and biologically similar peptides binding the same receptor, plays an important role in gastroduodenal protection and repair. In addition to peptides, the polyamines spermidine and spermine, and their precursor putrescine, are likely important intracellular modulators of cell proliferation and differentiation.[5]

Cell Renewal in Ulcer Disease

Whether or not impaired cell renewal of the epithelium plays a primary role in peptic ulcer disease is not known. However, the maintenance of gastroduodenal mucosal integrity is a dynamic balance between cell loss and cell production.[6] Either excessive cell loss or decreased new cell production, or a combination of both, may lead to a loss of epithelial integrity and result in mucosal erosions and ulcers. For example, NSAIDs are well known to cause gastric erosions or ulcers and it has been reported that NSAIDs increase exfoliation of epithelial cells. On the other hand, steroids do not increase cell exfoliation but have been found to depress epithelial proliferation. Although it is still controversial whether steroids are a cause of peptic ulcer disease, it is possible that steroids may retard ulcer healing via a depressive effect on epithelial cell proliferation. Finally, it is well known that physiological stress predisposes to gastroduodenal mucosal lesions. Stress has been shown to increase cell loss accompanied by depressed epithelial proliferation, well before the development of mucosal lesions. Thus, many agents and conditions affect normal cell renewal of the gastroduodenal epithelium (Fig. 2).[6]

Whatever the cause of mucosal ulceration, cell proliferation is a crucial step in tissue repair. The time required for reepithelialization is dependent on the depth, rather than the surface area, of mucosal injury. When the damage is limited to the mucosal layer, it is called an erosion. There are two types of erosions, superficial and deep.[7] A superficial erosion is a mucosal defect limited to surface mucus neck cells. This type of damage is accompanied by little or no inflammation and will be repaired within 1 day by cell migration (restitution). On the other hand, a deep erosion is a mucosal defect extending to the proliferative zone. Because of lost proliferative cells within the gastric gland, the epithelial defect must be replaced by cells from neighboring glands. Deep erosions are usually accompanied by a moderate inflammatory response. Inflammatory cells such as macrophages and monocytes may be an important source of growth-related peptides and

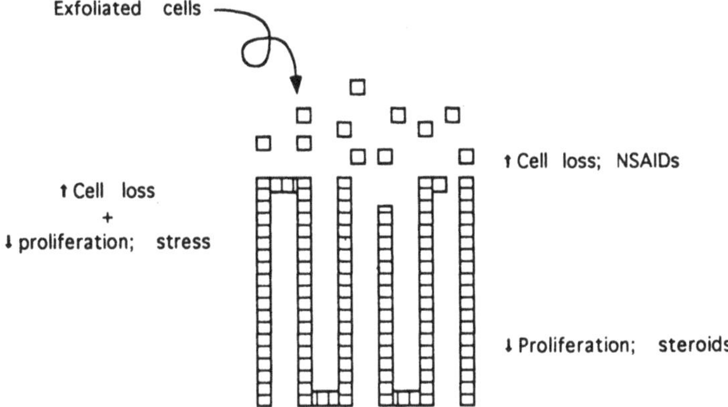

Figure 2. Effects of NSAIDs, steroids, and stress on cell renewal.

cytokines in accelerating tissue repair. Finally, ulcers are mucosal defects involving the muscularis layers. Ulceration is accompanied by a marked inflammatory response and the mucosal defect is temporarily replaced with granulation tissue before reepithelialization. Therefore, healing of ulcers requires many types of cells to be regenerated, not only epithelial cells but also nonepithelial cells such as fibroblasts and endothelial cells, and therefore takes much longer than erosions.

Effect of Sucralfate on Cell Proliferation

Sucralfate, which contains eight sulfate and aluminum molecules attached to a sucrose nucleus, protects against acute mucosal injury by noxious agents such as ethanol and aspirin and accelerates ulcer healing without inhibiting acid secretion. The mechanism of sucralfate protection has been studied extensively in acute gastroduodenal mucosal damage and it is now apparent that sucralfate does not protect surface epithelial cells but stimulates rapid cell migration (restitution), similarly to prostaglandins. This process does not necessarily involve cell proliferation, although it is likely that a decrease of the mature cell compartment as a result of desquamation of surface epithelial cells (superficial erosion) may lead to an eventual increase in cell proliferation by loss of negative feedback suppression. On the other hand, the mechanism by which sucralfate accelerates ulcer healing would likely involve cell proliferation. This is a new insight into sucralfate's action and recent reports of sucralfate's potential activities include enhancement of epithelial, endothelial, and fibroblast cell proliferation. Working hypotheses of sucralfate's action in accelerating superficial and deep erosions and ulcer healing are illustrated in Fig. 3. Experimental evidence shows that long-term sucralfate administration stimulates gastric epithelial proliferation in the rat. The mechanism by which sucralfate stimulates epithelial proliferation is not known, but is probably not a direct effect because short-term administration (up to 10 days) has no effect on epithelial

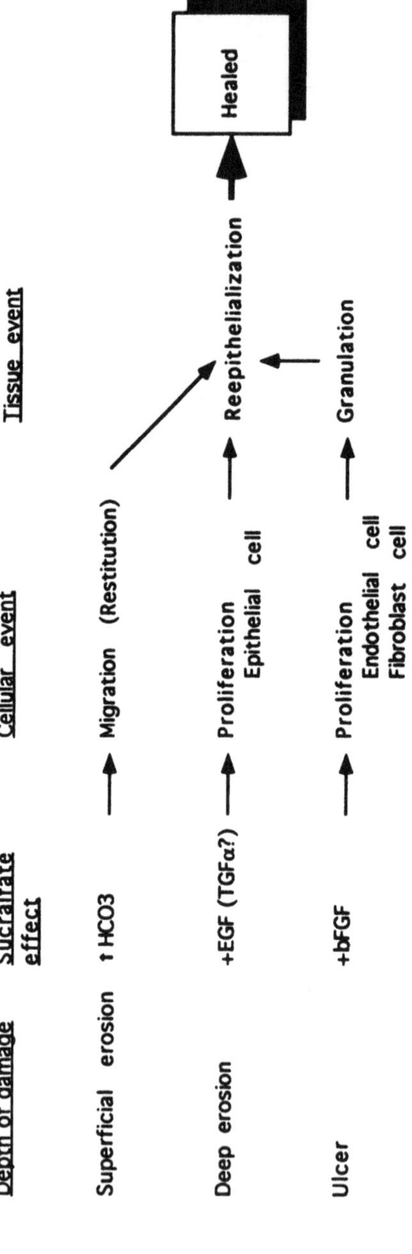

Figure 3. Potential actions of sucralfate on cell renewal with increasing levels of mucosal damage.

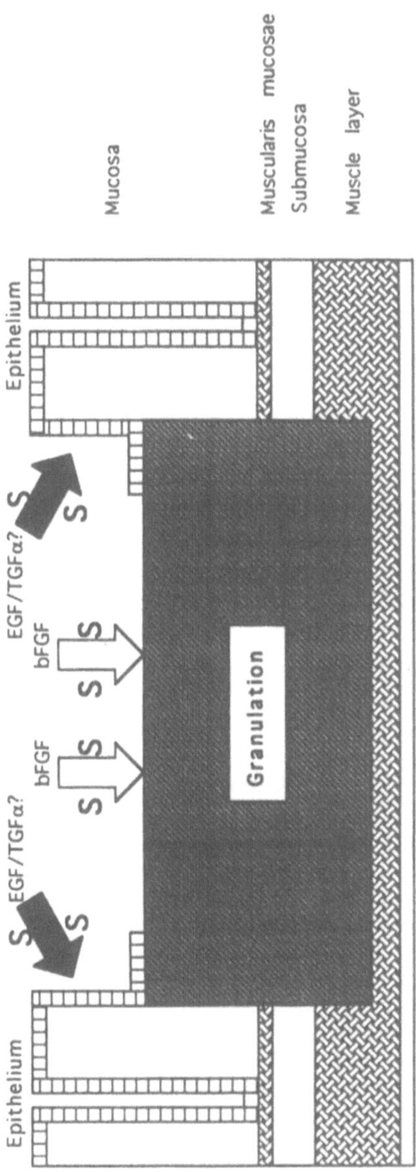

Figure 4. Possible mechanism of acceleration of ulcer healing by sucralfate.

proliferation. It is possible that sucralfate binds EGF, a potent mitogen for gastric epithelial cells, and thereby stimulates epithelial proliferation. In support of this hypothesis, the induction of increased expression of EGF receptor by sucralfate has been shown in rat stomach. However, recent studies have suggested that TGFα is more likely to be the actual ligand for the EGF receptor. The effects of sucralfate on TGFα and EGF binding to EGF receptor need to be studied. Sucralfate has also been reported to bind basic FGF and promote angiogenesis, which is an important element of granulation (Fig. 4). The peptide basic FGF was initially postulated as a potent stimulant of fibroblast proliferation. Recent studies have shown that basic FGF also stimulates endothelial cell proliferation.[8] Basic FGF is produced by many other cell types including gastric mucosal cells, but basic FGF is an acid-sensitive peptide. Thus, basic FGF bound to sucralfate may be protected from acid degradation and released slowly as the sucralfate dissolves. These findings enhance our understanding of how sucralfate may accelerate the healing of chronic peptic ulcers, but need further confirmation.

Future Perspectives

Although many studies of sucralfate's action have been conducted, most available information is based on acute, typically single-dose administration. It is important to realize that this is an unlikely clinical situation. We are just beginning to learn how sucralfate may accelerate ulcer healing on the cellular level. Ulcer healing is a complex process and requires cell regeneration, and possibly involves many growth factors such as PDGF, EGF, FGF, and TGFα and β. It is possible that not only EGF and FGF but also other peptides are involved in sucralfate's action in accelerating ulcer healing. Additional studies will be needed to elucidate the exact mechanisms of sucralfate's action.

References

1. Eastwood GL: Gastrointestinal epithelial renewal. *Gastroenterology* **72**:962–965, 1977. Comprehensive review of gastrointestinal epithelial renewal, which also covers basic methods and concept of epithelial renewal. Excellent for those who are interested in epithelial renewal.
2. Lacy E: Epithelial restitution in the gastrointestinal tract. *J Clin Gastroenterol* **10**(suppl 1):S72–S77, 1988. Rapid restitution after superficial injury, which is originally found in the gastric mucosa, is a phenomenon occurring throughout the gastrointestinal mucosa including esophagus.
3. Kuwayama H, Matsuo Y, Eastwood G: Gastroduodenal mucosal injury by nonsteroidal antiinflammatory drugs. *Drug Invest* **2**(suppl 1):22–26, 1990. Brief review of gastroduodenal mucosal injury by nonsteroidal antiinflammatory drugs with special reference to effects on epithelial renewal.
4. Barnes D: Growth factors involved in repair processes: An overview. *Methods Enzymol* **163**:707–715, 1988. Detailed review including methodology of growth factors in tissue repair. These are many growth factors that may stimulate or inhibit tissue repair process.
5. Luk GD: Polyamines in intestinal growth. *Biochem Soc Trans* **18**:1090–1091, 1990. An updated brief review of role of polyamines in intestinal growth. Readers can find the significance of polyamines in cellular growth as well as differentiation.
6. Eastwood G: Epithelial renewal in protection and repair of gastroduodenal mucosa. *J Clin Gastroen-*

terol **13**:S48–S53, 1991. This review summarizes changes in epithelial renewal of the gastroduodenal mucosa in response to different conditions or mucosal damaging agents.
7. Yeomans N: Repair and healing of established gastric mucosal injury. *J Clin Gastroenterol* **13**(suppl 1):S37–S41, 1991. A good review of the morphological process during repair of the gastric mucosa.
8. Folkman J, Szabo S, Stovroff M, *et al*: Duodenal ulcer. Discovery of a new mechanism and development of angiogenetic therapy that accelerates healing. *Ann Surg* **214**:414–425, 1991. This review introduces mechanism of healing ulcers focusing on FGF which can be achieved by either suppression of gastric acid secretion or sucralfate binding to FGF.

15

Vascular Factors
Mucosal Vasoprotection and Angiogenesis

ZSUZSA SANDOR and SANDOR SZABO

Introduction

Vascular factors refer to acute endothelial damage and protection, regulation of blood flow, and generation of new blood vessels (angiogenesis). The investigation of vascular factors is a relatively new subject in ulcer research.[15] Historically, most of the experimental work on the stomach was related to the structure and function of epithelial cells (e.g., gastric secretion) (Table I). This was in part the result of conceptual focus on epithelial cells and availability of methods. Subsequently, blood flow was investigated *per se* in relation to gastric secretion, mucosal injury, and ulcer localization in the stomach and duodenum. If ischemia was considered, it was ascribed to external or internal (e.g., thrombosis) narrowing and not to active involvement of endothelial cells (e.g., in regulating vascular permeability).

The present interest in vascular factors coincides with the introduction of the concept of gastric cytoprotection.[14] Namely, the early studies on the phenomenon and mechanism of the prevention of acute hemorrhagic mucosal lesions induced by ethanol revealed that alcohol causes a rapidly developing and early endothelial injury in the gastric mucosa (Table I). It was also soon revealed that this early vascular injury is nonspecific, i.e., also induced by HCl, NaOH, aspirin, and indomethacin which are the most frequently used damaging agents in ulcer research.[7,10,11,20] Furthermore, endothelial injury was associated with functional impairment of microcirculation in gastric mucosa, and gastroprotective agents such as prostaglandins and sulfhydryls were found to decrease vascular damage *and* maintain blood flow.[10,11] The most recent insight into the mechanisms of acute gastric mucosal protection thus holds that maintenance of blood flow and the energy-dependent

---

ZSUZSA SANDOR and SANDOR SZABO • Chemical Pathology Research Division, Department of Pathology, Brigham & Women's Hospital, and Harvard Medical School, Boston, Massachusetts 02115; *present address*: Department of Pathology and Laboratory Medicine, Veterans Affairs Medical Center, Long Beach, California, 90822.

Sucralfate: From Basic Science to the Bedside, edited by Daniel Hollander and G. N. J. Tytgat. Plenum Press, New York, 1995.

Table I. Vascular Factors in Ulcer Research[a]

History
Focus on epithelial, especially parietal and chief cells
Lack of adequate methods
Importance of blood flow *per se*
Ischemia
External narrowing (e.g., compression, spasm)
Internal obstruction (e.g., thrombosis, embolism)
Present
Ethanol: rapidly developing and early vascular injury
Endothelial damage is nonspecific: HCl, NaOH, aspirin, indomethacin
Vascular injury: associated with functional impairment of microcirculation
Gastroprotective agents decrease vascular damage and maintain blood flow
Maintenance of blood flow: essential for epithelial restitution and regeneration
Future
Mechanisms of vascular injury: direct and indirect etiologic factors
Endogenous mediators of vascular damage: monoamines, LT, TX, PAF, ET, etc.
Endogenous vasoprotectors: NO, prostacyclin, glucocorticoids, etc.
Protection and healing
Pharmacological targeting

[a]Modified from Ref. 15.

epithelial restitution are the key elements in gastric cytoprotection.[12,14,15,20] New methods like the *in vivo* microscopy of gastric capillaries, blood flow measurement by laser-Doppler, and the hydrogen clearance techniques also helped to demonstrate that rapid functional impairment of microcirculation follows the structural endothelial lesions and that these interactions are crucial in acute gastroprotection.

The recognition of the importance of angiogenesis in mucosal repair and ulcer healing is an even more recent development.[5,16,18] This was first investigated in elucidating the mechanisms of potent ulcer healing effects of basic fibroblast growth factor (bFGF) and platelet-derived growth factor (PDGF), although angiogenesis may play a role in the mechanism of action of epidermal growth factor (EGF) as well. Since sucralfate binds bFGF[4,5] and probably EGF as well, review of vascular factors is also warranted in analyzing the stimulation of chronic ulcer healing by sucralfate.[16,21]

Sucralfate is one of the few locally acting antiulcer drugs which exerts both acute gastroprotection and accelerates the healing of chronic gastric and duodenal ulcers without substantial suppression of gastric acidity.[16,19] Although sucralfate exerts numerous effects, its mechanism of action is still not completely understood, despite major advances during the last 15 years. Since reduction of early vascular injury and stimulation of angiogenesis are important in the mechanisms of acute gastroprotection and chronic ulcer healing, we will review both acute and chronic vascular factors related to the mechanism of action of sucralfate.

Acute Vascular Injury and Vasoprotection

Acute vascular injury and vasoprotection in the gastric mucosa are important elements in the mechanisms of action of gastroprotective agents such as sucralfate. Furthermore, maintenance of blood flow is essential for all protective mechanisms of the gastrointestinal tract.[12,14,15] As stated above, detailed investigations of vascular injury and protection and their role in the development of gastric mucosal injury and protection are relatively recent developments in ulcer research.

The mechanisms of early vascular injury and protection are not clearly understood. In these processes, however, *direct* and *indirect* effects are important. Direct effects are produced by the damaging exogenous chemicals while the indirect actions are exerted by endogenous chemicals and their metabolites as a result of liberation or modification of vasoactive products, such as monoamines, leukotrienes, thromboxanes, platelet activating factor, and as very recently recognized, endothelins and proteases (Fig. 1 and Table II).[6,9,15] Among the endogenous chemicals that may cause vascular injury, leukotrienes and platelet activating factor are about 10–100 times more potent than monoamines such as histamine, while endothelins are about 10–100 times more potent in causing microvascular injury in the gastric mucosa than leukotrienes.[9] The important role of vasoactive compounds is further reinforced by results showing that the development of ethanol-induced hemorrhagic erosions in the stomach is accompanied by mast cell degranulation and release of leukotrienes and biogenic amines such as histamine and serotonin.

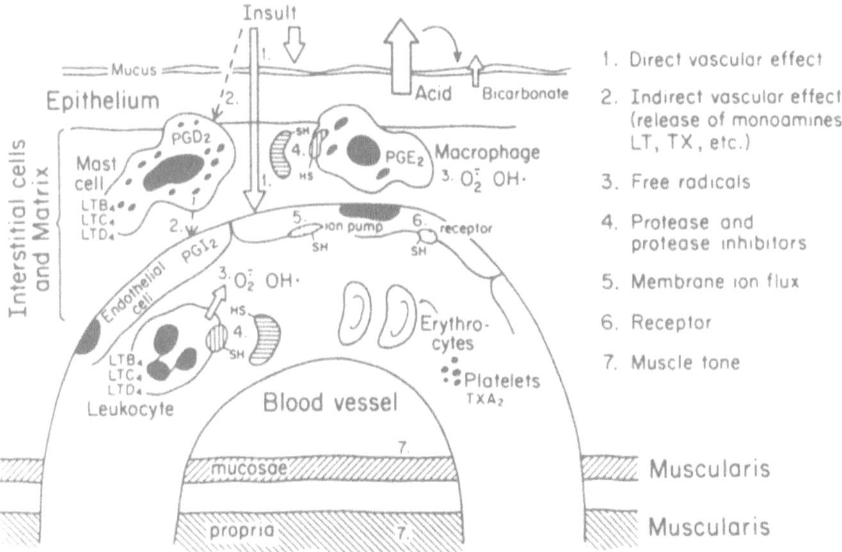

Figure 1. Interactions in gastric mucosal injury and protection, with special reference to the role of blood vessel and microcirculation.

Table II. Microcirculatory Stasis and Density of Hemorrhagic Mucosal Lesions after Topical Application of Necrotizing Agents to the Rat Gastric Mucosa

	Microcirculatory stasis		Mucosal lesions	
Treatment	Incidence (positive/total)[a]	Time until stasis (sec)	Incidence (positive/total)	Area (% of chamber surface)
Saline	0/5	NS[b]	0/5	0
Ethanol (100%)	12/12*	54 ± 5	12/12*	34.2 ± 4.2
HCl (0.6 N)	9/9*	81 ± 12	9/9*	78.8 ± 9.1**
NaOH (0.2 N)	9/9*	61 ± 6	9/9*	48.2 ± 6.5

[a]Positive = number of rats showing microcirculatory stasis or mucosal lesions.
[b]NS, no stasis.
*$p < 0.005$ (Fischer exact test) of control versus experimental groups.
**$p < 0.001$ (Student's t test) for ethanol versus HCl. Ethanol versus NaOH was not significantly different.

Furthermore, the ethanol-induced gastric mucosal injury was significantly decreased in a strain of mouse that is genetically deficient in mast cells.

The first *vascular tracers*, which revealed the early endothelial injury by labeling damaged capillaries and venules in the gastric mucosa, were colloidal carbon (India ink) and monastral blue which were injected intravenously (i.v.) 3 min before autopsy. One milliliter of either ethanol (100%), 0.2 N NaOH, or 0.6 N HCl was administered intragastrically and the animals were killed after 5, 15, 30 sec, 1–12 min later. Extravasation of another i.v. injected vascular tracer, Evans blue, into the gastric wall and into luminal contents was used as an indicator of vascular permeability. The areas of deposition of colloidal carbon or monastral blue and the hemorrhagic mucosal lesions were measured by stereomicroscopic planimetry.[20] *In vivo* microscopy of microcirculation to measure the movement of erythrocytes in the superficial mucosal capillaries of the transilluminated gastric wall was also employed.[10]

After administration of ethanol, NaOH, or HCl, the distribution of vascular labeling involving predominantly subepithelial capillaries and a few venules was anatomically similar. Time wise, vascular injury after the intragastric administration of alcohol and base developed very rapidly (e.g., in 5–15 sec), while acid caused a slightly delayed development of vascular injury and hemorrhagic erosions. Subsequently, markedly increased vascular permeability was found within 1–3 min after intragastric exposure to concentrated solutions of ethanol, acid, or base. These results, initially obtained in animal models and subsequently confirmed in human studies, clearly show that vascular injury is detectable before occurrence of hemorrhagic lesions.

These results and implications have also been confirmed with *in vivo* microscopy of rat gastric mucosal circulation. Namely, luminal application of damaging chemicals onto the chambered gastric mucosa first slowed and then stopped circulation in superficial gastric mucosal capillaries. Subsequently, dilation of mucosal arterioles and submucosal arteries was seen and vasodilation was maximal 1–3 min after application of damaging agents.[10] The congestion of capillaries and venules is probably caused by endothelial injury and compression of mural veins. Luminal hemorrhage was a late event in the *in vivo* microscopy studies as well.

All of these vascular studies demonstrated a significant inverse correlation between the severity of hemorrhagic mucosal lesions and gastric mucosal blood flow measured 10, 15, and 20 min after ethanol exposure. Namely, blood flow determined 15 min after 50% ethanol would predict the area of hemorrhagic mucosal lesions.[10]

The most severely affected tissues by hypoxia are the organs with end arteries and which cannot regenerate (e.g., brain, heart, kidney). Although gastric mucosal cells have not been studied extensively, the sensitivity of these cells to hypoxia is probably similar to that of myocardium.[3] The structural and functional integrity of microvasculature, on the other hand, ensures the delivery of nutrients and oxygen which are essential for energy-dependent processes such as epithelial restitution and rapid repair of superficial mucosal damage.[11,15,22]

Most of these vascular events have been investigated after pretreatment with gastroprotective agents including sucralfate, which do not markedly and directly alter the initial epithelial injury after administration of damaging agents. These drugs, however, diminish or prevent the early microvascular injury and maintain blood flow in the gastric mucosa. This vasoprotection leading to gastroprotection can be studied at both structural (e.g., light and electron microscopy) and functional levels (e.g., blood flow, vascular permeability). Several studies demonstrate that the absence of normal mucosal microvascular perfusion markedly increases the extent of damage by ethanol and that in the absence of microvascular flow, the protective effects of sucralfate are not expressed.[2,8,17] Comparative studies on gastric mucosal blood flow measured by laser-Doppler flowmetry and gastric mucosal injury induced by ethanol revealed that sucralfate, misoprostol, and omeprazole, but not cimetidine increased gastric mucosal blood flow in a dose-dependent manner and protected the mucosa against ethanol damage. The peak and summation blood flow were significantly greater with sucralfate than with misoprostol or omeprazole, but the degree of mucosal protection was similar[8] (Fig. 2). Sucralfate pretreatment antagonized the ethanol-induced depression of mucosal blood flow[8] (Fig. 3).

The sucralfate molecule contains eight oxidized SH groups (i.e., sulfates). Our laboratory found that sulfates are one of the most active components of the drug.[17] Vascular and gastroprotective studies were performed after pretreatment of fasted rats with sucralfate, equimolar amounts of potassium sucrose octasulfate, sodium sulfate, or aluminum chloride administered 30 min before ethanol. The results demonstrate that within 1 min, ethanol-induced vascular injury involved about 40% of the glandular stomach, and hemorrhagic lesions of the mucosa were hardly detectable at that time (Fig. 4).[17] Pretreatment with sucralfate or its components significantly decreased the extent of vascular injury and diminished the hemorrhagic mucosal lesions. If the stomach was removed 1 hr after ethanol exposure, there was no major difference between the component of sucralfate, but in the 1-hr experiment the most potent component of sucralfate was sulfate, hence sucrose octasulfate. This is in agreement with the demonstration that sulfate was the most active component in diminishing the HCl-induced esophageal damage in rabbits (Orlando, personal communication).

Blood flow was measured in anesthetized rats with direct visualization of transillumi-

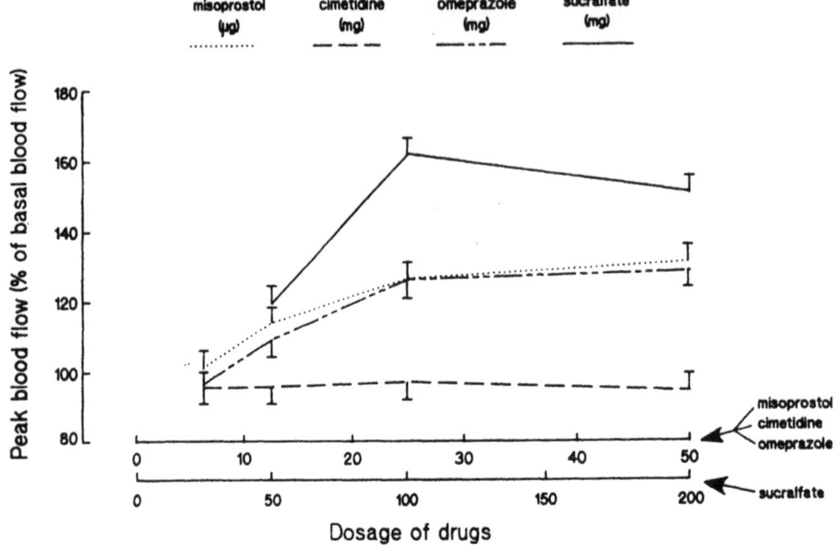

Figure 2. Relationship between peak gastric mucosal blood flow and doses of misoprostol, omeprazole, cimetidine, and sucralfate. A direct correlation was observed between the peak blood flow and misoprostol ($r = 0.7$, $p < 0.001$), omeprazole ($r = 0.74$, $p < 0.001$), and sucralfate ($r = 0.50$, $p < 0.01$), but not cimetidine (nonsignificant; $r = 0.18$, $p < 0.18$). (Reproduced with permission from: Hui WM, Chen BW, Cho CH, *et al*: Digestion **48:**113–120, 1991.)

nated subepithelial capillaries. Addition of 0.5 ml 100% ethanol to the chambered gastric mucosa led to complete cessation of red blood cell movements. If sucrose octasulfate was added to the chamber before the application of alcohol, the cessation of erythrocyte movements was prevented and blood flow was maintained.[10,15]

Thus, sucralfate and its components, especially sucrose octasulfate and sodium sulfate, decreased or prevented the ethanol-induced microvascular injury and maintained blood flow, allowing the rapid epithelial restitution to cover the superficial mucosal damage. These data also indicate that sucralfate, like other gastroprotective agents, protects against vascular injury, which is a target of the interaction of diverse mucosal damaging and protective agents.

Angiogenesis

Angiogenesis or neovascularization refers to proliferation and migration of vascular endothelial cells which eventually form a tube for new capillaries. This process normally occurs in wound healing. Angiogenesis is regulated by locally produced cytokines and growth factors (e.g., interleukins, prostaglandins, bFGF, TGFβ, PDGF) and circulating hormones (e.g., angiogenic steroids, glucocorticoids), in concert with the local environ-

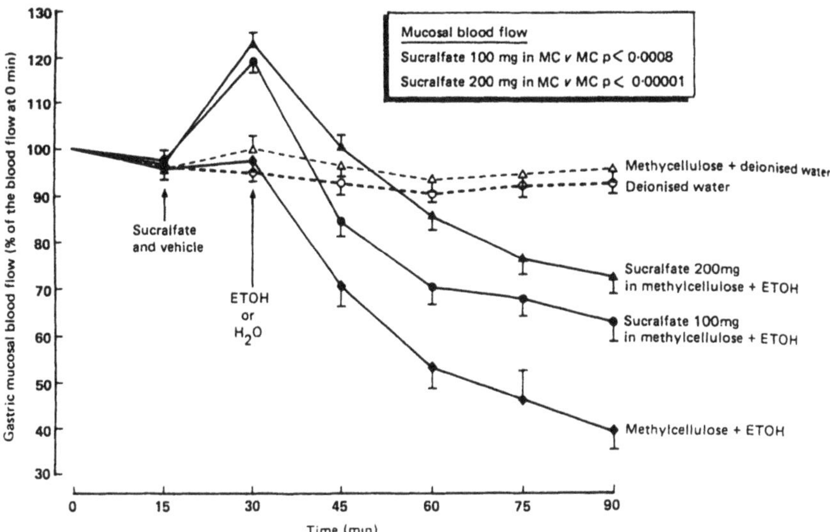

Figure 3. Effect of sucralfate on gastric mucosal blood flow in fasted rats treated with ethanol (EtOH) or deionized water (H_2O). Summation flow and peak flow (at 30 min) were significantly higher in rats pretreated with sucralfate than in those without pretreatment. (Reproduced with permission from: Chen BW, Hui WM, Lam SK, *et al*: *Gut* **30**:1544–1551, 1989.)

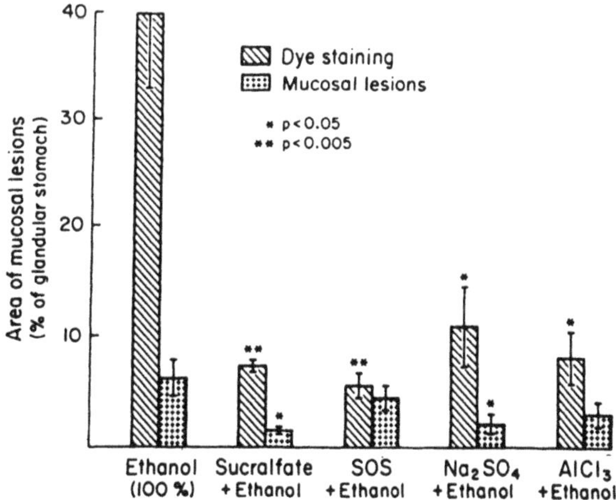

Figure 4. Influence of sucralfate (50 mg/100 g) and equimolar amounts of its components on vascular injury as revealed by monastral blue staining of damaged blood vessels and gastric mucosal hemorrhagic lesions 1 min after ethanol exposure in fasted rats. SOS, sucrose octasulfate. (Adapted from: Szabo S, Vattay, P, Scarbrough E, *et al*: *Am J Med* **91**(suppl 2A):158–160, 1991.)

ment (e.g., heparin, aminoglycans, proteases).[5,13,18] Among these, bFGF is the most potent endothelial mitogen which also stimulates the proliferation of other cells such as fibroblasts, smooth muscle cells, epithelial cells, and neurons. EGF exerts a weak angiogenic response while TGF derivatives often demonstrate biphasic effects, i.e., inhibition and stimulation of angiogenesis under certain conditions.

Angiogenesis is crucial in the generation of granulation tissue and wound/ulcer healing processes. Granulation tissue consists of growing capillaries, proliferating fibroblasts, collagen, and chronic inflammatory cells such as lymphocytes, plasma cells, and macrophages. The budding capillaries create the granular appearance of the bottom of the wound, hence the name granulation tissue. The healing of chronic gastrointestinal ulcers seems to be controlled by a few processes that govern wound healing, such as angiogenesis and proliferation of fibroblasts during the generation of granulation tissue. Recently, we performed a series of experiments to test the hypothesis that angiogenesis and granulation tissue formation stimulated by factors such as bFGF might accelerate the healing of experimental chronic duodenal ulcers.[18] In these rat experiments the cysteamine model of chronic duodenal ulcer was used, i.e., rats with penetrating ulcers (as determined by laparotomy) were randomized into vehicle control and treatment groups which were given 100 ng/100 g of the wild-type recombinant human bFGF, the acid-resistant mutein CS23, or, for comparison, the histamine H_2-receptor antagonist cimetidine (10 mg/100 g) by gavage twice daily until autopsy on day 21, when ulcers were measured and histologic sections taken.

The results revealed that the prevalence, i.e., rats with ulcers, was decreased only by bFGF–CS23 during the 3-week treatment. The ulcer crater was reduced marginally by cimetidine, and markedly by bFGF–w and the acid-resistant bFGF–CS23. Histology of bFGF-treated rats revealed prominent angiogenesis, mild mononuclear cell infiltration, dense granulation tissue in the ulcer bed, and healed ulcers which were completely epithelialized. Morphometric analysis of angiogenesis in histologic sections after immunohistochemical staining for endothelial cell-specific factor VIII revealed hypovascular ulcer craters in comparison with adjacent normal mucosa, and about a tenfold increase in angiogenesis in ulcer craters of rats treated with CS23.

Additional studies in fasted rats revealed that bFGF at 100 or 500 ng/100 g by gavage did *not* decrease gastric acid and pepsin secretion.[18]

From these experiments we concluded that oral administration of an angiogenic polypeptide made acid-stable by recombinant site-specific mutagenesis significantly accelerated the healing of chronic duodenal ulcers produced by cysteamine. Treatment with bFGF–CS23 caused a tenfold increase in angiogenesis in the ulcer bed. These findings demonstrate the important role of angiogenesis in ulcer healing and the possibilities of its new pharmacologic modulation.

We also examined whether sucralfate and its active components might stimulate angiogenesis and fibroblast proliferation *in vivo*.[21] Round, sterile (8×3 mm) sponges which contained 5 or 50 mg of sucralfate, sucrose octasulfate, or bFGF mutein CS23, 20 or 200 ng (as a positive control), were implanted subcutaneously in the rat. One week after the implantation the animals were killed, the sponges were removed, fixed in formalin, and processed for histologic and histochemical evaluation and morphometry. Under high (×200) power, the number of blood vessels and the area (mm^2) of granulation tissue surface were measured and the total number of blood vessels was calculated (Table III).

The results of the control group and sponges treated with low doses of sucrose octasulfate were similar. However, both sucralfate and sucrose octasulfate in the high doses increased the number of blood vessels, but only sucralfate enlarged the granulation tissue surface. The total number of blood vessels was 449% of controls in sucralfate sponge and 170% after sucrose octasulfate. The positive control bFGF was more active on a molar basis in all of the studied parameters. Since sucralfate increased the surface of granulation tissue, it was more active than sucrose octasulfate in increasing the total number of blood vessels (angiogenesis).

These results are in agreement with other *in vitro* and *in vivo* studies demonstrating that sucralfate induces proliferation of dermal fibroblasts and keratinocytes in culture and granulation tissue formation in full-thickness skin wounds in rats.[1] These results revealed that sucralfate induced proliferation of cultured dermal fibroblasts and keratinocytes, and also enhanced PGE_2 synthesis in basal keratinocytes, in interleukin-1-stimulated keratinocytes and dermal fibroblasts. Basal interleukin-1 and -6 release were not affected by sucralfate, but the agent enhanced interleukin-1-stimulated interleukin-6 release from fibroblasts. When applied daily to full-thickness wounds in rats, sucralfate increased the thickness of granulation tissue when assessed at day 12 (Fig. 5).

Our other recent studies show that sucralfate binds bFGF *in vitro* with high affinity and stabilizes the locally available bFGF.[4,5,16] Thus, endogenous bFGF might be one of the mediators of stimulation of angiogenesis and ulcer healing by sucralfate. Our very recent *in vivo* and *in vitro* experiments indeed demonstrate that sucralfate exposed to bFGF is much more potent in stimulating angiogenesis than sucralfate alone. Furthermore, under *in vivo* conditions, concentration of FGF measured in the duodenal ulcer crater is higher in sucralfate-treated than untreated rats. Thus, sucralfate seems to act as a sponge bringing in

Table III. Effect of Sucralfate, SOS, and bFGF on Angiogenesis and Granulation Tissue in Subcutaneously Implanted Sponges[a]

	Blood vessels		Granulation tissue surface		Total No. of blood vessels
Treatment	No./HPF[b]	%	mm^2	%	%
Controls	30.6 ± 2.1	100	2.9 ± 0.2	100	100
Sucralfate	67.6 ± 2.5*	221	5.9 ± 0.7*	203	449
Controls	35.8 ± 2.3	100	2.6 ± 0.1	100	100
SOS	58.7 ± 6.6**	164	2.7 ± 0.2	104	170
Controls	40.5 ± 2.9**	100	3.6 ± 0.5	100	100
bFGF-CS23	75.9 ± 3.7	187	7.6 ± 0.7*	211	396

[a]Adapted from Ref. 21.
[b]HPF denotes high-power field.
*$p < 0.001$.
**$p < 0.005$.

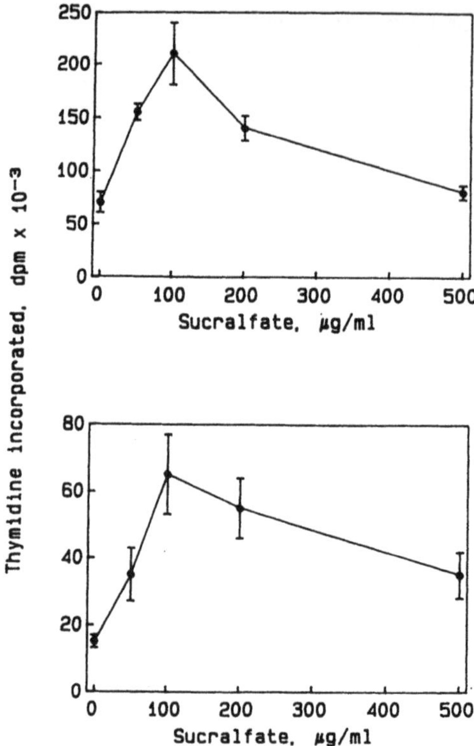

Figure 5. Sucralfate induces proliferation of cultured human dermal fibroblasts (upper panel) and human keratinocytes (lower panel). (Reproduced with permission from: Burch RM, McMillan BA: *Agents Actions* **34**:229–231, 1991.)

naturally occurring bFGF in the duodenal ulcer crater. Since bFGF is the most potent mitogen for endothelial cells, fibroblasts, and smooth muscle cells, ulcers treated with bFGF or sucralfate should have a prominent and well-vascularized granulation tissue, which provides a framework for reepithelialization to complete the healing process.

Summary

This chapter reviews the role of vascular factors such as acute endothelial damage and protection, regulation of blood flow and angiogenesis as they relate to the mechanisms of action of sucralfate. The maintenance of proper blood flow is essential for rapid epithelial restitution and is the most important element in acute gastroprotection. Preservation of microvascular integrity and the maintenance of mucosal blood flow seem to be important mechanisms of acute gastroprotection by sucralfate. Several *in vivo* and *in vitro* experiments revealed that sucralfate stimulated fibroblast and keratinocyte proliferation, and both sucralfate and sucrose octasulfate stimulated angiogenesis, whereas only sucralfate increased the area of granulation tissue. Thus, vascular factors seem to have a role in the mechanisms of acute gastroprotection and chronic ulcer healing by sucralfate.

References

1. Burch RM, McMillan BA: Sucralfate induces proliferation of dermal fibroblasts and keratinocytes in culture and granulation tissue formation in full-thickness skin wounds. *Agents Actions* **34**:229–231, 1991. Sucralfate has direct effects on wound healing in the skin; it increases the thickness of granulation tissue and induces the proliferation of keratinocytes and fibroblasts in culture.
2. Chen BW, Hui WM, Lam SK, *et al*: Effect of sucralfate on gastric mucosal blood flow in rats. *Gut* **30**:1544–1551, 1989. Sucralfate increases gastric mucosal blood flow and lessens the fall in blood flow after ethanol treatment in a dose-dependent manner in rats. This action may contribute to the gastroprotective effect of the drug.
3. Cotran RC, Kumar V, Robbins SL: *Robbins Pathologic Basis of Disease*, ed 4. Philadelphia, WB Saunders, 1989. One of the best textbooks of pathology.
4. Folkman J, Szabo S, Shing, Y: Sucralfate affinity for fibroblast growth factor. *J Cell Biol* **111**:223A, 1990. The first demonstration of bFGF binding to sucralfate *in vitro*, in comparison with heparin.
5. Folkman J, Szabo S, Stovroff M, *et al*: Duodenal ulcer: Discovery of a new mechanism and development of angiogenic therapy that accelerates healing. *Ann Surg* **214**:414–426, 1991. Extensive *in vitro* and *in vivo* studies on sucralfate binding of bFGF, and the demonstration of elevated levels of bFGF in chronic duodenal ulcers treated with sucralfate in rats.
6. Galli SJ, Bose R, Szabo S: Mast cell dependent augmentation of ethanol-induced acute gastric damage in mice. *Dig Dis Sci* **30**:375, 1985. Demonstration of role of mast cells and vascular factors in acute mucosal injury using mouse strains deficient in mast cells.
7. Guth PH, Poulsen G, Nagata H: Histologic and microcirculatory changes in alcohol-induced gastric lesions in the rat: Effect of prostaglandin cytoprotection. *Gastroenterology* **87**:1083–1090, 1984. This paper documents the stages of congestion in histologic sections of the rat stomach soon after administration of ethanol.
8. Hui WM, Chen BW, Cho CH, *et al*: Role of gastric blood flow in cytoprotection. *Digestion* **48**:113–120, 1991. Comparative study on the effects of misoprostol, omeprazole, cimetidine, and sucralfate on gastric mucosal blood flow. Sucralfate, misoprostol, and omeprazole but not cimetidine increased gastric mucosal blood flow in a dose-dependent manner. The blood flow was significantly greater after sucralfate in comparison with other drugs.
9. Morales RE, Johnson BR, Szabo S: Endothelin induces vascular and mucosal lesions, enhances the injury by HCl/ethanol, and the antibody exerts gastroprotection. *FASEB J* **6**:2354–2360, 1992. Intra-arterial infusion of endothelin caused vascular injury as revealed by monastral blue deposition and markedly aggravated the chemically induced gastric mucosal injury.
10. Pihan G, Majzoubi D, Haudenschild C, *et al*: Early microcirculatory stasis in acute gastric mucosal injury in the rat and prevention by 16,16-dimethyl prostaglandin E2 or sodium thiosulfate. *Gastroenterology* **91**:1415–1426, 1986. This paper describes the functional detection of congestion by laser-Doppler technique. The ethanol-induced decrease in blood flow was counteracted both by prostaglandins and by sulfhydryl derivatives despite the fact that these two protective agents, given alone, have differential effects on mucosal blood flow.
11. Pihan G, Szabo S, Trier JS: The role of microvasculature in acute gastric mucosal damage and protection, in Szabo S, Pfeiffer CJ (eds): *Ulcer Disease: New Aspects of Pathogenesis and Pharmacology*. Boca Raton, Fla, CRC Press, 1989, pp 135–145. A general review on the functional and structural, including electron-microscopic alterations in blood vessels and supply during acute gastric mucosal injury and protection.
12. Robert A: On the mechanism of cytoprotection, in Szabo S, Pfeiffer CJ (eds): *Ulcer Disease: New Aspects of Pathogenesis and Pharmacology*. Boca Raton, Fla, CRC Press, 1989, pp 417–421. A historic review by the discoverer of "cytoprotection" on the mechanisms of acute gastric mucosal

protection, concluding that one of the key events is the maintenance of mucosal blood flow by protective agents.

13. Sandor Z, Szabo S: Steroids and ulcers, in Braga PC, Guslandi M (eds): *Drug-Induced Injury to the Digestive System*. Berlin, Springer-Verlag, 1993 (in press). A modern review on the effect of all types of steroids on the gut, synthesizing both human and animal data. Special emphasis is placed on glucocorticoids and the recently discovered angiosteroids, i.e., angiogenic and angiostatic naturally occurring and synthetic steroids.
14. Szabo S: Critical and timely review of the concept of gastric cytoprotection. *Acta Physiol Hung* **73**:115–127, 1989. A critical and historical review that covers not only prostaglandins but other gastroprotective agents as well, and emphasizes the vascular factors as key elements in the mechanisms of mucosal protection.
15. Szabo S: Pharmacological modulation of cellular, vascular and motility factors, in Garner A, Whittle BJR (eds): *Advances in Drug Therapy of Gastrointestinal Ulceration*. New York, John Wiley & Sons, Ltd, 1989. An in-depth and analytic review of mucosal protection through separate discussion of cellular, vascular, and motility factors.
16. Szabo S: The mode of action of sucralfate: The 1×1×1 mechanism of action. *Scand J Gastroenterol* **26**(suppl 185):7–12, 1991. This is a detailed and critical review of the mechanisms of actions of sucralfate, emphasizing that not all actions of the drug are equally important for acute gastroprotection and healing of chronic ulcers. It is proposed that prevention of vascular injury, maintenance of mucosal blood flow allowing rapid epithelial restitution are key mechanisms for *acute* gastroprotection, in *both* acute and chronic action of sucralfate, while local binding and concentration of growth factors such as bFGF and EGF are the elements of stimulated *chronic* ulcer healing by sucralfate.
17. Szabo S, Brown A: Prevention of ethanol-induced vascular injury and gastric mucosal lesions by sucralfate and its components: Possible role of endogenous sulfhydryls. *Proc Soc Exp Biol Med* **185**:493–497, 1987. This rat study demonstrated that the gastroprotective action of sucralfate is mediated by a sulfhydryl-sensitive process, which is counteracted by the sulfhydryl alkylator *N*-ethylmaleimide. It was also shown that sulfate and sucrose octasulfate are the most potent gastroprotective components of sucralfate, and that the early ethanol-induced vascular injury is preventable not only by sucralfate but by its components as well, especially sulfates.
18. Szabo S, Folkman J, Vattay P, *et al*: Duodenal ulcerogens: Effect of FGF on cysteamine-induced duodenal ulcer, in Halter F, Garner A, Tytgat GNJ (eds): *Mechanisms of Peptic Ulcer Healing*. London, Kluwer Academic Pub, 1991, pp 139–150. Review of animal models of duodenal ulceration, and the first overview of the very potent ulcer healing properties of bFGF in rats with experimental duodenal ulcer.
19. Szabo S, Hollander D: Pathways of gastrointestinal protection and repair: Mechanism of action of sucralfate. *Am J Med* **86**(suppl 6A):23–31, 1989. Detailed overview of the processes of gastrointestinal protection and repair with special emphasis on the mechanism of sucralfate in acute gastroprotection and chronic ulcer healing.
20. Szabo S, Trier JS, Brown A, *et al*: Early vascular injury and increased vascular permeability in gastric mucosal injury caused by ethanol in the rat. *Gastroenterology* **88**:228–236, 1985. This is the first paper in a peer-reviewed journal describing the rapidly developing vascular tracers, monastral blue and colloidal carbon after administration of ethanol in rat. The lesions were prevented by prostaglandins and sulfhydryl derivatives.
21. Szabo S, Vattay P, Scarbrough E, *et al*: Role of vascular factors, including angiogenesis, in the mechanism of action of sucralfate. *Am J Med* **91**(suppl 2A):158–160, 1991. Demonstration of enhanced angiogenesis and granulation tissue production in s.c.-implanted sponges in rats: sucralfate was more potent than the water-soluble sucrose octasulfate.
22. Tarnawski A, Hollander D, Stachura J, *et al*: Prostaglandin protection of the gastric mucosa against alcohol injury—A dynamic time-related process. Role of the mucosal proliferative zone. *Gastroenterology* **88**:334–352, 1985. This paper compares the protective effect of prostaglandins and emphasizes the importance of preserving the proliferative zone for rapid restitution.

16

Sucralfate

Role of Endogenous Sulfhydryls and Basic Fibroblast Growth Factor (bFGF)

SANDOR SZABO, JUDAH FOLKMAN, Y. SHING, STEFANO KUSSTATSCHER, ZSUZSA SANDOR, and MIKI NAGATA

Introduction

Sucralfate is a locally acting gastroprotective and antiulcer drug that exerts its effect *in situ* without substantial absorption into the systemic circulation. Nevertheless, endogenous mediators seem to play a role in the mechanism of action of sucralfate.

Historically, the first endogenous mediators of sucralfate were related to aggressive factors, e.g., absorption of pepsin and binding of bile acids.[1,2] Prostaglandins were the first endogenous protective compounds suggested to have a role in the mechanism of acute gastroprotection by sucralfate.[3] Subsequently, sulfhydryls were implicated in the acute mucosal protection by the drug.[4] The apparent binding and enhanced local concentration of epidermal growth factor (EGF) in sucralfate-treated ulcers were suggested to play a role in the mechanisms of both acute gastroprotection and chronic ulcer healing by sucralfate.[5] Nevertheless, no rational and chemical basis has yet been identified that would explain an *in vitro* binding of EGF to sucralfate, and the elimination of bioavailable EGF has yet to be proven to affect the acute mucosal protection and chronic ulcer healing by sucralfate.

Among the latter two criteria, the first one has been satisfied by the interaction of sucralfate and basic fibroblast growth factor (bFGF). Namely, because of the similarity of

---

SANDOR SZABO, STEFANO KUSSTATSCHER, ZSUZSA SANDOR, and MIKI NAGATA • Department of Pathology, Brigham & Women's Hospital, and Harvard Medical School, Boston, Massachusetts 02115; *present address of* Sandor Szabo and Zsuzsa Sandor: Department of Pathology and Laboratory Medicine, Veterans Affairs Medical Center, Long Beach, California, 90822. JUDAH FOLKMAN and Y. SHING • Department of Surgery, Children's Hospital, and Harvard Medical School, Boston, Massachusetts 02115.

Sucralfate: From Basic Science to the Bedside, edited by Daniel Hollander and G. N. J. Tytgat. Plenum Press, New York, 1995.

sucrose to heparin, the "heparin-binding bFGF" was found to bind with great affinity to sucralfate both *in vitro* and *in vivo*.[6,7] Since bFGF is the most potent angiogenic polypeptide[8] and directly acting antiulcer drug which is on a molar basis 7 million times more potent than cimetidine,[9,10] bFGF has been strongly implicated in the mechanism of ulcer healing by sucralfate.[11,12]

The aim of this chapter is to summarize the pharmacologic and biochemical data on the role of sulfhydryls in mediating the acute gastroprotection by sucralfate, as well as the recent results on the binding of bFGF to sucralfate in the mechanism of chronic ulcer healing by the drug.

Sulfhydryls

Sulfhydryls, especially nonprotein sulfhydryls such as glutathione, are powerful antioxidants, and present in large concentration in the gastric mucosa and the liver.[13] In addition, protein sulfhydryls control membrane permeability, enzyme functions, and the tertiary structure of proteins. Unlike prostaglandins, sulfhydryls are *directly* and chemically involved in protective mechanisms such as the scavenging of free radicals, modulating enzyme activity, and membrane integrity which all might be relevant to the mechanism of acute mucosal protection. Prostaglandins, on the other hand, always exert their effect indirectly, and these molecules have not been directly implicated in any direct chemical mechanism of protection.

After describing the role of sulfhydryls in gastric mucosal protection,[14] we realized that the sucrose molecule contains eight oxidized sulfhydryls, i.e., sulfates, and we tested the hypotheses that sulfhydryls might mediate the action of sucralfate. These studies were very encouraging, especially after learning that virtually all of the gastroprotective agents can be counteracted by the subcutaneous injection of the sulfhydryl alkylator *N*-ethylmaleimide. We thus review here our relevant pharmacologic and biochemical experiments with sucralfate.

Pharmacology

The first experiments were related to investigating the most active component of sucralfate in acute gastric mucosal protection. Since the molecule of sucralfate contains eight oxidized sulfhydryls (i.e., sulfates), and our earlier work demonstrated that sulfhydryl-containing compounds and certain metals that influence mucosal sulfhydryls offer gastroprotection,[15] we tested the hypothesis that sulfate and aluminum might be the most active parts of sucralfate.

We administered equimolar doses of components of sucralfate, i.e., potassium sucrose octasulfate (SOS), inorganic sulfate, or aluminum salts, to rats in doses equimolar to 50 or 10 mg/100 g of sucralfate in the standard acute ethanol gastroprotection assay.[4] These studies revealed that the most potent gastroprotection was demonstrated by sulfate and aluminum molecules, e.g., in doses equimolar to 10 mg of sucralfate, pretreatment with only sodium sulfate afforded acute mucosal protection (Fig. 1). It was also apparent from these results that none of the components provided gastroprotection equal to

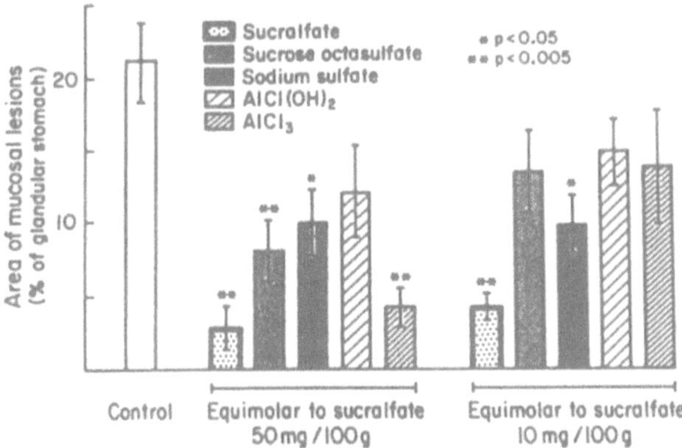

Figure 1. Effect of sucralfate and its components on ethanol-induced gastric erosions. Fasted rats were given sucralfate, 50 or 10 mg/100 g, or equimolar amounts of its components i.g. 30 min before ethanol. The animals were killed 1 hr after alcohol. (Reprinted with permission from Szabo and Brown.[4])

sucralfate (Fig. 1), implying a possible additive or synergistic interaction among the molecular components in inducing acute mucosal protection.

We also tested the hypothesis that sucralfate decreases ethanol-induced early vascular injury and the development of hemorrhagic mucosal lesions through a sulfhydryl-sensitive process which can be counteracted by sulfhydryl alkylators such as *N*-ethylmaleimide.[4] The postulated mechanism has been that sulfhydryls which can be alkylated by *N*-ethylmaleimide may represent a pathway in gastroprotection offered by sucralfate. In these experiments, sucralfate (10 mg/100 g) was given to the rats 30 min before ethanol. The alkylator *N*-ethylmaleimide (5 mg/100 g) was injected s.c. 10 min after sucralfate (i.e., 20 min before ethanol) and the animals were killed 1 hr after alcohol.[4] The results showed that sucralfate alone significantly decreased the area of ethanol-induced hemorrhagic mucosal lesions. When sucralfate administration was followed by s.c. injection of the sulfhydryl alkylator, the gastroprotection was abolished (Fig. 2).

These pharmacologic experiments indicate that sulfate is the most gastroprotective part of the sucralfate molecule, and suggest a sulfhydryl-sensitive process in the mucosal protection by this locally acting drug.

Biochemistry

In addition to pharmacologic implications of sulfhydryls, biochemical data are also available indicating the involvement of these endogenous protective antioxidants in the mechanism of action of sucralfate. Recent studies were designed to measure the concentration of gastric mucosal and hepatic nonprotein and protein sulfhydryls shortly after the administration of a gastroprotective dose of sucralfate in fasted rats.[16] In these experiments the concentration fractions of both protein and nonprotein sulfhydryls were measured by a

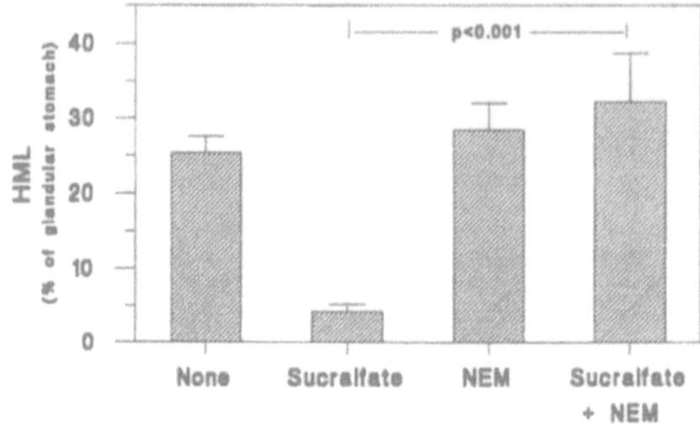

Figure 2. The effect of the sulfhydryl alkylator *N*-ethylmaleimide (NEM) on the gastroprotective effect of sucralfate against ethanol in the rat. Sucralfate (10 mg/100 g) was given i.g. 30 min before 100% ethanol (1 ml, i.g.) which was administered to rats of all groups. NEM (5 mg/100 g) was injected s.c. 10 min after sucralfate (i.e., 20 min before ethanol). Animals were killed 1 hr after alcohol.

recently modified enzyme-coupled spectrophotometric technique. Groups of fasted rats were pretreated with vehicle solvent or 50 mg/100 g of sucralfate, as in standard gastroprotective assays. Instead of receiving a damaging agent such as ethanol, after 30 min the rats were killed and the mucosa of the glandular stomach was scraped and a piece of the left lobe of the liver obtained.

The results revealed that the concentration of reduced glutathione was markedly increased in the gastric mucosa, but not in the liver (Table I). The levels of oxidized glutathione were also slightly enhanced in the stomach, while the protein sulfhydryls did not change in any of the organs examined. The biochemical data thus also implicate sulfhydryls in the mechanism of gastroprotection by sucralfate. Namely, in sucralfate-pretreated rats in the standard gastroprotection assay when ethanol is administered, the gastric mucosa contains an enhanced level of glutathione. This antioxidant neutralizes the

Table I. The Effect of a Gastroprotective Dose of Sucralfate on the Concentration of Sulfhydryls in the Gastric Mucosa

	Glutathione		PSH PSSG	
Treatment[a]	µmole/g tissue	µmole/mg protein	nmole/mg	protein
Controls	6.5 ± 0.5	1.1 ± 0.1	24 ± 1.1	173 ± 16.4
Sucralfate	11.0 ± 1.1*	1.8 ± 0.1*	20 ± 3.4	296 ± 3.5*

[a]Groups of fasted rats were given the vehicle solvent (controls) or sucralfate, 50 mg/100 g by gavage, and were killed 30 min later. Mucosa of the glandular stomach was scraped, homogenized, and processed for a spectrophotometric and enzyme-coupled determination of glutathione, protein sulfhydryls (PSH), and mixed protein and glutathione disulfides (PSSG).
*$p < 0.05$.

deleterious effect of free radicals which play a role in the mechanism of gastric mucosal injury induced by ischemia, stress, and several chemicals.

The enhanced antioxidant capacity of the gastric mucosa after sucralfate administration may thus be *one* of the mechanisms of gastroprotection of this locally acting drug.

bFGF

As stated above, bFGF is the most potent angiogenic molecule which also stimulates ulcer healing and its antiulcer effect is about 7 million times more potent on a molar basis than cimetidine. Because of the similarity of sucralfate to the repeating disaccharide structure of heparin and since bFGF is a heparin-binding growth factor, we tested the hypothesis that bFGF might bind to sucralfate.[6,7] To clarify the ensuing questions, both biochemical (*in vitro* and *in vivo*) and pharmacologic experiments were performed.

Biochemistry

In vitro and *in vivo* studies demonstrate that sucralfate binds to bFGF and protects it from proteolytic degradation. Namely, in the presence of sucralfate or SOS, bFGF showed increased resistance against degradation by acid and pepsin, and exerted enhanced angiogenesis.

The initial *in vitro* experiments demonstrated that bFGF bound to heparin immobilized on Sepharose beads and could be eluted with a high concentration of NaCl of approximately 1.5 M.[6] In the subsequent assay, however, when insoluble granules of sucralfate were mixed with Sepharose beads to form a chromatographic column and bFGF was loaded onto the column, the peptide bound so avidly to sucralfate that it could not be

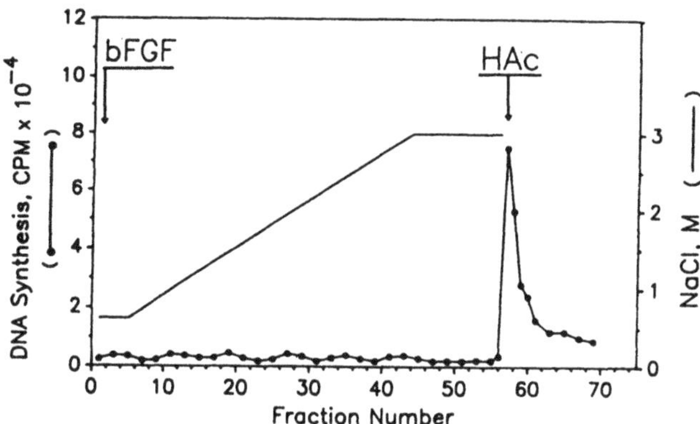

Figure 3. Elution of bFGF from a sucralfate–Sepharose column by acetic acid. The column was rinsed with a 10 ml Tris buffer and 0.6 M NaCl (80 ml) from 0.6 M to 3.0 M, (2) 20 ml of 3 M NaCl, and (3) 30 ml of 1.5 M acetic acid (pH 2.2). (Reproduced with permission from Folkman *et al.*[7])

removed by elution with up to 3 M NaCl (Fig. 3).[7] Thus, sucralfate had a higher affinity for bFGF than heparin, and bFGF was recovered from this column only by elution with 1.5 M acetic acid (pH 2.2). Acetic acid apparently dissolved the sucralfate and bFGF came out in the acidic solution. After this eluate was neutralized, diluted, and added directly to cultures of 3T3 fibroblasts, the eluted bFGF was highly mitogenic and retained its full biologic activity. Thus, although bFGF is normally degraded and inactivated by acid conditions, sucralfate protects bFGF at low pH.[7] The water-soluble SOS also protected the biologic activity of bFGF against acid degradation (Fig. 4). If bFGF was denatured by acid conditions before incubation with potassium SOS, however, bFGF biologic activity could not be recovered by addition of the SOS to the treated samples.[7] SOS (up to /200 μg/ml) neither increased nor decreased the mitogenic effect of bFGF under neutral pH conditions.

Thus, these *in vitro* biochemical experiments demonstrate that both sucralfate and its water-soluble variant SOS strongly bind bFGF which nonetheless can still exert its biologic effect.

In our animal experiments, the concentration of bFGF was also measured in the cysteamine model of duodenal ulceration with sucralfate.[7] After induction of duodenal ulcer by cysteamine-HCl (25 mg/100 g) three times on the first day, rats received oral sucralfate by gavage, 20 mg/100 g, twice daily for 7 days. These and control rats receiving the vehicle were killed on day 8. Sucralfate was gently washed away from the ulcer bed, and 1 g of stomach was then incubated in 5 ml NaCl 2.0 M (e.g., 500 mg stomach in 2.5 ml NaCl), plus 10 mM Tris at pH 7.0 to extract FGF from the tissues at 4°C for 12 hr. The extractant was centrifuged at 3000*g* for 30 min, and the supernatant was diluted fourfold with 10 mM Tris buffer to lower the salt concentration. The diluted supernatant was then applied to a heparin-affinity column. The column was rinsed with 0.6 M NaCl and eluted with 2.0 M NaCl, and the fractions were assayed for mitogenic activity on 3T3 fibroblasts. All of the mitogenic activity was in the 2.0 M NaCl fraction. The results demonstrate a significant increase of bFGF in the ulcer bed of sucralfate-treated rats compared with the control animals ($p < 0.001$) (Fig. 4). Furthermore, the ulcer beds of untreated animals had significantly more bFGF than normal duodenal or stomach mucosa ($p < 0.005$). The identity of the bFGF in the ulcer bed and in the mucosa was confirmed by Western blot analysis (Fig. 4).

These *in vivo* biochemical data demonstrate that sucralfate binds bFGF in the rat model of chronic duodenal ulceration as well. Furthermore, the bound bFGF is biologically active since it stimulated the proliferation of cultured fibroblasts.

Pharmacology

Following the *in vitro* and *in vivo* chemical binding studies with bFGF and sucralfate, we wanted to test if the combination of bFGF and sucralfate was more active in healing of experimental gastric and duodenal ulcers than either of the agents alone. We also tested the hypothesis that one of the mechanisms of this synergistic ulcer healing is the enhanced stimulation of angiogenesis by sucralfate and bFGF.

In the *in vivo* pharmacologic studies, animal models of chronic erosive gastritis and duodenal ulceration were used. We found, as a follow-up to our investigations on the gastroprotective role of sulfhydryls,[14,15] that ingestion of low concentrations of sulfhydryl

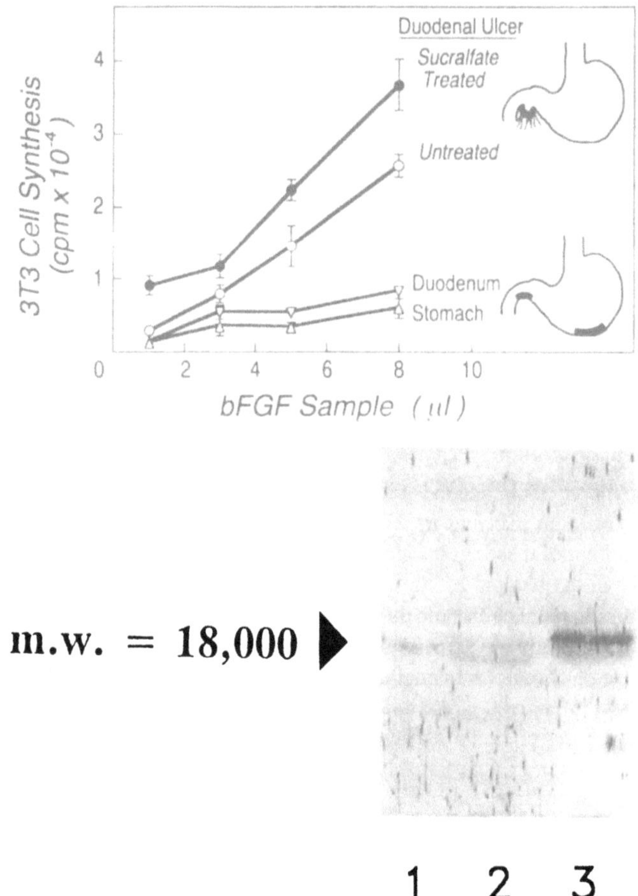

Figure 4. (Top) Effect of sucralfate on endogenous bFGF activity in the rat gastric mucosa. Duodenal ulcers were induced by cystamine and sucralfate was given by gavage (20 mg/100 g, twice daily for 7 days); animals were killed on day 8. One gram of stomach was then incubated in 5 ml NaCl 2.0 M to extract bFGF from the tissues at 4°C for 12 hr. The extractant was centrifuged and the supernatant was diluted fourfold with 10 mM Tris buffer to lower the salt concentration. The diluted supernatant was then applied to a heparin-affinity column. The column was rinsed with 0.6 M NaCl and eluted with 2.0 M NaCl, and the fractions were assayed for mitogenic activity on 3T3 fibroblasts. All of the mitogenic activity was in the 2.0 M NaCl fraction.

(Bottom) Western blot analysis of bFGF in rat stomach and duodenum. Fractions that eluted from the heparin-affinity column at approximately 1.5 M NaCl, which coincides with elution for pure bFGF, were then analyzed by Western blot analysis using a polyclonal antibody produced against the internal synthetic peptide of bFGF. Lane 1 shows bFGF control (18,000 molecular weight). Lane 2 is bFGF extracted from the duodenal ulcer of an untreated rat. Lane 3 is bFGF isolated from the ulcer bed of a sucralfate-treated rat. (Reproduced with permission from Folkman *et al.*[7])

alkylators (e.g., 0.1% iodoacetamide) in the drinking water induced severe, diffuse acute and chronic erosive gastritis in rats.[17] The lesions in the mucosa of the glandular stomach contain initially acute inflammatory cells such as leukocytes, mostly replaced by lymphocytes, plasma cells, and macrophages in the chronic stage of gastritis, which resembles the human alcoholic gastritis. We used this new animal model of gastritis to investigate the additive or synergistic therapeutic interaction of bFGF and sucralfate.

In these experiments, after induction of gastritis by the sulfhydryl alkylator 0.1% iodoacetamide in drinking water for 1 week, 60 rats were randomized to receive either (a) native bFGF–w (25 ng/100 g), (b) a site-specific mutated acid-stable bFGF–CS23 (25 ng/100 g), (c) low-dose sucralfate (5 mg/100 g), or (d) combinations of these agents by gavage twice daily. Untreated rats received vehicle only. All of the rats except controls remained on drinking water containing iodoacetamide for one more week. At autopsy on the 14th day macroscopic and histologic involvement of gastric glandular mucosa was quantified, and wet and dry stomach weights were obtained.[18]

The results (Table II) demonstrate that only acid-resistant bFGF was effective ($p < 0.05$). Neither native bFGF nor sucralfate had any effect at that low dose on chronic gastritis. Both native bFGF and the acid-resistant mutein in combination with sucralfate at a low dose were more efficient in the repair of mucosal injury and significantly more effective than either of these agents alone ($p < 0.001$). Thus, bFGF and sucralfate may act synergistically in the healing of chronic erosive gastritis.

In the animal model of chronic duodenal ulcer induced by cysteamine, sucralfate at 5 mg/100 g p.o. twice daily for 3 weeks was ineffective, while at 20 mg/100 g it significantly reduced the size of chronic duodenal ulcer by about 50%. Addition of a partially active dose of bFGF–w (50 ng/100 g p.o. twice daily for 3 weeks) resulted in a significant ulcer healing even by 5 mg of sucralfate, and marked improvement of the effect of 20 mg of sucralfate. Thus, our preliminary results with cysteamine-induced chronic duodenal ulcer demonstrate that sucralfate and bFGF exert additive, probably synergistic interaction.

One of the likely mechanisms of these interactions of sucralfate plus bFGF is the enhanced angiogenesis which is a key element in granulation tissue production and in ulcer healing. Angiogenesis can be quantitatively evaluated *in vivo* in sterile sponges

Table II. Effect of Oral Administration of bFGF and Sucralfate on the Chronic Gastritis Induced by Iodoacetamide in Rats[a]

Treatment	Chronic gastritis	Wet weight of stomach (g/100 g)
Control	Absent	0.66 ± 0.01
Vehicle	Extensive	0.84 ± 0.01
Sucralfate (5 mg/100 g)	Extensive	0.82 ± 0.03
bFGF–CS23 (25 ng)	Mild/healed	0.77 ± 0.02**
bFGF–wild (25 ng)	Extensive	0.82 ± 0.02
bFGF–wild + sucralfate	Mild/healed	0.70 ± 0.02*
bFGF–CS23 + sucralfate	Hardly detectable/healed	0.64 ± 0.02*

[a]Reproduced with permission from Szabo *et al.*[18]
*$p < 0.001$ versus vehicle; **$p < 0.005$ versus vehicle.

which contain the test compounds, and are implanted under the abdominal skin of rats. In our studies, six rounded sterile sponges (8×3 mm) which contained vehicle, sucralfate and/or bFGF (added in 100 μl to the sponges before implantation) were placed under the abdominal skin of Sprague–Dawley rats. The rats were killed on the 7th day, the sponges removed and fixed in 10% buffered formalin, cut and stained with hematoxylin and eosin and for the endothelial specific factor VIII. The number of newly developed blood vessels were counted in the ingrowing part of the sponges in at least seven areas where dense vessels (No./mm^2) were seen: vehicle 40.4 ± 4.3, sucralfate (5 mg) 59.4 ± 7.0*, bFGF (25 ng) 46.9 ± 5.1, bFGF (250 ng) 137.1 ± 5.3**, sucralfate + bFGF (25 ng) 162.2 ± 10.1**(++), sucralfate + bFGF (250 ng) 281.1 ± 12.2**(++), *$p < 0.05$, **$p < 0.001$ versus vehicle, $^{(++)}p < 0.001$ versus sucralfate.

We conclude from these assays that sucralfate alone accelerated angiogenesis which was significantly enhanced by combination with an ineffective dose of bFGF. The same dose of sucralfate combined with an angiogenic dose of bFGF also resulted in synergistic stimulation (e.g., more than five fold) of angiogenesis. We thus postulate that this synergistic enhancement of angiogenesis and granulation tissue production by sucralfate and bFGF may have a role in the mechanisms of ulcer healing by sucralfate.

Summary

Sulfhydryls were the second endogenous mediators, after the prostaglandins, implicated on the basis of pharmacologic studies in the mechanism of acute gastroprotection by sucralfate. Recent biochemical experiments confirmed these implications since a gastroprotective dose of sucralfate elevated the concentration of glutathione in the gastric mucosa, but not liver of fasted rats. New *in vitro* and *in vivo* experiments also demonstrate that sucralfate, because of its chemical similarity to heparin, avidly binds bFGF and delivers it in large concentrations to the site of experimental duodenal ulceration. Administration of natural or synthetic bFGF not only rapidly accelerated the healing of cysteamine-induced chronic duodenal ulcers, but joint treatment with low doses of bFGF plus sucralfate resulted in synergistic ulcer healing and stimulation of angiogenesis. Thus, mucosal sulfhydryls, especially glutathione, are one of the endogenous mediators of acute mucosal protection by sucralfate, while bFGF contributes to the chronic ulcer healing by this locally acting drug.

References

1. Nagashima R: Mechanisms of action of sucralfate. *J Clin Gastroenterol* **3**:117–127, 1981. A good general overview of the mechanisms of action, emphasizing the early stages of research which are usually not covered in contemporary reviews.
2. Koba H, Yamamoto R, Nakano H: History of the development of sucralfate. *Dig Dis Sci* **35**:A10, 1990. A brief summary of discovery and early development of sucralfate.
3. Hollander D, Tarnawski A: Protective effect of sucralfate on the gastric mucosa mediated by endogenous prostaglandins, in Szabo S, Mózsik G (eds): *New Pharmacology of Ulcer Disease: Experimental and New Therapeutic Approaches*. Amsterdam, Elsevier, 1987, pp 404–412. First

review of the experimental data implicating mucosal prostaglandins in the acute gastroprotective effect of sucralfate.

4. Szabo S, Brown A: Prevention of ethanol-induced vascular injury and gastric mucosal lesions by sucralfate and its components: Possible role of endogenous sulfhydryls. *Proc Soc Exp Biol Med* **185:** 493–497, 1987. Rat study demonstrating that the gastroprotective action of sucralfate is mediated in part by a sulfhydryl-sensitive process counteracted by the sulfhydryl alkylator *N*-ethylmaleimide. It was also shown that sulfate and sucrose octasulfate are the most potent gastroprotective components of sucralfate, and that the early ethanol-induced vascular injury is preventable not only by sucralfate, but by its components as well, especially sulfates.
5. Nexo E, Poulsen SS: Does epidermal growth factor play a role in the action of sucralfate? *Scand J Gastroenterol* **22:**45–49, 1987. First implications that epidermal growth factor may mediate part of the acute gastroprotection by sucralfate.
6. Folkman J, Szabo S, Shing Y: Sucralfate affinity for fibroblast growth factor. *J Cell Biol* **111:**A203, 1990. Brief summary of first *in vitro* data demonstrating that bFGF binds not only to heparin, but also to sucralfate which structurally resembles heparin.
7. Folkman J, Szabo S, Stovroff M, *et al*: Duodenal ulcer: Discovery of a new mechanism and development of angiogenic therapy that accelerates healing. *Ann Surg* **214:**414–426, 1991. Extensive *in vitro* and *in vivo* studies on sucralfate binding of bFGF, and demonstration of elevated level of bFGF in chronic duodenal ulcers treated with sucralfate in rats.
8. Folkman J, Klagsbrun M: Angiogenic factors. *Science* **235:**442–447, 1987. Review of peptides, steroids, and other molecules that influence angiogenesis.
9. Szabo S, Vattay P, Morales RE, *et al*: Orally administered bFGF mutein: Effect on healing of chronic duodenal ulcers in rats. *Dig Dis Sci* **34:**1323, 1989. First brief summary of experimental data demonstrating the potent ulcer healing effect of bFGF in the cysteamine-induced duodenal ulcer model.
10. Szabo S, Folkman J, Vattay P, *et al*: Duodenal ulcerogens: Effect of FGF on cysteamine-induced duodenal ulcer, in Halter F, Garner A, Tytgat GNJ (eds): *Mechanisms of Peptic Ulcer Healing*. London, Kluwer Academic Publishers, 1991, pp 139–150. Review of animal models of duodenal ulceration, and the first overview of the very potent ulcer healing properties of bFGF in rats with experimental duodenal ulcer.
11. Szabo S: The mode of action of sucralfate: The 1 × 1 × 1 mechanism of action. *Scand J Gastroenterol* **26:**7–12, 1991. Detailed and critical review of the mechanisms of actions of sucralfate emphasizing that not all actions of the drug are equally important for acute gastroprotection and healing of chronic ulcers. It is proposed that prevention of vascular injury, maintenance of blood flow allowing rapid epithelial restitution are key mechanisms for *acute* gastroprotection, while local binding and concentration of growth factors such as bFGF and EGF are the key elements of stimulated *chronic* ulcer healing by sucralfate.
12. Szabo S, Vattay P, Scarbrough E, *et al*: Role of vascular factors, including angiogenesis, in the mechanisms of action of sucralfate. *Am J Med* **91:**158S–160S, 1991. Demonstration of enhanced angiogenesis and granulation tissue production in subcutaneously implanted sponges in rats: sucralfate was more potent than the water-soluble sucrose octasulfate, and less potent than pure bFGF.
13. Meister A: On the antioxidant effects of ascorbic acid and glutathione. *Biochem Pharmacol* **44**(suppl 10)**:**1905–1915, 1992. General review of protective effect of sulfhydryls such as glutathione and vitamin C.
14. Szabo S, Trier JS, Frankel PW: Sulfhydryl compounds may mediate gastric cytoprotection. *Science* **214:**200–202, 1981. First *in vivo* demonstration that administration of sulfhydryls exerts acute gastroprotection in rats, while subcutaneous injection of sulfhydryl alkylators counteracted the "cytoprotection" by prostaglandins.
15. Dupuy D, Szabo S: Protection by metals against ethanol-induced gastric mucosal injury in the rat. Comparative biochemical and pharmacologic studies implicate protein sulfhydryls. *Gastroenterol-*

ogy **91**:966–974, 1986. First demonstration that not only glutathione but protein sulfhydryls may have a role in the protection of gastric mucosa.

16. Nagata M, Sandor Z, Kusstatscher S, *et al*: Selective increase in glutathione concentration in gastric mucosa after sucralfate administration. *Gastroenterology* 1994 (in press). An abstract describing the selective elevation of mucosal glutathione concentration after a gastroprotective dose of sucralfate in rats.
17. Szabo S, Trier JS, Brown A, *et al*: Sulfhydryl blockers induce severe inflammatory gastritis in the rat. *Gastroenterology* **86**:1271, 1984. Brief report on the induction of diffuse chronic erosive gastritis by ingesting sulfhydryl alkylators such as iodoacetamide in drinking water in rats.
18. Szabo S, Kusstatscher S, Stovroff M: Role of bFGF and angiogenesis in ulcer healing and the treatment of gastritis, in Domschke W, Konturek SJ (eds): *The Stomach: Physiology, Pathophysiology and Treatment*. Berlin, Springer-Verlag, 1993, pp 193–197. Brief review on the effect of oral treatment with bFGF and/or sucralfate in the treatment of experimental chronic gastritis induced by iodoacetamide in rats.
19. Sandor Z, Kusstatscher S, Karaoli T, *et al*: Synergistic angiogenesis after joint administration of sucralfate and bFGF in rats. *FASEB J* 1994 (in press). Abstract describing the first results on the synergistic angiogenesis by sucralfate and bFGF in the subcutaneous sponge assay in rats.

17

Effects of Sucralfate on Growth Factor Availability

STANISLAW J. KONTUREK, JAN W. KONTUREK, TOMASZ BRZOZOWSKI, BRONISLAW L. SLOMIANY, and AMELIA SLOMIANY

Introduction

The maintenance of gastric mucosal integrity under an adverse environment of luminal contents depends on the delicate balance of numerous factors that control the mucosal defense lines such as mucus–alkaline secretion, mucosal hydrophobicity, rich mucosal blood flow, maintenance of mucosal sulfhydryls, rapid restitution of epithelial cells, proliferation of mucosal cells, and tissue repair.

Primary among these are epidermal growth factor (EGF), transforming growth factor alpha (TGFα), platelet-derived growth factor (PDGF), and basic fibroblast growth factor (bFGF). These factors have been identified in the gastric mucosa and found to exhibit the protective, mitogenic, and angiogenic activities that appear to be essential for the proliferation in the normal mucosa as well as for the reepithelialization, repair, and healing processes occurring in the damaged or ulcerated mucosa.

Although growth factors differ in structure, origin, and sensitivity to luminal degradation, the common mechanism of their action on target cells is the interaction with specific high-affinity membrane receptors. The binding of growth factors to their receptors generates a signal that is amplified and transduced to activate cytoplasmic regulatory proteins which then alter gene expression and induce the biological responses. In case of EGF and TGFα, the ligands bind to the same receptors and this results in the activation of intrinsic receptor tyrosine kinase and autophosphorylation of receptor that appears to be a central event in mediating the biological affects of EGF and TGFα (Fig. 1).

STANISLAW J. KONTUREK, JAN W. KONTUREK, and TOMASZ BRZOZOWSKI • Institute of Physiology, University School of Medicine, Krakow, Poland. BRONISLAW L. SLOMIANY and AMELIA SLOMIANY • Research Center, University of Medicine and Dentistry, Newark, New Jersey.

Sucralfate: From Basic Science to the Bedside, edited by Daniel Hollander and G. N. J. Tytgat. Plenum Press, New York, 1995.

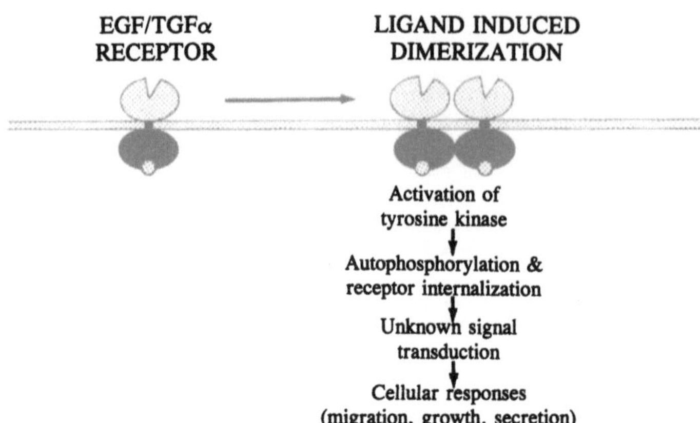

Figure 1. The action of growth factors such as EGF or TGFα includes the binding to a common receptor, activation of tyrosine kinase, and autophosphorylation of receptor with subsequent intracellular signal transduction and final cellular responses.

The pharmacological agents that are capable of protecting the growth factors from their degradation by acid–pepsin secretion in the gastric lumen, influencing their binding to the receptors or affecting the expression of these receptors, may alter the biological action of growth factors on the gastric mucosa. Among the agents of this category is sucralfate, the therapeutic effects of which until recently have been linked to the formation of a protective "barrier" over the eroded mucosa and binding of aggressive factors such as pepsin and bile acid. Recent findings indicate that sucralfate affects numerous mucosal functions including the mucus–alkaline secretion, strengthening of apical mucosal barrier, mucosal blood flow, prostaglandin biosynthesis, proliferation of mucosal cells, repair and healing of mucosal lesions and ulcerations. These effects depend, in part, on the prolongation of the luminal bioavailability of growth factors and increased expression of their receptors in the mucosa. Sucralfate may also bind bFGF and protect it from the acid degradation to allow for its accumulation in the area of gastric lesions and the acceleration of angiogenesis and repair of the mucosa (Fig. 2).

In this review we describe the biochemical and physiological mechanisms underlying the protective and ulcer healing effects of sucralfate with special emphasis placed on the implication of growth factors present in the stomach.

Growth Factors in the Gastric Mucosa—Origin and Spectrum of Biological Action

Gastric Mucosal Growth and Its Control

Gastric mucosa is one of the most rapidly proliferating tissues in the body. Migration, proliferation, and growth of mucosal cells are balanced by continuous cell loss through

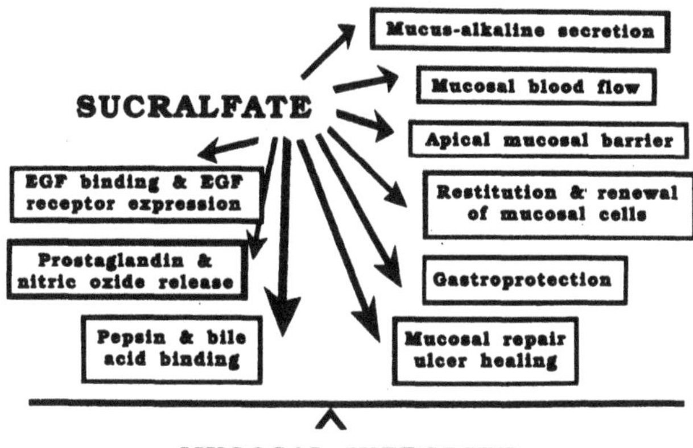

Figure 2. The spectrum of biological effects of sucralfate (on right) and its possible mechanisms of action (on left) resulting in the maintenance of mucosal integrity.

exfoliation so that under normal conditions, the population of mucosal cells is maintained by a dynamic steady state. Because of the rapid turnover of mucosal cells, any imbalance between cell growth and cell loss, e.g., after exposure to topical irritants, may lead to mucosal injury, erosions, or ulcerations.

The growth of the mucosa is controlled by a variety of factors including nongastrointestinal hormones such as growth hormone and gut hormones such as gastrin and somatostatin and polypeptide growth factors, particularly EGF, TGFα, PDGF, and bFGF that may be brought into play especially following mucosal damage to facilitate mucosal cell restitution, repair and healing through endocrine or local paracrine or exocrine (luminal) pathway.

Certain antiulcer drugs may also affect the mucosal growth either by stimulation of the release of growth-promoting gut hormones such as gastrin (e.g., histamine H_2-receptor antagonists or proton pump inhibitors) or by enhancing the release and receptor expression of EGF and other polypeptide growth factors (e.g., sucralfate).

EGF, TGFα, PDGF, and bFGF in the Gastric Mucosa

EGF is a 53-amino-acid polypeptide that was originally discovered by Cohen[1] in mouse salivary glands and then found to resemble urogastrone (extract of urine from pregnant women showing a beneficial effect on healing of experimental ulcers) in chemical structure and the spectrum of biological action; hence, the common name EGF/URO has been proposed.[2–4]

In the digestive system, EGF has been detected in large quantities in the salivary glands, Brunner's glands, and the pancreas. It is stored in the tubular or ductal cells and released into saliva and duodenopancreatic secretion so the EGF present in the gastric lumen originates mainly from the salivary secretion.

EGF-like immunoreactivity has also been detected in the gastric mucosa but it is not clear whether it is normally produced locally in the mucosa or simply taken up from the gastric lumen. Several studies reported that chronic gastrointestinal ulcerations are accompanied by an increased expression of EGF and EGF receptors, especially within the area of mucosal lesions and ulcers.[3] Certain drugs, especially sucralfate, were reported to enhance the accumulation of EGF in the ulcer area to promote cell proliferation, angiogenesis, and healing. Wright *et al.*[5] showed that the ulceration of epithelium anywhere in the gastrointestinal mucosa induces the development of a novel cell lineage from the stem cells and this lineage contains and secretes abundant immunoreactive EGF/URO. It was proposed that a principal *in vivo* role for EGF is the local regeneration and ulcer healing. Other studies showed, however, only negligible EGF-immunoreactivity and the absence of EGF mRNA expression either in intact or injured gastric mucosa indicating that the gastric mucosa has no ability to express EGF and that EGF observed in the ulcer area may be simply taken up from the gastric lumen.[6]

The major form of growth factor in the gastric mucosa was found to be TGFα, which is a 50-amino-acid polypeptide showing about 35% sequence homology, a common receptor, and nearly identical spectrum of biological activity with EGF. Mucosal damage markedly increased the TGFα mRNA expression and the local production and release of TGFα into the gastric lumen suggesting that TGFα, not EGF, is the major growth factor produced in the intact and injured gastric mucosa.

Another growth factor that may be implicated in the maintenance of mucosal integrity is PDGF, a glycoprotein composed of two peptide chains (A and B) linked by disulfide bonds. It constitutes the major mitogenic activity in platelets and shows a similar spectrum of biological action to EGF including direct stimulation of growth of connective tissue cells and endothelial and epithelial cells, mucosal repair, and wound or ulcer healing. It may be the first growth factor released locally in the area of gastric lesions by platelets and macrophages.

bFGF, a 146-amino-acid polypeptide, was also demonstrated in intact and damaged mucosa and proposed to participate in mucosal repair, particularly when this labile peptide is protected from acid degradation in the gastric lumen by antiulcer agents such as sucralfate or antacids.[7] This peptide is produced by a variety of cells including fibroblasts, endothelial cells, and smooth muscle cells and is stored in extracellular matrix to be released on tissue damage or remodeling and to stimulate locally the proliferation of these cells. The role of bFGF in mucosal repair has yet to be proven but recent studies of Folkman *et al.*[7] suggest that bFGF plays a crucial role in angiogenesis in the granulation tissue at the ulcer bed. The relative contribution of each of the growth factors encountered in the stomach in the maintenance of mucosal integrity, growth, repair, and healing requires further studies.

Involvement of Growth Factors in the Function and Integrity of Gastric Mucosa

EGF, TGFα, and PDGF administered parenterally *in vivo* are very potent inhibitors of gastric acid secretion; however, receptors involved in this inhibition are located on the basolateral membrane of parietal cells so they may not be available for these factors present in the gastric lumen. EGF and other growth factors have been detected only in minute concentrations in the blood present partly as a free plasma peptide and partly bound to platelets. Studies *in vitro* on the isolated gastric glands or parietal cells confirmed that EGF is a direct inhibitor of acid production induced by histamine and other secretagogues. The inhibition of acid production is very rapid and does not require continuous exposure to EGF as in the case of stimulation of cell proliferation suggesting that the transduction of signal from the receptors of the acid transport system in the parietal cells is very rapid.

Since it is unlikely that EGF and other growth factors are released in physiologically important amounts to affect gastric acid secretion, there is considerable interest in the luminal effects of endogenous EGF delivered to the stomach in saliva or local effects of TGFα, PDGF, and bFGF released in the gastric mucosa. EGF, TGFα and PDGF are acid-stable and relatively resistant to pepsin degradation so they are attractive candidates to participate in mucosal integrity, even without affecting gastric acid secretion. The spectrum of their biological effects includes the stimulation of mucus–alkaline secretion, strengthening of the apical mucosal barrier to acid and pepsin backdiffusion, the increase in mucosal blood flow, stimulation of rapid restitution of and renewal of mucosal cells, gastroprotection against various topical irritants and ulcerogens, and the acceleration of healing of acute and chronic gastric ulcerations (Fig. 3).

All biological effects of EGF and related peptides are mediated by specific receptors on the target cells. It is of interest that the activation of EGF receptors in the mucosal cells leads to the stimulation of calcium channel activity through the phosphorylation of channel proteins.[8] Calcium is an important regulatory element for many cellular processes including cell integrity and secretion so certain biological effects of EGF could be related to the activation of calcium channel by this peptide (Fig. 4). The influx of calcium into the mucosal cells caused by the exposure to ethanol may result in the calcium imbalance and

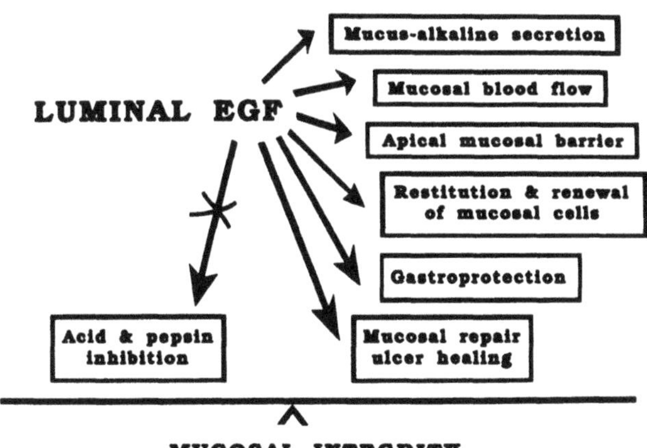

Figure 3. Luminal EGF in the stomach does not affect gastric acid secretion but results in various biological effects on the gastric mucosa similar to those observed after administration of sucralfate.

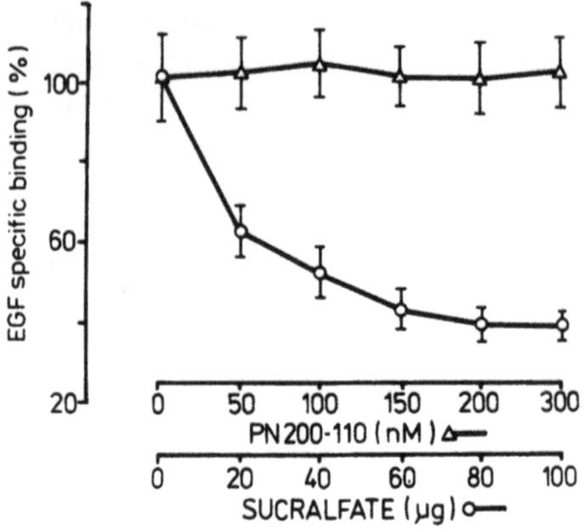

Figure 4. Effect of sucralfate on the EGF binding to gastric mucosal calcium channel protein. Sucralfate exerts an inhibitory effect on the EGF binding to receptor and reduces dose-dependently calcium uptake whereas the calcium channel receptor antagonist PN200-110 had no effect on EGF binding.

cell damage. The ability of sucralfate to reduce calcium uptake through the inhibition of EGF-stimulated gastric mucosal calcium channel may explain, at least in part, the protective activity of this drug (Fig. 5).

Role of Growth Factors in Gastroprotection

The hypothesis that salivary EGF participates in the repair and healing of gastric mucosal injury is suggested by studies in salivectomized rats. These rats have atrophic gastric mucosa and show the absence of adaptive cytoprotection to mild irritants and delayed healing of acute and chronic gastric ulcerations that may be reversed by oral or parenteral EGF as well as by TGFα and PDGF but not bFGF. Salivectomy increases the susceptibility of gastric mucosa to the formation of acute lesions by various irritants and to abolish the adaptive cytoprotection.[3] These studies suggest a close link between the

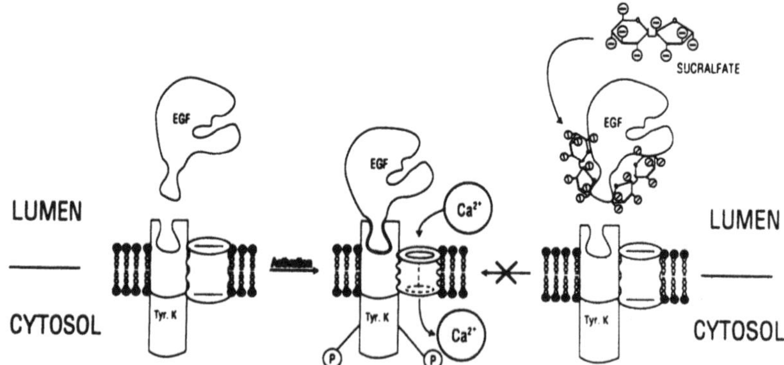

Figure 5. Schematic presentation of the binding of EGF to calcium channel protein and the inhibitory influence of sucralfate on this binding.

salivary EGF and gastric mucosal biosynthesis of prostaglandins that have been implicated in this cytoprotection. Furthermore, removal of salivary glands reduced the ability of the gastric mucosa to adapt to various ulcerogens such as aspirin. The reduction in gastric EGF after salivectomy was accompanied by a decrease in DNA synthesis and DNA contents suggesting that the decrease in mucosal growth-promoting action of EGF is responsible for the increased sensitivity of the mucosa to damaging agents and the loss of gastric adaptation.

The importance of endogenous EGF, TGFα, or PDGF in the protection of gastric mucosa has been emphasized by numerous investigators. EGF given parenterally prevented the formation of acute mucosal lesions induced by various ulcerogens such as absolute ethanol, acidified aspirin, bile acids, or stress (Fig. 6). This protection was also observed by some investigators after intragastric administration of these growth factors but it was less pronounced and occurred when gastric lesions were produced by less severe ulcerogens such as acidified aspirin, taurocholate, or stress but not necrotizing agents such as absolute ethanol. Administration of bFGF failed to protect the mucosa against any topical irritant or ulcerogen.

The role of luminal EGF in gastroprotection is supported by studies reporting that the removal of salivary glands leads to a dramatic fall in EGF content in gastric lumen (Fig. 7).

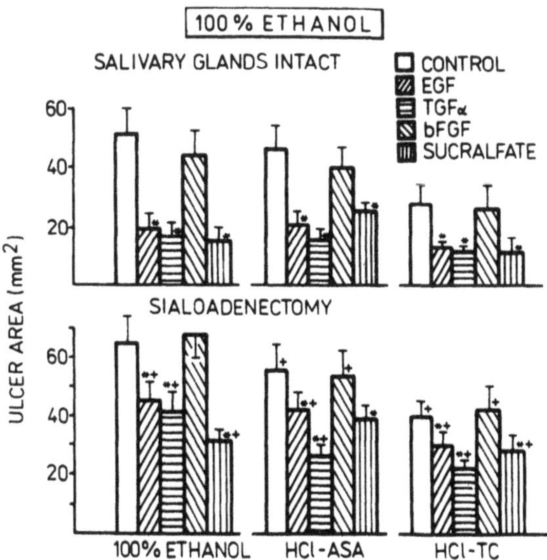

Figure 6. Effects of EGF, TGFα and bFGF (infused s.c. in a dose of 100 μg/kg per hr) or sucralfate (given in a dose of 100 mg/kg i.g.) on the area of acute gastric lesions induced by 100% ethanol (1.5 ml), acidified aspirin (ASA) (200 mg/kg in 1.5 ml of 0.15 mM HCl), or acidified taurocholate (80 mM taurocholate in 1.5 ml of 0.15 mM HCl) in rats with intact or resected salivary glands. Means ± S.E.M. of 8–10 rats. Asterisk indicates significant ($p < 0.05$) decrease below the vehicle control value. Cross indicates significant increase above the values obtained in similar experiments in rats with intact salivary glands.

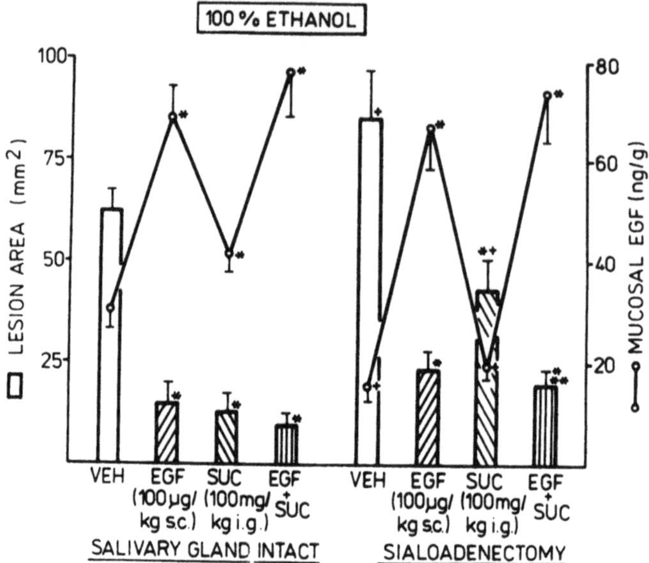

Figure 7. Effects of EGF (100 μg/kg per hr s.c.), sucralfate (100 mg/kg i.g.), or their combination on the area of ethanol-induced gastric lesions and mucosal content of immunoreactive EGF in rats with intact or excised salivary glands. Means ± S.E.M. of 8–10 rats. Asterisk indicates significant decrease below the vehicle control value. Cross indicates significant increase above the value obtained in similar experiments in rats with intact salivary glands. Double asterisks indicate significant decrease below the value obtained with sucralfate alone in rats with resected salivary glands.

Such salivectomy did not produce spontaneous gastric lesions but greatly augmented the formation of the ulcerations induced by various ulcerogens (cysteamine) and topical irritants (aspirin, bile acids, 100% ethanol). Because the intragastric application of saliva-containing EGF or EGF alone prevented the formation of the lesions, it has been postulated that EGF in saliva is an active gastroprotective component. Addition of sucralfate enhanced the protective action of EGF only in salivectomized rats but not in animals with intact salivary glands. This suggests that under normal conditions, the amount of EGF released into the stomach is sufficient for sucralfate to exhibit its maximal protective activity.

Role of Growth Factors in Healing of Chronic Gastric Ulcerations

As mentioned previously, the beneficial action of urogastrone on healing of chronic peptic ulcerations was recognized long ago and it was clearly dissociated from the gastric inhibitory effect of this substance. More recently, it was shown that EGF also accelerates the healing of chronic duodenal ulcers induced by cysteamine in rats. This acceleration was comparable to that of cimetidine but not accompanied by any change in gastric secretion (unlike cimetidine) suggesting that EGF acted directly on the mucosa via promotion of mucosal growth and reepithelialization. EGF and other growth factors enhanced ulcer healing while salivectomy delayed the healing process and this could be reversed by the addition of growth factors to salivectomized rats (Fig. 8). The finding that EGF and other growth factors administered orally enhanced ulcer healing and reversed the delay of healing in salivectomized animals as well as normalized mucosal growth emphasizes an important role of cell renewal in EGF-induced promotion of the healing process. We showed that the induction of ODC activity is probably involved because blocking of ODC by DFMO almost completely reversed the acceleration of ulcer healing by EGF. As EGF accumulates in the ulcer area either by adsorption of the peptide from the gastric contents or by local production related to novel EGF-secreting cells, it is likely that it promotes local cell renewal and proliferation in the ulcer bed.

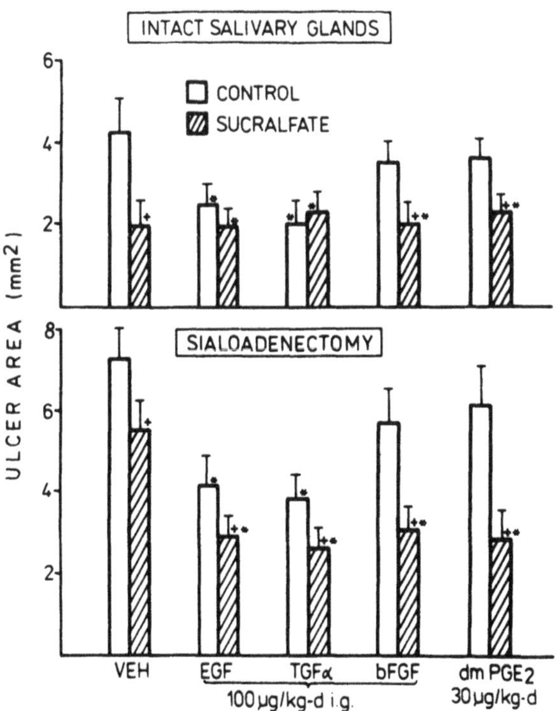

Figure 8. Effects of intragastric (i.g.) administration of EGF, TGFα or bFGF (100 μg/kg per day) or dimethyl PGE_2 (30 μg/kg per day) without (control) or with concurrent sucralfate (400 mg/kg per day) on the area of chronic gastric ulcers induced by acetic acid in rats with intact or resected salivary glands. Initial area of gastric ulcer was about 28 mm^2 and the examination of the effects of tested substances was made after 7 days of treatment. Asterisk indicates significant decrease below the vehicle control value. Cross indicates significant decrease below the value obtained in tests without administration of sucralfate.

Interaction of Growth Factors with Sucralfate

Sucralfate as Mucosoprotectant and Ulcer Healing Agent

Sucralfate, a basic aluminum salt of the sulfated disaccharide sucrose, is widely used as an antiulcer drug because it accelerates ulcer healing but does not reduce gastric acid secretion nor neutralize luminal acid. Its mechanism of action is not clear except that it is known to bind to the ulcer bed. After acidification such as occurs following intragastric administration, sucralfate becomes a viscous and adhesive substance tightly bound to eroded or ulcerated mucosa. In eroded areas the surface epithelial cells are lost and positively charged uncovered tissue proteins attract the negatively charged sucralfate particles.

Formation of a protective barrier by sucralfate over injured, eroded, or ulcerated mucosa together with the inhibition of pepsin activity and adsorption of pepsin and bile salts was initially postulated as the major mechanisms for the healing action of sucralfate. The main site of sucralfate action was claimed to be the eroded or ulcerated areas of the mucosa.

The concept of a "Band-Aid" action of sucralfate cannot explain, however, the ability of this drug to prevent the formation of acute mucosal injury induced by a variety of topical irritants and necrotizing substances because in all of these instances sucralfate is given before the development of mucosal lesions or ulcerations. Indeed, pretreatment with sucralfate reduces in a dose-dependent manner the formation of acute mucosal lesions induced by acid-dependent (e.g., aspirin, bile acids, stress) and acid-independent (e.g., absolute ethanol) ulcerogens (see Fig. 6). This protective activity depends on the presence of an acidic pH in the gastric lumen and the acidification of sucralfate or active stimulation of acid secretion greatly augments the protective properties of sucralfate while the inhibition or neutralization of gastric acid attenuates this protection.

Implication of Prostaglandins, Nitric Oxide, and Growth Factors in Gastroprotective Activity of Sucralfate

Sequential analysis of the mucosal changes showed that sucralfate did not prevent the excessive exfoliation of surface epithelium caused by topical irritants but protected deeper mucosal layers including the proliferative zone cells and mucosal microvessels. The morphological and functional features of sucralfate's protection of the gastric mucosa against ethanol-induced necrosis are similar to those obtained with prostaglandin (PG) suggesting that endogenous PG mediate, at least in part, the protective action of sucralfate. This is supported by the observations that (1) the pretreatment with indomethacin, an inhibitor of PG biosynthesis, reduced the protective effect of sucralfate and (2) sucralfate increased significantly mucosal generation and luminal release of PG both in animals and in humans.

If the protective action of sucralfate is mediated entirely by the release of mucosal PG, which play a key role in gastric mucosal protection, then the mucosal damage induced by nonsteroidal anti-inflammatory agents (NSAID) such as aspirin or indomethacin, which almost completely inhibit PG biosynthesis, should abolish the protective action of sucralfate. Although sucralfate cannot induce the release of PG from a mucosa in which PG biosynthesis has been blocked by NSAID, it displayed the mucosal protection against NSAID damage both in animals and in humans. Furthermore, the augmented gastroprotective action of acidified sucralfate cannot be reversed by the treatment with indomethacin. The PG independence of the mucosal protection afforded by acidified sucralfate is also evident from the fact that the mucosal lesions induced by aspirin that caused almost complete suppression of PG were also attenuated by acidified sucralfate. Also, stress-induced mucosal lesions, which are accompanied by a marked decrease in mucosal generation of PG, were found to be prevented by acidified sucralfate. These findings indicate that there may be other mechanisms of action of sucralfate which obviously are independent of PG or that some of its protective activity is mediated by other mechanisms.

The mucosal microvasculature plays a vital role in supplying the mucosa with oxygen and nutrients. Sucralfate was reported to increase gastric mucosal blood flow in both normal and injured mucosa. Although the protection of gastric microvasculature and increased blood flow to the mucosa by sucralfate could be partly reversed by the pretreatment with indomethacin and, therefore, attributed to the endogenous PG, recent studies suggest that these effects of sucralfate may also be mediated by endogenous nitric oxide (NO), another locally acting hyperemic and mucosoprotective substance. Blocking of NO synthase by L-nitro-arginine analogue reversed the gastroprotective and hyperemic effects of sucralfate at its native and acidic pHs (Fig. 9). Concurrent administration of

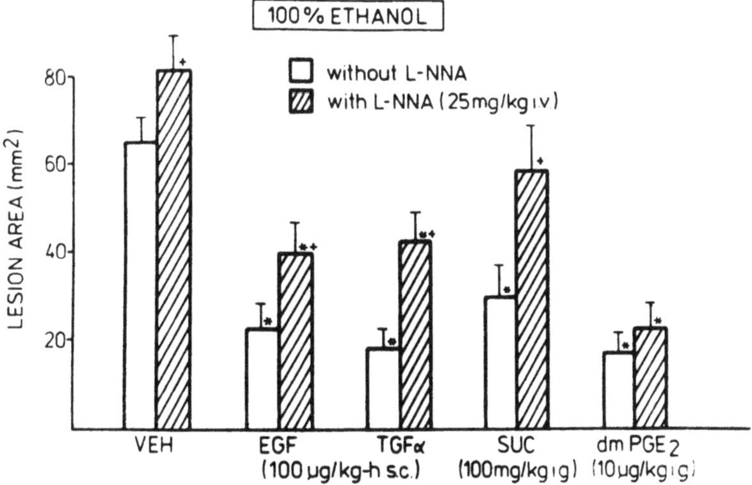

Figure 9. Effects of EGF (100 μg/kg per hr s.c.), TGFα (100 μg/kg per hr s.c.), sucralfate (200 mg/kg i.g.), or 16,16-dimethyl PGE_2 (10 μg/kg i.g.) on ethanol-induced gastric lesions in rats without or with administration of L-NNA (25 mg/kg i.v.) 15 min before the administration of EGF, TGFα sucralfate, or $dmPGE_2$. Means ± S.E.M. of 8–10 rats. Asterisk indicates significant decrease below the vehicle control value. Cross indicates significant increase above the value obtained in rats without administration of L-NNA.

L-arginine but not D-arginine restored the protective activity of acidified sucralfate against ethanol damage.[9] The suppression of both the PG system with indomethacin and the NO system with L-nitro-arginine completely eliminates the protective activity of sucralfate, suggesting that these two systems closely interact on the integrity of gastric mucosal cells and the maintenance of mucosal circulation. It is of interest that the NO system seems to participate also in the gastroprotection by growth factors such as EGF or TGFα, indicating again that the protective mechanism of growth factors on the gastric mucosa involves similar mediators as sucralfate. In contrast to growth factors, the gastroprotection induced by exogenous methylated PGE_2 analogue does not appear to be mediated by the NO system.

The gastroprotective activity of sucralfate as well as growth factors against ethanol damage can also be eliminated by pretreatment with *N*-ethylmaleimide (NEM), the sulfhydryl alkylator (Fig. 10). Since this agent reversed the protection by exogenous PG, it is likely that the first biological effect of sucralfate is binding to endogenous sulfhydryls which could be considered as common final mediator in the mucosal protection by other agents.

Interaction of Sucralfate and Growth Factors in Mucosal Repair and Ulcer Healing

Experimental studies in animals demonstrated that more prolonged exposure of the gastric mucosa to sucralfate produces the functional and morphological changes in normal or ulcerated mucosa that are indistinguishable from those evoked by growth factors, especially EGF and TGFα.

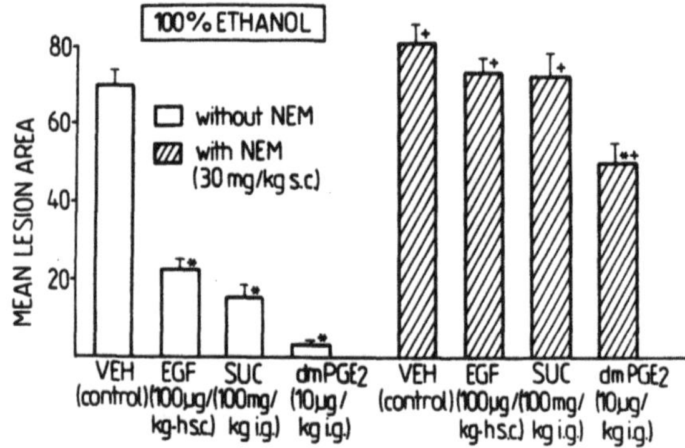

Figure 10. Effects of EGF (100 µg/kg per hr s.c.), sucralfate (100 mg/kg i.g.), or 16,16-dimethyl PGE_2 (10 µg/kg i.g.) on ethanol-induced gastric lesions in rats without or with administration of *N*-ethylmaleimide (NEM) (30 mg/kg s.c.). Means ± S.E.M. of 8–10 rats. Asterisk indicates significant decrease below the vehicle control value. Cross indicates significant increase above the value obtained in corresponding experiments in rats without administration of NEM.

New data of the mucus secretion indicate that sucralfate, similarly as EGF or TGFα, is capable of initiating a chain of events linking extracellular signals to intracellular responses. They activate a cascade of regulatory protein phosphorylation, the process closely associated with cellular proliferative activities. Slomiany *et al.*,[8] who first provided evidence of the presence of EGF receptors in gastric mucosa, also demonstrated that the administration of sucralfate results in the increase in gastric expression of EGF and TGFα receptors (Fig. 11). Gastric mucosal cell membranes isolated from the stomach of rats receiving sucralfate twice daily for 3 consecutive days (200 mg/kg per day) revealed over 50% increase in specific EGF and TGF binding as compared with vehicle-treated controls. Examination of protein tyrosine phosphorylation patterns using antiphosphotyrosine antibody revealed that EGF, TGFα, and PDGF caused a marked increase in protein phosphorylation and the phosphoprotein profiles obtained with EGF were quite similar to those obtained with TGFα or PDGF. This indicates that these growth factors exert their action through a common receptor in gastric mucosal cells.

The demonstration that the gastric mucosal cell membranes from the stomach exposed to sucralfate show a significant increase in EGF, TGFα and PDGF specific receptor binding attests to the effect of sucralfate on the mucosal cell proliferation. This effect until now has been attributed solely to the drug's ability to bind growth factors and to prolong their luminal availability. Indeed, sucralfate was found to be capable of coprecipitating with EGF, TGFα, PDGF, and bFGF in a pH-dependent manner so that with the decrease of pH below 4.5 such as occurs in the gastric lumen, most luminal growth factors are bound to sucralfate (Fig. 12). This binding of luminal EGF (delivered to the stomach in saliva) or TGFα, PDGF, and bFGF (produced and released by gastric mucosa) seems to be an important factor since sucralfate also chelates selectively with proteinaceous material in the eroded or ulcerated mucosa to form a dense coating on the base of the injured mucosa. This is supported by the observation that radiolabeled EGF or TGFα introduced into the stomach accumulates in severalfold higher amounts that in the intact mucosa. Thus, high concentrations of EGF and other growth factors in the injured or ulcerated mucosa treated with sucralfate originate from the expression of a higher number of specific receptors for these growth factors as well as from the accumulation of these

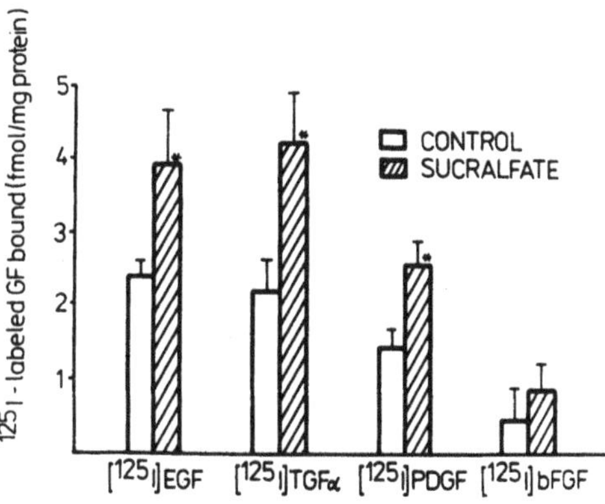

Figure 11. Effects of prolonged administration of sucralfate on gastric mucosal receptor expression for EGF, TGFα, PDGF, or bFGF. Gastric mucosal cell membranes were prepared from the stomachs of groups of rats receiving sucralfate for 3 days (200 mg/kg per day). Means ± S.E.M. of five experiments performed in duplicate. Asterisk indicates significant increase above the vehicle control values.

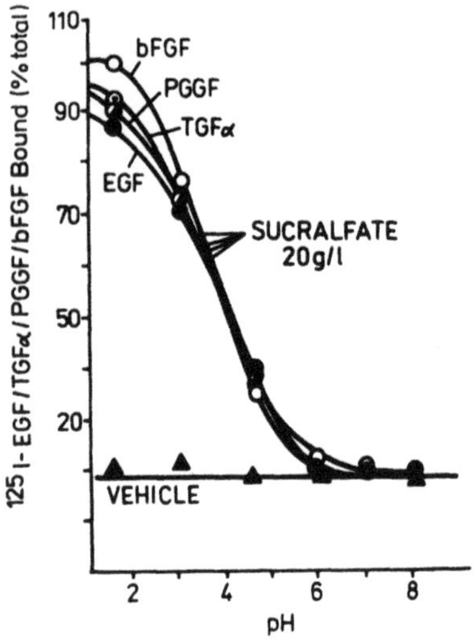

Figure 12. Binding of labeled EGF, TGFα, PDGF, or bFGF by sucralfate (20 g/liter) or vehicle solution adjusted to pH ranging from 1.5 to 8.0. The results are expressed in percent of total labeled growth factor added to the solution.

factors in the mucosa because of their physical adsorption to sucralfate and the binding with proteins in the eroded or ulcerated mucosa. An important role of interaction of sucralfate and EGF is evidenced by the finding that salivectomy reduced the ulcer healing effect of sucralfate and the addition of EGF restored the healing effect of sucralfate in salivectomized rats.

Role of Growth Factors and Sucralfate in Angiogenesis at the Ulcer Bed

Angiogenesis and neovascularization is a central event in wound healing and gastric erosions and ulcerations are not dissimilar from chronic wounds. Studies of healing of wounds show that the production of granulation tissue composed of a delicate matrix of fibroblasts and capillaries start with the release of a variety of growth factors originating first from the platelets in the form of PDGF and then from the macrophages. Fibroblasts and capillaries develop together stimulated by locally released growth factors. Among these factors, bFGF appears to be the most potent stimulant of proliferation of endothelial cells. It may be released from its store in extracellular matrix as a result of tissue damage and act locally to enhance angiogenesis and fibroplasia.

bFGF is a very labile polypeptide and may quickly undergo degradation in the gastric lumen by acid and pepsin. Sucralfate has a high affinity to bFGF and protects bFGF from degradation in the acid milieu that would be normally found in the stomach. This protective property of sucralfate for EGF probably explains intense angiogenesis observed in the chorioallantoic membrane of the chick embryo or rabbit cornea with implanted sucralfate or sucralfate–bFGF pellets.

Folkman *et al.*[7] provided evidence that bFGF is present in significantly higher amounts in the ulcer bed of sucralfate-treated rats compared with the vehicle-treated animals. They also showed that other antiulcer drugs such as cimetidine result in an increase in the level of bioactive bFGF by virtue of reducing gastric acid content and the degradation of bFGF in the ulcer bed. A unified concept was proposed that endogenous bFGF has a central role in ulcer healing and various antiulcer drugs accelerate the healing process presumably by longer survival of endogenous bFGF. It should be emphasized that bFGF should first be released from its storage in the extracellular matrix before interaction with its receptors on target cell plasma membrane and the stimulation of proliferation of fibroblasts and endothelial cells. No direct evidence was provided that such release occurs at the ulcer bed during the healing process and, therefore, it is not clear when sucralfate could interact with bFGF in the time course of ulcer healing.

References

1. Cohen S: Isolation of mouse submaxillary gland protein accelerating incisor eruption and eyelid opening of newborn animals. *J Biol Chem* **237**:1155–1159, 1962. Paper providing first evidence that EGF is produced and released by salivary glands.
2. Burgess AW: Epidermal growth factor and transforming growth factor. *Br Med Bull* **45**:410–424, 1989. Review article describing the biochemistry and physiology of EGF and TGF.
3. Konturek SJ: Role of growth factors in gastroduodenal protection and healing of peptic ulcerations. *Gastroenterol Clin North Am* **19**:41–65, 1990. Review article describing the distribution and protective and healing effects of EGF on the gastric and duodenal mucosa.
4. Konturek JW, Brzozowski T, Konturek SJ: Epidermal growth factor in protection, repair and healing of gastroduodenal mucosa. *J Clin Gastroenterol* **13**(suppl 1):S88–S97, 1991. Review of the gastroprotective and ulcer healing actions of EGF with emphasis on the involvement of polyamines and prostaglandins in this actions.
5. Wright NA, Pike C, Elia G: Induction of a novel epidermal growth factor-secreting cell lineage by mucosal ulceration in human gastrointestinal stem cells. *Nature* **343**:82–85, 1990. Paper demonstrating that EGF-producing cells may proliferate from the stem cells in the ulcer area to stimulate locally the repair and healing process.
6. Polk WH, Dempsey PJ, Russell WE, *et al*: Increased production of transforming growth factor alpha following acute gastric injury. *Gastroenterology* **102**:1462–1474, 1992. Paper providing evidence that the mucosal damage results in an increase in TGFα mRNA expression and TGFα release suggesting that this growth factor participates in gastric mucosal repair following acute gastric injury. EGF mRNA expression was not detected and little EGF was found, indicating that this growth factor does not originate from the intact or injured gastric mucosa.
7. Folkman J, Szabo S, Stovroff M, *et al*: Duodenal ulcer. Discovery of a new mechanism and development of angiogenic therapy that accelerates healing. *Ann Surg* **214**:414–425, 1991. The proposal of a model for ulcer healing by conventional therapy involving bFGF as the major factor in angiogenesis and healing of gastroduodenal ulcers.
8. Slomiany BL, Liu J, Yao P, *et al*: Characterization of the epidermal growth factor receptor in the gastric mucosa. *Digestion* **47**:181–190, 1990. Paper demonstrating the existence and binding characteristics of high-affinity receptor for EGF in the membranes of the gastric mucosa.
9. Tarnawski A, Erickson RA: Sucralfate—24 years later: Current concepts of its protective and therapeutic actions. *Eur J Gastroenterol Hepatol* **3**:795–810, 1991. A comprehensive overview of the basic and clinical research related to the gastroprotective and ulcer healing action of sucralfate and the concepts of the mechanisms of action of this drug on the gastric mucosa.

18

Duodenal Ulcer Therapy, "Acid Rebound," and Early Relapse

I. N. MARKS and G. O. YOUNG

Introduction

It is generally accepted that duodenal ulcers (DU) recur within a year in 75–90% of patients following healing with an H_2-receptor antagonist (H_2RA). Relapse rates following initial treatment with colloidal bismuth agents are appreciably, and often significantly, lower than those following initial treatment with an H_2RA, and a similar short-term advantage has been reported in most 3- to 6-month follow-up studies in patients healed initially with sucralfate. The reason for the trend toward lower relapse rates following ulcer healing with mucosal protective agents is not clear. Attention has been drawn to differences in the quality of ulcer healing following treatment with an H_2RA and the mucosal protective agents, and the antimicrobial effect of colloidal bismuth agents against *H. pylori*—and the possible effect of sucralfate on these organisms is clearly pertinent. A third possibility relates to the concept of increased parietal cell sensitivity following treatment with an H_2RA. This review will focus on acid secretory changes following DU healing with sucralfate and H_2RAs, and an attempt will be made to link these with the liability to early relapse.

Concept of Increased Parietal Cell Sensitivity, Upregulation, and "Acid Rebound"

Receptors may increase or decrease in number following treatment with different agents. Treatment with receptor antagonists usually results in an increase in number and/or

I. N. MARKS and G. O. YOUNG • Gastrointestinal Clinic and Department of Medicine, University of Cape Town and Groote Schuur Hospital, Observatory, South Africa.

Sucralfate: From Basic Science to the Bedside, edited by Daniel Hollander and G. N. J. Tytgat. Plenum Press, New York, 1995.

sensitivity of receptors, or upregulation, whereas treatment with receptor agonists tends to be linked with a decrease, or downregulation, of the receptors. This is not invariable since agonists such as gastrin, angiotensin, and prolactin may also cause upregulation. In general, however, treatment with a receptor antagonist leads to upregulation of the receptor with consequent rebound phenomena once treatment is withdrawn.

Apart from the upregulation of the H_2 receptors which may occur after prolonged treatment with an H_2RA, the high pH during such treatment may also cause an increase in serum gastrin levels with subsequent upregulation of the gastrin receptors. It may be argued that upregulation of both H_2 and gastrin receptors, with increased responsiveness to physiologic stimuli such as meals, leads to "acid rebound" following withdrawal of treatment and a possible increase in the liability to ulcer relapse. Receptor counts have not been carried out in this setting, however, and the cause of acid rebound following withdrawal of treatment with an H_2RA remains uncertain.

Measurement of Parietal Cell Responsiveness

The terms *parietal cell responsiveness* (PCR) and *parietal cell sensitivity* (PCS) define the sensitivity of the parietal cells in terms of the response to a low-dose stimulus. They are at best rather arbitrary. The stimuli may differ, the low dose employed by different workers is not necessarily the same, and the response may or may not be corrected for basal secretion. PCR may be measured, simply, as the response to a minimal or submaximal stimulus expressed in millimoles per hour, whereas PCS is derived from the ratio of a low-dose or submaximal response to the maximum acid output (MAO) or from dose–response curves. Transformation of the dose–response data may allow calculation of the ED_{50}, i.e., the dose required for producing 50% of the MAO. This provides yet another measure of PCR or PCS. Some workers have chosen to employ the now-fashionable 24-hr intragastric acidity or pH profiles in the assessment of acid secretory responses before and after ulcer therapy. The possible correlation between these qualitative measures and the more traditional quantitative ones has not been established (Table I).

Acid Secretory Changes following H_2-Receptor Antagonists in Health and Disease

Appreciation of the acid secretory changes following withdrawal of treatment with H_2RAs necessitates an understanding of the relationship between PCR and DU activity. There is good evidence to show that PCR in patients with an active DU is higher than in control subjects. The ED_{50} of pentagastrin has been shown to be significantly lower in DU patients than in controls, and the increased sensitivity of patients with an active DU to pentagastrin is now well established.[1] The evidence regarding the relationship between ulcer healing and decreased PCR is more controversial. Antral distension studies showed a fall in PCR on DU healing, and an early study[2] showed both basal and peak acid outputs to be significantly higher in an active DU group of patients than in a predominantly antacid-

Table I. Measurement of Parietal Cell Responsiveness

I. Response to minimal or submaximal stimulus (meq/hr)
  1. Antral distension
  2. Low dose: pentagastrin, tetragastrin, histamine, and impromidine
  3. Simulated test meal/chewing gum
  4. 24-hr intragastric pH or acidity
  5. Nocturnal acid secretion
  6. Basal acid secretion

II. Parietal cell sensitivity (PCS)
  A. Dose–response curves: pentagastrin, tetragastrin, histamine, impromidine
    1. Ratio of low or submaximal responses to MAO (%)
    2. ED_{50}—dose required for 50% MAO
  B. Other submaximal response MAO ratios (%)
    1. Antral distension versus MAO
    2. Chewing gum response versus MAO
    3. Nocturnal acid secretion versus MAO
    4. Basal acid secretion versus MAO

treated group of patients with a healed DU. The finding of a significant decrease in acid secretion following DU healing has since been confirmed in sucralfate-treated patients.

"Acid Rebound" after H_2-Receptor Blockade

The notion of "acid rebound" after withdrawal of treatment with an H_2RA is not a new one. The evidence for this is strong in control subjects, good in patients with healed DU, and seemingly less convincing in patients being treated for an active DU (Table II). A Scandinavian group reported a transient increase in PCR in *control subjects* following 4 weeks' treatment with full-dose cimetidine[3] and ranitidine,[4] respectively, and the Royal Free group showed rebound intragastric hyperacidity in healthy subjects after prolonged treatment with full-dose cimetidine, nizatidine, famotidine,[5] or ranitidine.[6] It should be noted that the duration of acid rebound was little more than 2–6 weeks.[3,4,6]

The effect of ranitidine on PCR in patients with *healed DU* may be dose-dependent. Jones and co-workers[7] reported increased responses to graded doses of impromidine following 3 months' maintenance treatment with ranitidine 150 mg nocte in a small group of DU patients in remission, but we were unable to confirm their findings in an almost identical study.[8] Fullarton and co-workers[9] found a convincing increase in nocturnal acid secretion in a similar group of patients 48 hr after stopping 4 weeks' treatment with full-dose nizatidine and, in a subsequent study,[10] showed a similar effect with full-dose ranitidine but not with famotidine. The authors conceded that the failure to demonstrate acid rebound with famotidine may have been related to its longer half-life. The Berne group,[11] interestingly, showed no change in acid response after 24 days' treatment with ranitidine 300 mg qid. The posttreatment study was carried out a mere 36–48 hr following the last dose and, again, a residual drug effect could not be excluded.

The demonstration of "acid rebound" following successful treatment of an *active DU*

Table II. Changes in Parietal Cell Responsiveness Following Treatment with H_2RAs in Health and Disease[a]

	Medication	Method	Effect
Controls			
Aadland and Berstad[3]	Cm 1 g/day 4 weeks	Pg/Hs D-R	+[b]
Frislid *et al.*[4]	Rn 150 mg BD 4 weeks	Meal	+
Nwokolo *et al.*[5]	Cm, Nz, Fm(FD) 35 days	24-hr I/G pH	+
Prewett *et al.*[6]	Rn 300 mg/day 25 days	24-hr I/G pH	+
Healed DU			
Jones *et al.*[7]	Rn 150 mg/day 3 months	Imp D-R	+
Johnston *et al.*[8]	Rn 150 mg/day 3 months	Imp D-R	Nil
Fullarton *et al.*[9]	Nz 300 mg/day 4 weeks	Nocturnal AO	+
Fullarton *et al.*[10]	Rn, Fm, Nz(FD) 4 weeks	Nocturnal AO	+
Wilder-Smith *et al.*[11]	Rn 1200 mg/day 34 days	24-hr I/G pH	Nil
Active DU			
Aadland and Berstad[12]	Cm 1 g/day 4 weeks	Pg D-R	Nil
Savarino *et al.*[13]	Nz 300 mg/day 4 weeks	24-hr I/G pH	Nil
Marks *et al.*[14]	Rn 300 mg/day 6 weeks	Pg/Hs D-R	Nil
Johnston *et al.*[15]	Rn 300 mg/day 6 weeks	MSF AO	Nil
Kummer *et al.*[16]	Rn 300 mg/day 6 weeks	Nocturnal AO	+
Johnston *et al.*[17]	Rn 300 mg/day 6 weeks	Pg D-R	Nil
Johnston *et al.*[17]	Rn 300 mg/day 6 weeks	Basal AO	Nil

[a]Abbreviations used: Cm, cimetidine; Rn, ranitidine; Nz, nizatidine; Fm, famotidine; FD, full dose; Pg, pentagastrin; Hs, histamine; Imp, impromidine; D-R, dose response; MSF, modified sham feeding; I/G, intragastric; AO, acid output.
[b]+, significant rise.

with H_2RAs has proved to be even more difficult. Aadland and Berstad[12] reported no consistent change in PCS before and following healing of an active DU with cimetidine, but theorized that a cimetidine-induced increase in PCS might have been masked by a decrease in PCS caused by healing. Others[13] found no significant difference in 24-hr intragastric pH studies in nizatidine-healed DU patients.

The Cape Town group attempted to resolve the dilemma as to whether DU healing with an H_2RA invites acid rebound by carrying out a series of comparative studies with ranitidine and sucralfate.[14–16] The duration of therapy and timing of the acid secretory studies and endoscopies were standardized throughout, but the acid secretory stimuli varied in the different studies. The assumption in the design of the studies was that sucralfate, with its mucosal protective rather than acid inhibitory mechanism of action, would cause little if any acid rebound following withdrawal of treatment. Healing with sucralfate was associated with a significant decrease in the various parameters of acid secretion in all three studies (Table III). No significant decrease was noted in the ranitidine-treated group in the first two studies,[14,15] and there was, indeed, a significant increase in nocturnal acid secretion in the third.[16] The failure of the acid secretory responses to fall, despite ulcer healing, in the ranitidine-treated groups in the first two studies[14,15] could be

Table III. Comparative Data in Ranitidine- and Sucralfate-Treated Patients with Duodenal Ulcer Disease[a]

	Medication	Method	Effect
Healed DU			
Johnston *et al.*[8]	Rn 150 mg/day 3 months	Imp D-R	Nil
	Sc 2 g/day 3 months	Imp D-R	Nil
Active DU			
Marks *et al.*[14]	Rn 300 mg/day 6 weeks	Pg/Hs D-R	Nil
	Sc 4 g/day 6 weeks	Pg/Hs D-R	–
Johnston *et al.*[15]	Rn 300 mg/day 6 weeks	MSF AO	Nil
	Sc 4 g/day 6 weeks	MSF AO	–
Kummer *et al.*[16]	Rn 300 mg/day 6 weeks	Nocturnal AO	+
	Sc 4 g/day 6 weeks	Nocturnal AO	–
Johnston *et al.*[17]	Rn 300 mg/day 6 weeks	Basal AO	Nil
	Sc 4 g/day 6 weeks	Basal AO	–

[a]Abbreviations used: Sc, sucralfate; Rn, ranitidine; Imp, impromidine; PG, pentagastrin; Hs, histamine; AO, acid output; MSF, modified sham feeding.
[b]+, significant rise; –, significant fall.

construed as evidence of a ranitidine-induced "acid rebound," while the results of the third[16] were clearly in keeping with this concept.

Nature of Therapy, "Acid Rebound," and Early Relapse

The protocol in the three Cape Town studies allowed for endoscopic assessment of relapse rates 4–6 weeks after documented healing and withdrawal of treatment.[17,18] The overall 4- to 6-week relapse rate was 40% in the 35 ranitidine-treated patients and only 9% in the 32 sucralfate-healed patients. The low incidence of early relapse in the sucralfate-treated groups was linked to decreased acid secretion on healing, while the higher incidence in the ranitidine-treated groups reflected the lack of such a decrease. Consideration of the relapse data in individual patients, irrespective of therapy, showed than an early relapse could be predicted in those in whom acid secretion increased, rather than decreased, on ulcer healing. This concept linking increased PCS following DU healing with early relapse was strongly supported by the findings in a Japanese study[19] of 65 patients followed for 2 years after documented DU healing.

Conclusion

Studies in DU patients show that acid secretion tends to fall on healing, and that the trend is more marked following treatment with sucralfate than H_2RAs. Failure of acid secretion to fall following ulcer healing may be construed as evidence of "acid rebound," and would appear to favor the development of early relapse.

ACKNOWLEDGMENT. We acknowledge support from the South African Medical Research Council.

References

1. Lam SK, Koo J: Gastrin sensitivity in duodenal ulcer. *Gut* **26**:485–490, 1985. Study confirming increased parietal cell sensitivity in patients with an active duodenal ulcer.
2. Achord JL: Gastric pepsin and acid secretion in patients with acute and healed duodenal ulcer. *Gastroenterology* **81**:15–18, 1981. Study suggesting that acid secretion decreases on duodenal ulcer healing.
3. Aadland E, Berstad A: Parietal and chief cell sensitivity to histamine and pentagastrin stimulation before and after cimetidine treatment in healthy subjects. *Scand J Gastroenterol* **14**:933–938, 1979.
4. Frislid K, Aadland E, Berstad A: Augmented post-prandial gastric secretion due to exposure to ranitidine in healthy subjects. *Scand J Gastroenterol* **21**:119–122, 1986.
5. Nwokolo CU, Smith JTL, Pounder RE: Rebound intragastric hyperacidity occurs following dosing with cimetidine, nizatidine and famotidine. *Gastroenterology* **96**:A369, 1989.
6. Prewett EJ, Hudson M, Nwokolo CU, *et al*: Nocturnal intragastric acidity during and after a period of dosing with either ranitidine or omeprazole. *Gastroenterology* **100**:873–877, 1991. Studies in control subjects showing acid rebound following treatment with various H_2-receptor blockers.
7. Jones DB, Howden CW, Burget DW, *et al*: Alteration of H_2-receptor sensitivity in duodenal ulcer patients after maintenance treatment with an H_2-antagonist. *Gut* **29**:890–893, 1988.
8. Johnston DA, Marks IN, Young GO, *et al*: Maintenance treatment with ranitidine and sucralfate does not affect acid secretory responses. *S Afr Med J* **78**:A353, 1990.
9. Fullarton GM, McLaughlan G, Macdonald A, *et al*: Rebound nocturnal hypersecretion after 4 weeks H_2-antagonist therapy. *Gut* **30**:449–454, 1989.
10. Fullarton GM, Macdonald AMI, McColl KEL: Rebound hypersecretion after H_2-antagonist withdrawal—A comparative study with nizatidine, ranitidine and famotidine. *Aliment Pharm Ther* **5**:391–398, 1991.
11. Wilder-Smith DH, Halter F, Merke HS: Tolerance and rebound hyperacidity in DU patients. *Gut* **31**:A600, 1990. Studies in patients with duodenal ulcer in remission using different parameters of acid secretion and showing conflicting results following treatment with variable doses of H_2RAs.
12. Aadland E, Berstad A: Parietal and chief cell sensitivity to pentagastrin stimulation before and after cimetidine treatment for duodenal ulcer. *Scand J Gastroenterol* **14**:111–114, 1979.
13. Savarino V, Mela GS, Zentilin P, *et al*: Lack of gastric acid rebound after stopping successful short-term course of nizatidine in duodenal ulcer patients. *Am J Gastroenterol* **86**:281–284, 1991.
14. Marks IN, Young GO, Tigler-Wybrandi NA, *et al*: Acid secretory response and parietal cell sensitivity in patients with duodenal ulcer before and after treatment with sucralfate or ranitidine. *Am J Med* **86**(suppl 6A):145–147, 1989.
15. Johnston DA, Marks IN, Young GO, *et al*: Duodenal ulcer healing and acid secretory responses to modified sham-feeding and pentagastrin stimulation. *Aliment Pharm Ther* **4**:403–410, 1990.
16. Kummer A, Johnston DA, Marks IN, *et al*: Changes in nocturnal acid secretion on duodenal ulcer healing with ranitidine and sucralfate. *Gut* **33**:175–178, 1992.
17. Johnston DA, Marks IN: Short-term relapse rates after duodenal ulcer healing. *S Afr J Cont Med* **8**:999–1002, 1990. Studies examining the effect of H_2RAs in patients with active duodenal ulcer using different parameters of acid secretion. Acid rebound was noted only in the study in which nocturnal acid secretion was measured.
18. Marks IN, Johnston DA, Young GO: Acid secretory changes and early relapse following duodenal ulcer healing with ranitidine or sucralfate. *Am J Med* **91**(suppl 2A):95–101, 1991.
19. Yanaka A, Muto H: Increased parietal cell responsiveness to tetragastrin in patients with recurrent duodenal ulcer. *Dig Dis Sci* **33**(11):1459–1465, 1988. Studies documenting the relationship between persistent elevation of parietal cell sensitivity on duodenal cell healing and early relapse.

19

Effect of Sucralfate on Experimental Ulcers

SUSUMU OKABE, YOSHIYASU OGIHARA, and HIROYUKI KOBA

Introduction

Sucralfate is one of the best-known drugs which is frequently used for the treatment of peptic ulcers.[1,2] The mechanisms of action of sucralfate have been described in the preceding chapters. In this chapter, a detailed account will be given of the results of experimental studies of sucralfate conducted to assess its effects in preventing and healing a variety of experimental ulcers induced in animals, and also of their correlation with the results of clinical use of the drug in humans.

Usefulness of Animal Ulcer Models in the Development and Evaluation of Antiulcer Drugs

There are various experimental ulcer models currently in use for testing drugs potentially useful in the treatment of peptic ulcers. It now seems generally accepted that the most promising drug should be determined by means of the following three-step testing program. For drug to be tested, it is relatively easier to perform primary screening tests in acute ulcer models (e.g., pylorus-ligated ulcers, stress ulcers, or drug-induced ulcers). If the drug survives this initial assessment of its potential usefulness, it must then be subjected to more time-consuming secondary screening tests with chronic ulcer models (acetic acid ulcers, cryo ulcers, or thermal ulcers). If these tests indicate that the specific pharmacologic action of the drug is worth pursuing, the drug is then submitted to tertiary screening tests designed to elucidate the mechanism of its antiulcer action.

SUSUMU OKABE and YOSHIYASU OGIHARA • Department of Applied Pharmacology, Kyoto Pharmaceutical University, Kyoto 607, Japan. HIROYUKI KOBA • Chugai Pharmaceutical Co., Ltd., Tokyo 104, Japan.

Sucralfate: From Basic Science to the Bedside, edited by Daniel Hollander and G. N. J. Tytgat. Plenum Press, New York, 1995.

The mechanism of action of antiulcer drugs, though inferable from measurements of various relevant factors in experiments involving acute and chronic ulcer models, is usually explored using separate experimental systems.

Historical Overview of Testing of the Efficacy of Sucralfate

In the 1960s when sucralfate was under development in Japan, animal ulcer models currently in widespread use for the screening of drugs for peptic ulcers, such as the ethanol and acetic acid ulcer models, were not available. Pylorus-ligated ulcers (Shay ulcers) were the only *in vivo* system for assessing the specific pharmacologic activity of the drug. Namekata *et al.*,[3] at the Research Institute of Chugai Pharmaceutical Co., in a search for an agent useful in treating peptic ulcers, screened a series of polysaccharide sulfates for antiulcer activity in terms of antipeptic activity in pylorus-ligated rats and for anticoagulant activity as potential unwanted side effects. As a result, they found that the shorter the carbohydrate chain of these compounds, the lower their potential for producing adverse effects was, and also that the higher the degree of sulfation, the more pronounced their antiulcer action was. The screening of sulfate mono-, di-, tri-, and tetrasaccharides led these investigators to identify, as the skeleton of the most suitable candidate for development, a sulfuric acid ester of sucrose containing in its molecule three sulfuric acid esters of primary alcohol that release a sulfate radical exhibiting antipeptic activity with relative ease. Substituting aluminum hydroxide (as in sucralfate) for sodium in the molecule of sucrose sulfate in expectation of an additional antacid action resulted in a compound that was proven to be markedly effective in inhibiting ulcer development, probably owing to its combined antipeptic and antacid actions observed on pylorus-ligated ulcers and histamine-induced ulcers.

Later on, sucralfate was shown to have a potent antiulcer action in studies carried out by Japanese investigators using a diversity of experimental ulcers (histamine ulcers, stress ulcers, steroid ulcers, reserpine ulcers, and clamping cortisone ulcers) and was put to clinical use as an antiulcer drug.

Sucralfate was virtually equipotent with H_2-receptor antagonists (H_2RAs) in its clinical effectiveness but was quite distinct from these drugs in that it facilitated ulcer healing without inhibiting gastric acid secretion. This difference between sucralfate and H_2RAs provided impetus for postmarketing investigations of the drug to elucidate its exact mechanism of action. In addition, with the progress of research work on the pathophysiology of peptic ulcers, various animal models of drug-induced ulcers were devised, with which in-depth studies of the antiulcer action of sucralfate were carried out. These postmarketing research efforts verified the therapeutic potency of the drug. At the present time, the drug is recognized to be representative of the so-called mucosa-protecting and defense factor-strengthening agents.

As is obvious from the above-mentioned studies, the testing of sucralfate as to its antiulcer efficacy has been continually performed in the light of updated knowledge, and the latest information at each stage of development and clinical usage. In view of its unique feature of acting directly on the gastric mucosa from the lumen of the stomach, it is likely that a novel pharmacologic activity will be added to the well-established mechanism of action of sucralfate, as the mechanisms of the underlying healing and recurrence of ulcers are clarified by new studies.

Experimental Ulcer Models and Effect of Sucralfate on Acute Ulcer Models

Pylorus-Ligated Ulcers

Since first reported in 1945 by Shay *et al.*, this classical peptic ulcer model has been employed for testing the potency of antiulcer drugs all over the world. This *in vivo* screening test is simple and easy to perform, assures a high incidence of ulceration, is evaluated as having an acceptable predictive value, and is employed as a primary specific screening method for anti-peptic ulcer activity. The cause of ulcer formation in this model is the aggressive action of gastric juice (acid and pepsin).

As mentioned earlier, sucralfate was developed after surviving the initial assessment of its potential usefulness by means of this test system. Our own testing of the drug using this model[4] showed that the preventive effect of sucralfate on ulcers, as expressed in terms of a percentage of the ulcer index value for controls at 14 hr after ligation of the pylorus, was 60% at 30 mg/kg, and above 90% at 100 and 300 mg/kg (Fig. 1).

However, there were no substantial differences in pepsin output between the control group, and the groups receiving 100 and 300 mg/kg of sucralfate. In addition, Nagashima[5] reported that the antipeptic action of sucralfate ceased within a short period of time. Therefore, the antiulcer effect of sucralfate can be construed to be due to protection of the

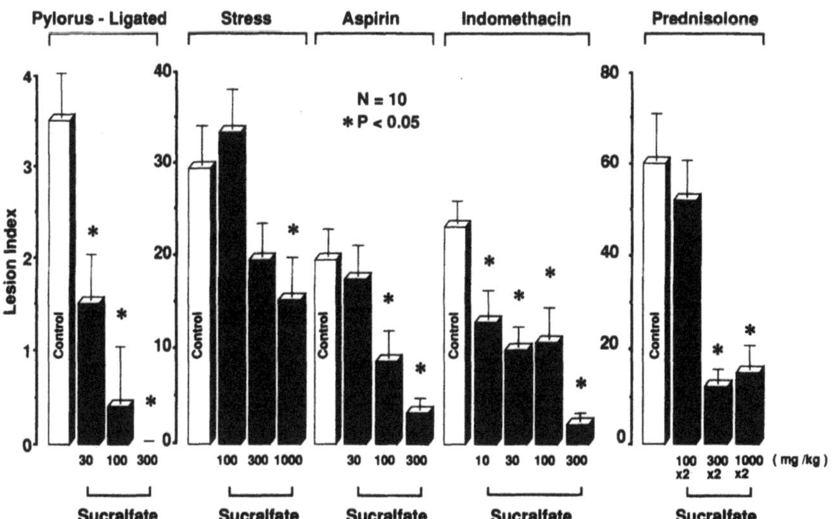

Figure 1. Effects of sucralfate on various acute gastric ulcers induced in rats. There was significant prevention of the development of gastric ulcers with sucralfate.

gastric mucosa against aggressive acid and pepsin secretion by the drug adhering to the glandular portions of the gastric walls, and not to an antipeptic action in the gastric lumen.

Propantheline (anticholinergic drug), when tested in parallel in a similar experimental design, showed 90% inhibition of ulcers at 30 mg/kg, a dose level effective in inhibiting gastric acid secretion, while cimetidine and antacids (at respective doses of 200 and 1000 mg/kg) proved entirely ineffective. This discrepancy may well be accounted for by the shorter duration of action of the latter drugs.

Stress Ulcers

Several kinds of stress, including restraint, water immersion-restraint, and cold-restraint, have been used as effective means of producing stress ulcers (pathologically superficial erosion) in animals. Of them, the water immersion-restraint stress ulcer model, in which rats are immersed up the xiphoid process in a water bath under restraint in a cage with wire netting, provides a simple test that gives a constant high yield of mucosal ulceration of constant severity. Therefore, this ulcer model is used commonly as a primary screening method for antiulcer drugs of potential benefit to humans. Sucralfate at 100 mg/animal proved effective in almost totally preventing the hemorrhagic erosion of the gastric mucosa occurring in the immersion of rats in cold water (19–23°C) for 10–12 hr.

In our study,[4] sucralfate at a dose of 1000 mg/kg had a significant (52%) inhibitory effect, as compared with a control, on the superficial erosions of the gastric mucosa caused by 7-hr immersion in cold water (23°C), although the drug at 100 or 300 mg/kg failed to provide significant protection against this form of stress-induced mucosal damage (Fig. 1). Propantheline and cimetidine tested in parallel both had a dose-dependent inhibitory effect on water immersion-induced stress ulcers, whereas an antacid proved ineffective even at 1000 mg/kg.

Increased gastric acid secretion, gastric hypermotility, and local circulatory disturbance occurring in association with excitation of the vagal nervous system have been implicated as the principal causes of stress ulcers. The beneficial effect of sucralfate on this particular type of experimental ulcer, like its effect on pylorus-ligated ulcers, seems to be the result of protection of the gastric mucosa against aggressive factors. Auguste *et al.*[6] in their experiment on cold stress ulcers (4°C, 2 hr) observed that sucralfate (at 35 mg/100 g body wt) inhibited ulcer development almost completely by inducing mucosal tissue levels of prostaglandin E_2. It thus seems valid to assume that the effect of sucralfate on stress ulcers can be explained at least partly by the stimulation of endogenous prostaglandins.

Drug-Induced Ulcers

Aspirin and many other drugs are known to give rise to ulceration of the gastric mucosa in animals. Experimental ulcers induced by anti-inflammatory drugs in particular are in widespread use both in Japan and abroad for screening the antiulcer activity of new drugs. These animal models of drug-induced ulcers bear resemblance to drug-induced gastritis and ulcerations in humans and thus will allow the prediction of the clinical efficacy of an antiulcer drug. Of all animal models of drug-induced ulcers, we will describe the five most commonly used models.

Aspirin Ulcers. Aspirin, when administered orally or parenterally to fasted rats or dogs, gives rise to an ulcer in the stomach several hours after its administration. These animal species are quite susceptible to this particular type of gastric mucosal injury. This makes aspirin ulcers suitable for assessing the antiulcer potency of a drug. The presence of gastric acid is a prerequisite for the production of gastric mucosal injury by aspirin allowing the efficient production of ulcerations by administration of aspirin orally to pylorus-ligated rats. The direct action of aspirin on the gastric mucosa and back diffusion of acid occurring in association with disruption of the gastric mucosal barrier caused by hydrochloric acid have been suggested to play roles in the pathogenesis of this particular type of ulcer.

Our experiments[4] demonstrated that ulcers induced by 100 mg/kg aspirin in pylorus-ligated rats were inhibited in a dose-dependent fashion by pretreatment with sucralfate, with 84.8% inhibition at a dose of 300 mg/kg. A similar dose-dependent antiulcer effect was produced by pretreatment of pylorus-ligated rats with propantheline, antacids, or cimetidine (Fig. 1).

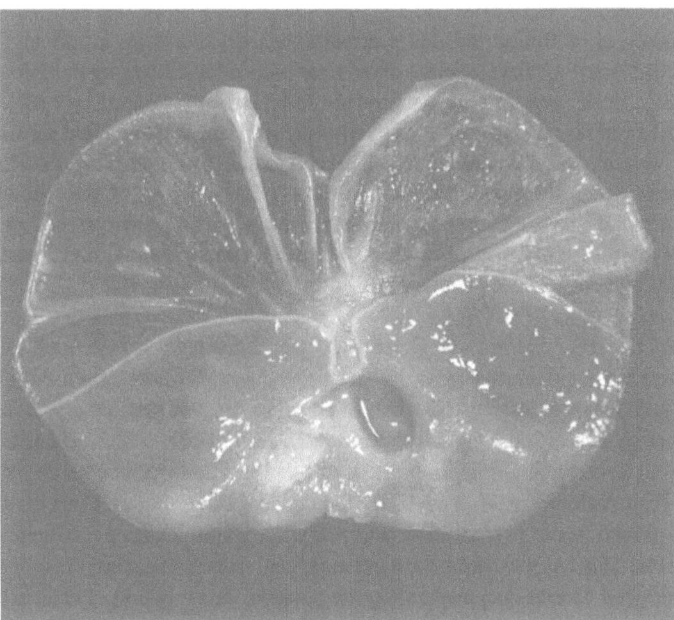

Figure 2. Gross appearances of an acetic acid-induced gastric ulcer in a rat. The ulcer was photographed 5 days after submucosal injection of acetic acid in the border of the antrofundic mucosa.

The role of pepsin in the production of aspirin-induced gastric injury is minimal, if any at all. The antiulcer effect of sucralfate could be attributed in part to its inhibitory action on back diffusion of acid. In fact, enhancement by sucralfate on the inhibitory action of mucus on acid back diffusion was suggested by Tasman-Jones[7] as being likely.

Endogenous prostaglandin-mediated cytoprotection has also been suggested as part of sucralfate's effect, although the drug cannot be anticipated to contribute greatly to this particular mechanism of cytoprotection inasmuch as the biosynthesis of endogenous prostaglandins is blocked, owing to inhibition of cyclooxygenase by aspirin. Shea-Donohue *et al.*[8] in their study involving rhesus monkeys found that sucralfate protects the gastric mucosa against aspirin-induced injury by augmenting the secretion of soluble mucus.

We have long assumed that sucralfate inhibits the formation of aspirin ulcers by increasing the blood flow through the gastric mucosa. This view is supported by the published study of Konturek *et al.*[9] who demonstrated that sucralfate acts to maintain gastric mucosal blood flow through the mediation of nitric oxide.

Indomethacin Ulcers. It is a well-known fact that long-term use of nonsteroidal anti-inflammatory drugs (NSAIDs) causes gastric mucosal injury associated with hemorrhage or even perforation. In animals, NSAIDs give rise to gastric ulcers within a short period of time and this makes NSAID-induced ulcers well-suited for experimental purposes. Mention will be made here only of ulcers induced by indomethacin, an NSAID currently in widespread clinical use.

Ligumsky *et al.*[10] reported that pretreatment with sucralfate at 125 mg/rat almost completely inhibited the development of an ulcer induced by 30 mg/kg indomethacin. In a parallel study, these investigators explored the influence of sucralfate on cyclooxygenase activity, PAF, and so on, but failed to obtain any data confirming these mechanisms.

Also in our study[4] sucralfate was demonstrated to inhibit the development of indomethacin ulcers in a dose-dependent fashion (Fig. 1). We are of the opinion that this beneficial effect of the drug is related in part to its actions on gastric mucus and mucosal blood flow, as in the case of aspirin ulcers. Antacid, propantheline, and cimetidine also significantly prevented the development of ulcers.

Steroid Ulcers. Steroids in general are well known to cause peptic ulcers or to aggravate an existing ulcerative lesion. These potential side effects limit the clinical use of these drugs. A drug that lessens these unwanted side effects of steroids would be useful in clinical practice. Steroid-induced ulcers are not an easy-to-perform screening test, taking 4 to 8 days to develop in animal models. It should be noted that sucralfate significantly prevented the development of prednisolone-induced gastric mucosal ulcers, suggesting that the combined use of prednisolone and sucralfate might lessen the adverse effects of corticosteroids (Fig. 1).[10,11] Both propantheline and cimetidine significantly prevented corticoid-induced ulcerations, suggesting the possible participation of acid in the pathogenesis of corticosteroid ulcerations.

Taurocholate Ulcers. Morris *et al.*,[12] using an *ex vivo* model, demonstrated that the development of gastric mucosal injury induced by 80 mM sodium taurocholate in an acid medium was effectively inhibited by both pre- and posttreatment with sucralfate. Based on the finding that this protective effect of sucralfate was not abolished by the addition of indomethacin, the same authors reasoned that the effect of sucralfate in this model would be related primarily to adherence of the drug to the mucosal surface, and increased secretion of mucus and anti-inflammatory factors rather than stimulation of endogenous prostaglandin secretions.

Ligumsky *et al.*[10] reported that pretreatment with sucralfate at 125 mg/rat proved effective in preventing gastric mucosal injury caused by exposure to 30 mM sodium taurocholate. They also found that sucralfate treatment caused the tissue levels of leukotriene C_4 and PAF to decrease. These findings, taken together, led the investigators to conclude that the drug prevents sodium taurocholate-induced gastric mucosal injury by inhibiting these gastric mucosal injury-aggravating factors.

Ethanol Ulcers. While ethanol at high concentrations has long been known to give rise to ulcerations of the gastric mucosa, it was not until recently that the usefulness of ethanol ulcers as a screen for antiulcer activity became an issue. Recent studies have shown that 100% ethanol administered orally can produce gastric mucosal ulcerations of uniform severity in 1 hr in a reliably high percentage of animals. This screening test, because of the simplicity and ease with which it can be performed, is now the most commonly used screening method. This type of ulceration is thought to be caused primarily by the direct damaging action of 100% ethanol on the gastric mucosa (particularly blood vessels). The extent to which gastric acid is involved in the ulcerogenic mechanism of alcohol is assumed to be minimal, if any at all. In fact, H_2RAs having an inhibitory action on gastric acid secretion have been proven to be entirely ineffective in the prevention of ethanol ulcers.

The effectiveness of sucralfate against ethanol ulcers has been established by Hollander *et al.*,[13] who demonstrated that pretreatment with sucralfate was effective in the prevention of ethanol ulcers. We also confirmed their findings in rats, i.e., thc ulcers were potentially prevented by sucralfate administered at 200 and 300 mg/kg. Since prior administration of indomethacin (which can inhibit the biosynthesis of prostaglandins) resulted in lessening of sucralfate's effect, it seems that sucralfate exerts its effect through the stimulation of endogenous prostaglandins and the drug is now believed to be capable of producing adaptive cytoprotection. It should be noted, however, that Coleman *et al.*[14] demonstrated that the effect of mild irritants which are also capable of providing adaptive cytoprotection ceases within about 1 hr, while that of sucralfate lasts for about 6 hr.

The mechanism underlying the persistent protective effect of sucralfate and the mechanisms whereby sucralfate induces endogenous prostaglandin secretion remain obscure. Chen *et al.*[15] have demonstrated that the gastric mucosal blood flow-maintaining effect of sucralfate accounts for part of its effect on ethanol ulcers, while Szabo and Brown[16] suggested a sulfhydryl-mediated mechanism for the antiulcer effect of sucralfate.

Chronic Gastric Ulcer Model

Numerous animal models currently in use for screening antiulcer drugs are those involving acute gastroduodenal ulcers. Here, a description will be given of experimental acetic acid ulcers devised by one of the present authors (S.O.).

Various screening tests permit evaluation of the effectiveness of an antiulcer drug in the prevention or development of an acute ulcer, but cannot assess the drug's potency in promoting the healing and preventing the recurrence of an ulcer once developed. In order for patients to be entirely freed from peptic ulcers, not only complete healing of the ulcers but also prevention of a possible recurrence must be accomplished and, to this end, it is necessary to elucidate the mechanisms underlying the healing and recurrence of ulcers, and thereby discover drugs that will serve these purposes. We have used acetic acid ulcers in our effort to accomplish these goals.

Acetic Acid Ulcers

Acetic acid ulcers are now in extensive use for screening the potency of antiulcer drugs, mainly because of the simplicity of the techniques involved and the acceptable persistence of the ulcers produced (Fig. 2). In this test, an ulcer is produced by either injecting acetic acid into the gastric wall, applying it to the serosal aspect of the stomach or duodenum, or its intraluminal application. The process of spontaneous healing of an acetic acid ulcer once developed bears a close resemblance to that of human ulcers, a feature that makes drug testing with acetic acid and other chronic ulcer models essential for the successful screening of an antiulcer drug. The acetic acid ulcer in its original form had disadvantages in that a test drug needed to be administered for a considerably long period of time (usually 2 to 4 weeks) and the ulcerative lesion thus produced tended to heal spontaneously, making it difficult to assess the therapeutic response. To overcome these difficulties, we modified the test by the addition of indomethacin (1 mg/kg for 2 to 4

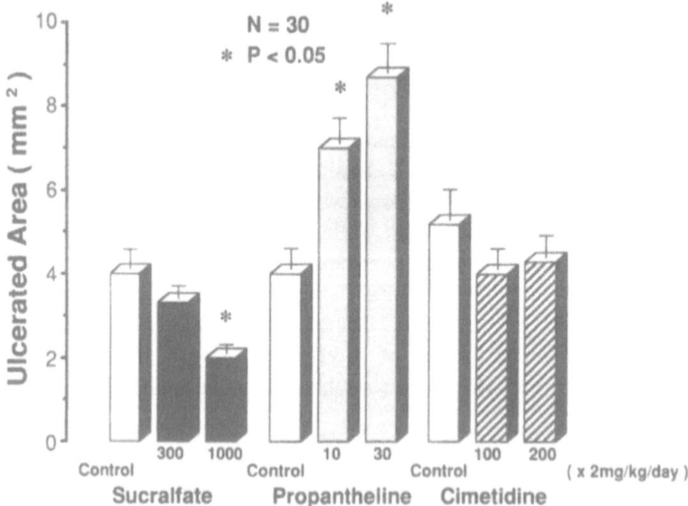

Figure 3. Effects of sucralfate, propantheline, and cimetidine on spontaneous healing of acetic acid-induced gastric ulcers in rats. Each drug or the vehicle (as the control) was administered orally (by gastric intubation) twice daily for 14 days.

weeks) following the development of an acetic acid ulcer so that the spontaneous healing of the ulcers could be delayed. With this modification, ulcerative lesions of control animals could be kept large enough to permit macroscopic observation for assessment of the therapeutic response even 4–8 weeks after their development.

Using the acetic acid ulcer model with delayed ulcer healing caused by indomethacin, we tested sucralfate as to its potency in accelerating ulcer healing. The results indicated that the drug promoted the spontaneous healing of ulcers (Fig. 3).[4,17,18] Although cimetidine had no effect on ulcer healing, propantheline significantly delayed the ulcer healing. It is most likely that the delayed emptying by propantheline might be involved in the delay in ulcer healing. It should be noted that sucralfate apparently prevented the delayed healing of ulcers in a dose-related manner when administered three times a day for 4 weeks (Fig. 4). In contrast, both propantheline and cimetidine had no or little effect on delayed ulcer healing.

The prostaglandin levels in the gastric mucosa were found to be significantly decreased with indomethacin administration (the decrease was not prevented by sucralfate) in the delayed ulcer healing model, while they were not significantly increased in the control acetic acid ulcer model. In pylorus-ligated rats, treatment with sucralfate was followed by a significant increase in both the volume and the pH of the gastric contents. Based on these findings, we surmise that the effect of sucralfate in promoting ulcer healing is partly related to elevation of gastric pH and perhaps stimulation of prostaglandins. The observed significant increase in the gastric contents may be construed as indicating a contribution of the increased mucus secretion and delivery of FGF to sucralfate's effect.

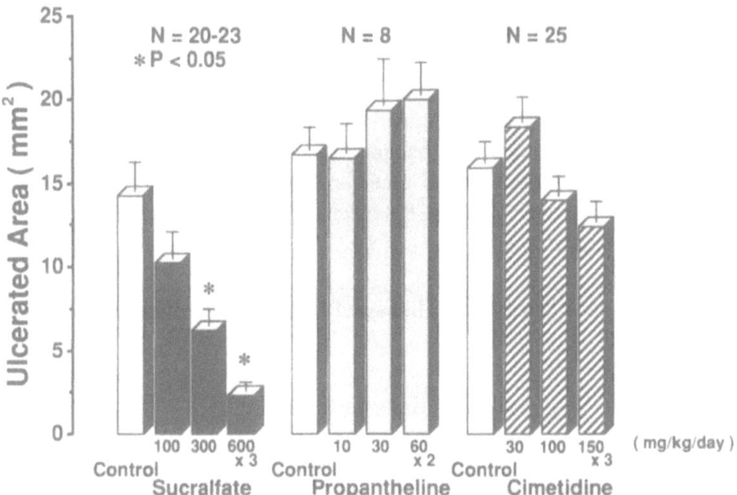

Figure 4. Effects of sucralfate, propantheline, and cimetidine on delayed healing (caused by repeated administration of indomethacin) of acetic acid-induced gastric ulcers in rats. Each drug or the vehicle (as the control) was administered orally (by gastric intubation) two or three times a day for 28 days.

These issues remain to be resolved by further studies. Kuwayama *et al.*[19] reported that sucralfate also significantly prevented the delay in healing of acetic acid ulcers induced in rats by repeated administration of hydrocortisone.

These results strongly suggest that the combined treatment with NSAIDs or steroidal drugs and sucralfate will greatly mitigate the adverse effect of the former drugs on the healing process of preexisting ulcers.

Conclusion

A few of the most illustrative potency tests for sucralfate that have so far been performed in Japan and abroad, with various experimental ulcer models, were presented with special reference to assessment of the drug's potency and action. Sucralfate was shown to have a powerful inhibitory action on acute ulcer models and to have a healing-promoting effect on chronic ulcer models. The test results, the clinical effects and mechanism of action of sucralfate, as well as the future outlook for the drug, can be briefly summarized as follows:

1. Not all drugs that have been proved to be effective in animal models will manifest a therapeutically adequate antiulcer action. Sucralfate can safely be said to be among those that exert a reliable therapeutic effect on both experimental and human ulcers.
2. Sucralfate has been shown to have inhibitory effect on the development of experimental drug-induced ulcers, but its clinical usefulness in human NSAID gastritis remains to be established.
3. Sucralfate has been demonstrated in clinical studies to promote the healing of peptic ulcers to essentially the same degree as H_2RAs.
4. Efforts to elucidate new mechanisms of the protection of the mucosa provided by sucralfate will increase our understanding of the mechanisms involved in the activities of this drug which has multiple mechanisms of action.
5. Studies of the mechanisms of ulcer healing and prevention of recurrence will prove of help in understanding the mechanisms whereby sucralfate promotes the healing of peptic ulcers.

ACKOWLEDGMENT. We thank N. J. Halewood for critical reading of the manuscript.

References

1. Thomson ABR, Mahachai V: Medical management of uncomplicated peptic ulcer disease, in Berk JE (ed): *Gastroenterology*. Philadelphia, Saunders, 1985, p 1132–1133. A review of the medical approach to the therapy of peptic ulcer disease.
2. Hunt RH: The treatment of peptic ulcer disease with sucralfate: A review. *Am J Med* **91**(suppl 2A):102–106, 1991. A recent review of the therapy of peptic ulcer disease with sucralfate.
3. Namekata M: Studies on oxidized starch sulfates for medical purposes. IV. Protective effect of sulfates of oxidized starch and its reduced products on experimental peptic ulceration. *Chem Pharm*

Bull **10:**177–181, 1962. One of the original articles dealing with the effects of sucralfate on experimental ulcers.

4. Okabe S, Takeuchi K, Kunimi H, *et al*: Effects of an antiulcer drug, sucralfate (a basic aluminum salt of sulfated disaccharide), on experimental gastric lesions and gastric secretion in rats. *Dig Dis Sci* **28:**1034–1042, 1983. An article dealing with the antiulcer activity of sucralfate on various experimental ulcer models.
5. Nagashima R: Development and characteristics of sucralfate. *J Clin Gastroenterol* **3**(suppl 2):103–110, 1981. A review article about the development of sucralfate.
6. Auguste LJ, Shamash F, Stein TA, *et al*: Effect of sucralfate on the gastric mucosal levels of prostaglandin E_2. *Curr Surg* **44:**127–132, 1987. An article dealing with the effects of sucralfate on endogenous prostaglandins.
7. Tasman-Jones C: Gastric mucus. Physical properties in cytoprotection. *Med J Aust* **142**(suppl): S5–S6, 1985. An article dealing with the effect of sucralfate on gastric mucus.
8. Shea-Donohue T, Steel L, Montcalm E, *et al*: Gastric protection by sucralfate. Role of mucus and prostaglandins. *Gastroenterology* **91:**660–666, 1986. An article dealing with the effect of sucralfate on gastric mucus and PGs.
9. Konturek SJ, Brzozowski T, Majka J, *et al*: Nitric oxide in gastroprotection by sucralfate, mild irritants and nocloprost. *Gastroenterology* **102**(p 2):A101, 1992. An article dealing with the mechanisms of gastroprotective action of sucralfate.
10. Ligumsky M, Karmeli F, Rachmilewitz D: Sucralfate protection against gastrointestinal damage: Possible role of prostanoids. *Isr J Med Sci* **22:**801–806, 1986. An article dealing with the mechanisms underlying the gastroprotection of sucralfate.
11. Nobuhara Y, Takeuchi K, Okabe S: Effects of various agents on prednisolone-induced gastric lesions in rats. *Jpn J Pharmacol* **38:**219–222, 1985. An article dealing with the effects of various drugs, including sucralfate, on experimental gastric ulcers induced by prednisolone.
12. Morris GP, Keenan CM, MacNaughton WK, *et al*: Protection of rat gastric mucosa by sucralfate. Effects of luminal stasis and of inhibition of prostaglandin synthesis. *Am J Med* **86**(suppl 6A):10–16, 1989. An article dealing with the mechanisms of gastroprotective action of sucralfate.
13. Hollander D, Tarnawski A, Krause WJ, *et al*: Protective effect of sucralfate against alcohol-induced gastric mucosal injury in the rat. Macroscopic, histologic, ultrastructural, and functional time sequence analysis. *Gastroenterology* **88:**366–374, 1985. An article dealing with the mechanisms of gastroprotective action of sucralfate.
14. Coleman JC, Lacz JP, Browne RK, *et al*: Effects of sucralfate or mild irritants on experimental gastritis and prostaglandin production. *Am J Med* **83**(suppl 3B):24–30, 1987. An article dealing with the mechanism of gastroprotective action of sucralfate in relation to endogenous PGs.
15. Chen BW, Hiu WM, Lam SK, *et al*: Effect of sucralfate on gastric mucosal blood flow in rats. *Gut* **30:**1544–1551, 1989. An article dealing with the effect of sucralfate on gastric mucosal blood flow.
16. Szabo S, Brown A: Prevention of ethanol-induced vascular injury and gastric mucosal lesions by sucralfate and its components: Possible role of endogenous sulfhydryls. *Proc Soc Exp Biol Med* **185:**493–497, 1987. An article dealing with the gastroprotective mechanism of sucralfate in relation to endogenous sulfhydryls.
17. Okabe S, Ogihara Y: Effects of sucralfate on delayed healing of acetic acid-induced gastric ulcers in rats (Abstract). *Jpn J Pharmacol* (suppl) **49:**191, 1989. An article dealing with the preventive effect of sucralfate on delayed healing of experimental gastric ulcers caused by indomethacin.
18. Konturek SJ, Brzozowski T, Drozdowicz D, *et al*: Role of acid milieu in the gastroprotective and ulcer-healing activity of sucralfate. *Am J Med* **91**(suppl 2A):20–29, 1991. An article dealing with the mechanism of gastroprotective action of sucralfate.
19. Kuwayama H, Matsuo Y, Eastwood GL: Effects of sucralfate, lansoprazole, and cimetidine on the delayed healing by hydrocortisone sodium phosphate of chronic gastric ulcers in the rat. *Am J Med* **91**(suppl 2A):15–19, 1991. An article dealing with the mechanism of action of sucralfate on delayed healing of experimental gastric ulcers by hydrocortisone.

20

Effect on Experimental Esophageal Injury

ROY CHARLES ORLANDO

Introduction

Gastroesophageal reflux occurs in everyone and in the large majority it remains a benign event, producing neither symptoms nor signs of disease. The reason for this is the presence of a three-tiered esophageal defense that is poised to: (1) minimize the frequency of reflux events (antireflux barriers such as the lower esophageal sphincter), (2) minimize the duration of contact between esophageal epithelium and noxious elements in the refluxate (luminal clearance mechanisms), and (3) minimize the impact and damage to the tissue during the time of contact with the noxious elements in the refluxate (Fig. 1).

In about 10% of subjects, gastroesophageal reflux is pathologic, producing symptoms (e.g., heartburn) and damage to tissue; most commonly that tissue is the esophageal epithelium. Damage from reflux is caused by the presence within the stomach of high concentrations of gastric (hydrochloric) acid (pH of gastric contents daily falling as low as 0.8–1). Further experimental studies have shown that the rate and/or degree of mucosal damage to esophageal epithelium is markedly accelerated if pepsin or conjugated bile salts are present within an acidic refluxate, although the importance of these additives relative to the development of reflux esophagitis is clinically uncertain. Nonetheless, given that the presence of these three factors in a refluxate is responsible for most of the damage, drugs that reduce the noxious quality of one or more of them would be anticipated to be efficacious for the treatment of reflux esophagitis.

Sucralfate, the basic salt of aluminum hydroxide and sucrose octasulfate, is a poorly absorbed oral agent that has been reported to reduce symptoms and heal lesions in patients with reflux disease (see Chapter 26). Although the mechanisms by which sucralfate exerts its beneficial effects are complex and still poorly understood, data from experimental studies with animal tissue have provided insight into some of its unique qualities. Interest-

ROY CHARLES ORLANDO • Tulane University School of Medicine, New Orleans, Louisiana 70112.

Sucralfate: From Basic Science to the Bedside, edited by Daniel Hollander and G. N. J. Tytgat. Plenum Press, New York, 1995.

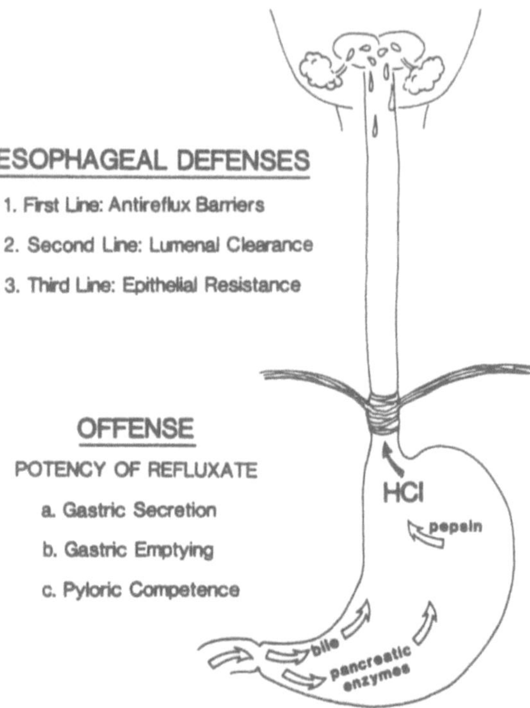

Figure 1. The determinants of reflux injury to esophageal mucosa are shown. Esophagitis develops when the noxious contents accumulated within the stomach (offensive force) exceed the protective capacity of the three-tiered defensive system. (Reprinted with modifications from Orlando RC: Reflux esophagitis, in Yamada T (ed): *Textbook of Gastroenterology*. Philadelphia, J B Lippincott Co, 1991.)

ingly, sucralfate as constituted in pill form is insoluble in water.[1,2] When in contact with acid, however, it initially polymerizes into a white viscid substance through the creation of intermolecular and intramolecular hydrogen bonds. On continued exposure to an acidic environment, the molecule undergoes further change releasing both aluminum and the water-soluble and tissue-reactive sulfated sugar, sucrose octasulfate. In Table I the actions by which sucralfate and its components protect against injury to the esophageal epithelium are listed and these are discussed in more detail below.

Benefits of Sucralfate in Experimental Esophagitis

Intraluminal Buffering

Since it has been well documented that acid is highly damaging to the esophageal mucosa, agents with the capacity to buffer hydrogen ions clearly have the potential for

Table I. Sucralfate: Mechanisms of Protection in Esophagitis

1.	Intraluminal buffering
2.	Intraluminal binding of pepsin
3.	Intraluminal binding of bile salts
4.	Creation of a preepithelial diffusion barrier
5.	Enhanced tissue resistance to acid

therapeutic benefit in reflux disease. In this respect, sucralfate contains aluminum hydroxide, a buffer commonly employed in over-the-counter antacids. However, the amount of aluminum hydroxide in sucralfate is small and its buffering capacity is only slowly realized on placement of the compound in acid solution. Therefore, it is generally acknowledged that sucralfate is an ineffective buffer and one, in fact, that is incapable of raising the pH of gastric contents. However, in circumstances where the volume of acid is low, as for example within the esophageal lumen after the bolus of the refluxate has been cleared by peristalsis and gravity (residual volume approximately 1 ml of acid), even the modest buffering capacity in sucralfate may be beneficial. Orlando and colleagues have in fact documented such a scenario in experimental studies using Ussing chamber-mounted sheets of rabbit esophageal epithelium.[3] In these studies, tissues treated with sucralfate can be shown to raise pH sufficiently to protect (both morphologically and functionally, the latter by prevention of the decline in tissue electrical resistance) against injury from exposure to small noxious concentrations of acid.

Intraluminal Binding of Pepsin

The addition of pepsin to an acidic solution is known to increase the solution's noxious potential for damaging the esophageal epithelium. Therefore, agents with the capacity to reduce peptic activity should also possess therapeutic benefit. Sucralfate is a molecule that has been shown to possess pepsin-binding properties, a function that appears to reside in both its aluminum hydroxide and sucrose octasulfate moieties. In this respect the experiments by Schweitzer and colleagues using *in vivo* acid-perfused rabbit esophagi are of interest.[4] They perfused the rabbit esophagus with a nondamaging concentration of acid, but converted the solution to a damaging one by the addition of pepsin. Subsequently, the administration of sucralfate to a group of acid–pepsin-perfused animals was observed to be protective, a finding consistent solely with the propensity for sucralfate to bind pepsin and so reduce its activity in solution.

Intraluminal Binding of Bile Salts

Like pepsin, the addition of conjugated bile salts to an acidic solution is known to increase the solution's potential to damage the esophageal epithelium. Therefore, agents such as sucralfate that possess the capacity to reduce their concentration in solution should be of therapeutic benefit in those cases of reflux esophagitis in which bile salts play a role. Currently, it remains uncertain as to what role bile salts play in the pathogenesis of esophagitis for subjects in whom the refluxate is acidic. Nonetheless, it is generally accepted that deconjugated bile salts do play an important role in many cases of "alkaline" esophagitis in which the pH of the refluxate is from 7 to 8.

Creation of a Preepithelial Diffusion Barrier

To produce damage to the esophageal epithelium, noxious elements within the refluxate must first diffuse from the aqueous luminal environment to the epithelial cell surface. This process (of diffusion), however, can be altered by changing the nature of the milieu through which the ions and molecules must pass. Sucralfate, by virtue of its polymerization to a viscid material in an acidic medium and subsequent adherence to the epithelial cell surface, does in effect create a physical barrier to diffusion both for hydrogen ions and for pepsin.[4] However, it is important to note that the degree to which this property as opposed to others possessed by sucralfate contributes to its therapeutic benefit remains unclear, because protection by sucralfate against acid injury can be demonstrated without the formation of this visible substance (see below).

Enhanced Tissue Resistance to Acid

As noted above, the polymerization of sucralfate and its adherence to mucosal surfaces can protect by creating a physical barrier to diffusion of ions and molecules; however, studies by Orlando and colleagues have shown that sucralfate can exert a protective effect against acid injury to esophageal epithelium even without it.[3] The reason for this is the liberation in an acidic environment of the water-soluble and tissue-reactive molecule, sucrose octasulfate. Although forming no visible barrier, sucrose octasulfate has been clearly shown to alter the ability of rabbit esophageal epithelia to withstand the damaging effects of acid (Fig. 2).[3,5] The precise mechanism by which sucrose octasulfate produces a more resistant tissue has yet to be determined, but it is clear that, unlike gastric tissues, the protective effect is not related to the release of tissue prostaglandins.[6] Prostaglandins in experimental esophagitis appear to have no protective role and in fact some studies have suggested that their administration may lead to worsening of acid- or radiation-mediated disease.

Summary

Sucralfate can improve symptoms and lesion healing in subjects with reflux esophagitis through multiple mechanisms. These mechanisms include both the ability to act within the lumen to reduce the activity of hydrogen ions (by buffering), pepsin and bile salts (by binding), and by the ability to interact with the epithelium to produce a physical (by polymerization) and chemical (by creation of sucrose octasulfate) barrier to hydrogen ions. Experimental studies have documented that the aluminum hydroxide moiety in sucralfate is responsible for its buffering capacity as well as for a significant component of its capacity to act as a binding agent. The sucrose octasulfate component of sucralfate also has the capacity to bind pepsin as well as to exert a unique action on the tissue that reduces

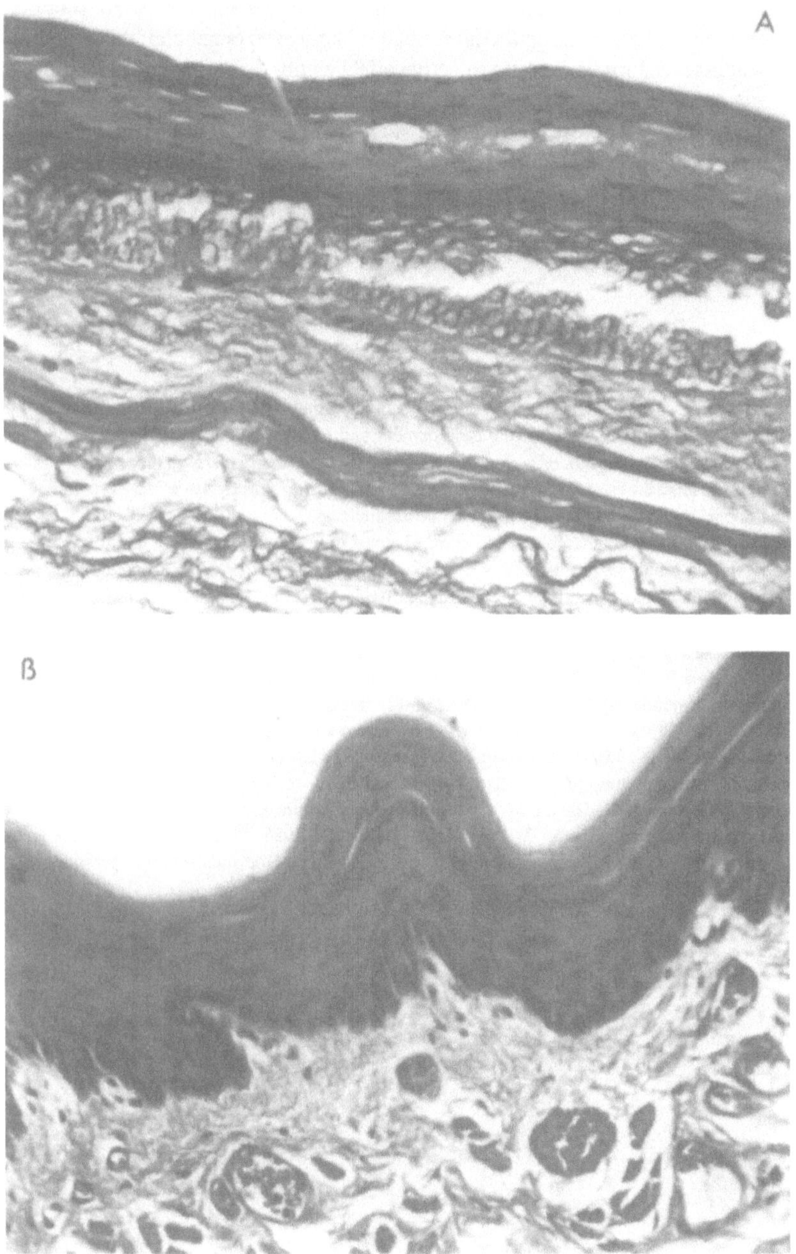

Figure 2. Esophageal epithelium 1 hr after *in vivo* perfusion with 120 mM HCl/120 mM NaCl (pH 1.1). Intracellular and intercellular edema is present throughout the tissue and the upper and lower layers have been separated by extensive necrosis in the midlayer.

the damaging effects of hydrogen ions. Further, though the ability of sucralfate to polymerize and adhere to the epithelial surface is likely to be beneficial, this property does not appear essential for its overall protective effect against experimental acid injury to the esophagus.

Finally, it is of interest that although sucralfate has many properties that appear to make it an ideal agent for the treatment of reflux disease, clinical trials have not been uniformly successful. Although the precise reasons for this are not clear (see Chapter 26), the problem appears to be related to sucralfate's water-insoluble nature and limited time of retention within the human esophagus after ingestion as a suspension.

References

1. Nagashima R: Development and characteristics of sucralfate. *J Clin Gastroenterol* **3**(suppl 2):103–110, 1981. This article describes the development and molecular characteristics of sucralfate.
2. Nagashima R: Mechanisms of action of sucralfate. *J Clin Gastroenterol* **3**(suppl 2):117–127, 1981. This article describes some of the early *in vitro* data supporting a protective effect of sucralfate against acid-peptic injury to epithelia of the gastrointestinal tract.
3. Orlando RC, Turjman NA, Tobey NA, *et al*: Mucosal protection by sucralfate and its components in acid-exposed rabbit esophagus. *Gastroenterology* **93**:352–361, 1987. This article demonstrates that the two components of sucralfate, aluminum hydroxide and sucrose octasulfate, contain very different protective properties against acid injury to the esophagus.
4. Schweitzer EJ, Bass BL, Johnson LF, *et al*: Sucralfate prevents esophagitis in rabbits. *Gastroenterology* **88**:611–619, 1985. This article demonstrates the ability of sucralfate to convert a damaging acid solution to a nondamaging one through its ability to bind pepsin.
5. Orlando RC, Tobey NA: Why does sucralfate improve healing in reflux esophagitis? The role of sucrose octasulfate. *Scand J Gastroenterol* **25**(suppl 173):17–21, 1990. This article demonstrates the protective effect of sucrose octasulfate against acid injury to human esophageal mucosa.
6. Katz PO, Geisinger KR, Hassan M, *et al*: Acid-induced esophagitis in cats is prevented by sucralfate but not synthetic prostaglandin W. *Dig Dis Sci* **33**:217–224, 1988. This article supports the protective properties of sucralfate against acid injury to the esophagus and indicates that prostaglandins are unlikely candidates to mediate its beneficial effects.

V

Safety and Drug Interactions

21

Safety of Sucralfate

DAVID R. MATHEWS and NICOLA G. DAHL

General Background Information

Sucralfate, the basic aluminum salt of a sulfated disaccharide, is an ulcer-healing drug that has been used worldwide for over 20 years. The drug is extremely well tolerated during acute and maintenance therapy, and has proven to have an excellent overall safety profile related in large part to its nonsystemic action.

In short-term[1,2] and long-term[3] double-blind clinical trials, the incidence of adverse events was similar in the sucralfate and placebo treatment groups. The most commonly reported adverse reactions associated with sucralfate can be attributed to local effects in the gastrointestinal tract.

Constipation, the most frequent complaint, occurs in about 2% of patients. The mechanism of constipation has not been clearly established, but aluminum has been shown to depress motility of gastrointestinal smooth muscle. The reduced gastrointestinal motility can lead to constipation.

Concern for aluminum absorption and accumulation during sucralfate therapy, especially with long-term use, has been expressed. Sucralfate is minimally absorbed after oral administration. The low systemic absorption of sucralfate may result from its low solubility and high polarity in the gastrointestinal tract. Studies indicate that only 3–5% of an oral dose reaches systemic circulation as sucrose sulfate,[4] whereas the amount of aluminum absorbed is less than 0.02%.[5] It has been demonstrated that the small amount of aluminum absorbed from sucralfate is rapidly eliminated through the kidney and does not appear to accumulate, except in chronic renal failure patients (data on file).

Some of the information discussed in this chapter has been derived from clinical studies performed or sponsored by Marion Merrell Dow Inc., where additional information is on file (i.e., "Human Toxicology" data, information on potential distribution of aluminum after absorption, intraluminal binding information).

DAVID R. MATHEWS and NICOLA G. DAHL • Marion Merrell Dow Inc., Kansas City, Missouri 64137.

Sucralfate: From Basic Science to the Bedside, edited by Daniel Hollander and G. N. J. Tytgat. Plenum Press, New York, 1995.

Clinical Trial Safety Data

In pre- and postmarketing clinical studies in the United States, adverse reactions to sucralfate were minor and rarely led to discontinuation of the drug. In studies involving over 2700 patients treated with sucralfate for up to 1 year, adverse effects were reported in 129 (4.7%) (data on file).

Constipation was the most frequent complaint (2%). Other gastrointestinal adverse effects reported in less than 0.5% of the patients included diarrhea, nausea, vomiting, gastric discomfort, indigestion, flatulence, and dry mouth. In addition, pruritus, rash, dizziness, sleepiness, vertigo, back pain, and headache were also reported in less than 0.5% of the patients.

Side effect comparisons with placebo during an acute (up to 8 weeks) sucralfate clinical trial are provided in Table I. Of the 116 sucralfate-treated patients, 15 (12.9%) had a complaint listed as a side effect. This was nearly identical to the incidence in the placebo group (14/116 patients; 12.1%). Neither sucralfate nor placebo had an effect on hematologic, renal, or hepatic function.[2]

In another premarketing study comparing maintenance (up to 1 year) sucralfate and placebo therapy in duodenal ulcer patients ($n = 61$), only three patients experienced drug-related side effects. One sucralfate-treated patient reported an episode consisting of

Table I. Side Effects Reported during a Premarketing Acute Duodenal Ulcer Study

	Sucralfate (n = 116) (No. of patients)	Placebo (n = 116) (No. of patients)
Constipation	3	0
Nausea	2	2
Headache(s)	2	1
Dry mouth	2	1
Indigestion	1	0
Pruritus, hives	1	0
Rash	1	1
Vertigo	1	0
Dizziness	1	1
Hypertension	1	1
Back pain	1	2
Diarrhea	0	3
Drowsiness	0	2
Vomiting	0	1
Hot spells	0	1
Nervousness	0	1
Nocturia	0	1
Desquamation	0	1
Fatigue	0	1
Increased appetite	0	1
Lightheadedness	0	1
	16	21

headache, nausea, tinnitus, amblyopia, and dizziness. Two placebo-treated patients experienced side effects, one with constipation and one with nausea. Results of clinical laboratory tests indicated that sucralfate had no effects on hematologic, hepatic or renal function, or electrolyte concentrations (including calcium and phosphorus).[3]

Postmarketing Surveillance Safety Data

Since the introduction of sucralfate to the U.S. market in 1981, the adverse events noted in the premarketing clinical trials above continue to be the most common reports.

In addition, there are postmarketing reports of hypersensitivity reactions, including urticaria (hives), angioedema, and rhinitis (data on file). A causal relationship between the hypersensitivity reactions and sucralfate has not been established and, most of the time, the reaction disappears without interruption of sucralfate therapy. Although the molecular structure of sucralfate includes a sulfur ion in the sulfate moiety, it is not chemically related to the sulfonamide compounds. The possibility of a cross-hypersensitivity reaction in patients with a documented "sulfa allergy" receiving sucralfate has never been investigated. However, because of the chemical differences, this possibility is remote.

Human Toxicology

As summarized below, no serious untoward effects were seen in healthy volunteers who received up to three times the recommended total daily dose of sucralfate for 4 weeks.

In order to evaluate human toxicologic effects of sucralfate, healthy men (18–49 years old, 54–86 kg) were given single daily oral doses of 4, 8, and 12 g (three subjects received 4 g, three received 8 g, and three received 12 g). In the multiple-dose portion of the study, 2 g was given qid (which is double the recommended 1-g qid dose for duodenal ulcer therapy) for 14 days, and 3 g was given qid (three times the recommended dose) for 28 days (data on file).

Three subjects reported nausea and/or vomiting, two in the 2-g qid group and one in the 3-g qid group. One subject given 2 g qid reported abdominal pain. No adverse effects of sucralfate administration were noted in results of the following tests/observations: hematology, blood chemistry, urinalysis, electrocardiogram, pulse rate, blood pressure, temperature, body weight, ophthalmic exam, audiogram, and stool guaiac.

Potential Aluminum Absorption and Toxicity

Overview

Sucralfate, although minimally absorbed, contains approximately 20% of elemental aluminum by weight. The aluminum moiety can dissociate at low pH and be released in the stomach. The maximum amount of aluminum available for absorption from a 4-g daily dose of sucralfate is approximately 800 mg.

Concern has been expressed about aluminum absorption and accumulation during sucralfate therapy, especially with long-term use. Based on the available information, however, sucralfate-treated patients with normal kidney function are not at risk for developing aluminum toxicity. The only reports of aluminum-related toxicity during sucralfate therapy have been described in patients with end-stage renal disease. Because the kidney is the primary route for elimination of aluminum, and because aluminum does not cross dialysis membranes, sucralfate should be used with caution in patients with chronic renal failure.

Until recently, understanding of the absorption, distribution, and excretion of aluminum after oral ingestion was limited because of the lack of sensitive analytical techniques to determine aluminum concentration. Information available concerning the pharmacokinetics and toxicity of aluminum in general, and sucralfate specifically, is summarized in the following sections.

Absorption

In a review article addressing aluminum absorption in general, Alfrey stated that over 98% of an oral aluminum load is excreted in the feces.[6] Based on data available from aluminum-containing antacid studies, the normal gastrointestinal uptake of aluminum is 0.1–0.3%.[5] This information suggests that only a very small percentage of aluminum from orally ingested sucralfate would be absorbed systemically.

There is one study that estimated the amount of aluminum absorbed from sucralfate. Haram *et al.*[5] compared aluminum absorption from sucralfate or an aluminum-containing antacid in a randomized, crossover study. Eleven volunteers with normal renal function received four doses of either 1 g sucralfate or 1100 mg aluminum hydroxide/magnesium carbonate gel (approximate 244 mg aluminum/tablet) over a 1-day period. The treatments were separated by at least 1 week. The daily urinary excretion of aluminum was measured for 4 days, beginning the day before each treatment was started. There was no significant difference in urinary aluminum excretion between the two treatments. There was also no significant difference in calculated median percentage aluminum absorption: 0.005% (range: 0.001–0.017%) from sucralfate and 0.006% (range: 0.002–0.060%) from aluminum-containing antacid.

Distribution

Based on autopsy reports, subjects with no evidence of kidney disease have low concentrations of aluminum in all tissues except the lung.[7] When renal function deteriorates, tissue aluminum concentrations increase (especially in the liver and bone). When sucralfate is used for up to 1 year, the small amount of aluminum absorbed does not appear to accumulate in bone or affect mineral metabolism in patients with normal kidney function.[3,8]

Excretion

With normal environmental exposure in subjects with normal renal function, the kidney appears to be capable of excreting all absorbed aluminum.[9] In addition, it has been demonstrated that subjects with normal kidney function can respond to an oral aluminum load (aluminum-containing antacids) by increasing urinary aluminum excretion by 30 to

40 times baseline values.[10] It should also be noted that this study reported a rapid decrease in urinary aluminum excretion when oral aluminum loading is discontinued.

Aluminum Toxicity and Plasma Aluminum Concentrations

In general, aluminum toxicity (encephalopathy, osteomalacia, microcytic hypochromic anemia, myopathy, or cardiac conduction defects) has been observed almost exclusively in dialysis patients. The symptoms of toxicity usually are manifest after months of systemic aluminum exposure. Most of the cases reported in the literature occurred in patients who received large aluminum loads through intravenous (dialysis treatments with aluminum-contaminated dialysate) and/or oral (aluminum-containing antacids to control hyperphosphatemia) routes of administration.[11]

Plasma aluminum concentrations may not correlate with intake or body load and should not be used as a sole determinant of aluminum toxicity. Although serum aluminum monitoring by itself is not adequate for evaluating aluminum intoxication, osteomalacia appears to be associated with aluminum concentrations between 100 and 200 μg/liter,[12] and neurotoxicity has been reported at serum aluminum concentrations greater than 300 μg/liter in dialysis patients.[13]

To date, there are six published case reports of aluminum-related toxicity during sucralfate therapy.[14–19] All six cases involved dialysis patients who received sucralfate for either prolonged periods (4 and 6 months) or in conjunction with other sources of aluminum.

In summary, although it is difficult to determine the extent of aluminum absorption from sucralfate administration, it appears that the amount of aluminum absorbed from sucralfate is similar to that from aluminum-containing antacids. The data available also suggest that aluminum does not accumulate in bone during short-term sucralfate administration or in serum during short- or long-term therapy in patients with normal kidney function. However, aluminum-related toxicity has been reported during sucralfate therapy in dialysis patients; therefore, the potential for aluminum accumulation in this patient population should be considered.

Aluminum Toxicity versus Alzheimer's Disease

There is no evidence that sucralfate administration is linked to Alzheimer's disease. Research has suggested that aluminum deposits are increased in persons with Alzheimer's disease. However, a recent review article stated that evidence indicates that Alzheimer's disease and aluminum toxicity are two different disease processes with distinct clinical, histologic, and neurochemical features.[20] Exposure to aluminum-containing medications does not increase the risk of Alzheimer's disease.

Bezoar Potential

Bezoars (indigestible concretions) form in the stomach or intestine of patients with impaired gastric emptying related to the effects of prior gastrointestinal surgery or other conditions associated with gastric stasis (e.g., diabetic gastroparesis). The presence of adhesions, diverticula, or other abnormalities may predispose a patient to the formation of bezoars. Along with various foodstuffs, certain medications may occasionally become impacted in the gastrointestinal tract.

Characteristics of sucralfate that may favor bezoar formation include the formation of an insoluble gelatinous substance in the presence of acid, and its tendency to delay gastric motility. These factors should be kept in mind when considering the use of this agent in patients prone to bezoar formation. It is also important to note that sucralfate may bind with other compounds administered through a nasogastric tube including antacids and proteins in enteral feedings.

There are infrequent reports of bezoar formation in patients receiving sucralfate.[21–26] These patients usually had other factors which may have contributed to, or been the primary cause of, the mass formation. Thus, a definitive causal relationship between bezoar formation and sucralfate therapy is yet to be established.

Intraluminal Binding

Phosphate-Binding Effects

Sucralfate has phosphate-binding activity comparable in potency to aluminum hydroxide antacids when equivalent amounts of aluminum are administered. Sucralfate has been used therapeutically as a phosphate-binding agent in dialysis patients.[27,28] The available data suggest that sucralfate doses, 2 to 4 g/day, have minimal effect on serum phosphorus in patients with normal kidney function. However, prolonged exposure to large doses of aluminum-containing medication, including sucralfate, has been associated with hypophosphatemia.[29]

It is not recommended that sucralfate be used as a phosphate-binding agent, since it offers no advantage over aluminum antacids.

Potential Binding with Nutrients

Direct incompatibilities between sucralfate and any dietary substances have not yet been demonstrated. However, since sucralfate is a locally active agent, it is recommended that this product be dosed on an empty stomach to prevent potential interaction with other materials (e.g., food) in the gastrointestinal tract. Based on an animal investigation, sucralfate will bind with food; however, the selective binding of sucralfate to the ulcer sites is not altered.[30] Since this study was done in animals, the extrapolation of these findings to humans who have highly variable diets is limited.

Studies evaluating the effect of sucralfate on nutrient absorption have not been conducted. But the absence of reports describing vitamin deficiency during short- or long-term sucralfate administration suggests that the potential for an interaction is minimal.

Safety Concerns Associated with Nasogastric Tube Administration of Sucralfate

Sucralfate suspension has been evaluated in critical care patients with nasogastric tubes in place. To avoid clogging of the tube and potential bezoar formation in this high-risk population, the following method of sucralfate suspension administration through the tube has been described[31]:

1. After administration of the sucralfate or antacid dose, the nasogastric tube is clamped for 1 hr.
2. If regurgitation occurred around the tube or the volume of aspirate exceeded 150 ml at the end of the 1-hr period, the tube is clamped for 30 min after each drug administration; intermittent suction is applied for 30 min of each hour until the aspirate is less than 150 ml.

Information concerning the administration of sucralfate in relation to tube feedings was not provided. As mentioned previously, it is desirable to have this product dosed on an empty stomach to prevent potential interaction with other products (e.g., food) in the gastrointestinal tract. To allow administration of sucralfate on an empty stomach (as recommended), it would be ideal to temporarily discontinue tube feedings when the sucralfate dose is given.

Flushing the tube before and after sucralfate administration may help prevent clogging and minimize the possible interaction with other administered compounds. It has been recommended that 10 ml of water be used as the flushing solution.[32]

Use in Special Populations

Use in Geriatric Patients

Peptic ulcer disease (PUD) is present in approximately 25% of elderly hospitalized patients and 12% of elderly outpatients.[33] Although some of the clinical aspects of PUD are unaffected by age, changes in the pathophysiology of the disease and in individual response to drug therapy can occur with increasing age. PUD can be a more serious disease in elderly (compared with younger patients) with a higher mortality rate and a greater incidence of complications.

The aging process is associated with reduced acid secretion and motor function, and a weakening of mucosal defenses, such as decreased mucosal thickness, gastric cell renewal, and mucosal blood flow.[33,34] Initially, there had been speculation that sucralfate required an acidic pH for activity and might not work as well in older patients because of reduced gastric acid output. However, subsequent studies suggest that gastric pH does not have a major influence on the binding of sucralfate to ulcerated mucosa or on sucralfate efficacy. In addition, the mechanism of antiulcer activity of sucralfate includes enhancing mucosal defense properties. Review articles discussing antiulcer management in the elderly include sucralfate as effective therapy.[34,35]

In general, side effects occur more frequently in geriatric patients than in younger patients. The higher incidence of adverse reactions in the elderly population may be the result of pharmacokinetic (absorption, distribution, or elimination) and/or pharmacodynamic (receptor responsiveness) differences that occur with age, or may be the result of multiple-drug therapy. The favorable side effect profile and the minimal systemic absorption of sucralfate have been recognized as beneficial features in older patients.

Studies that evaluate the efficacy and safety of sucralfate specifically in older patients have not been conducted. However, similar to the general population, about 30% of the duodenal ulcer patients in U.S. multicenter studies ($n = 271$) were 60 years or older. The outcome of these geriatric patients, in terms of ulcer healing and side effects, were similar to those of the entire study group. These data are supported by a retrospective survey of 196 geriatric patients with PUD. The healing rates with sucralfate [1 g four times daily or 2 g twice daily (38/48; 79.1%)] and H_2 antagonists [cimetidine or ranitidine; 75/94 (79.4%)] were similar; the side effect profiles were also similar (data on file).

Use during Pregnancy

Carafate (sucralfate) is placed in the Food and Drug Administration (FDA)-assigned pregnancy Category B. Category B denotes that animal reproduction studies have failed to demonstrate a risk to the fetus, and there are no adequate and well-controlled studies in pregnant women. Fetal or reproductive defects were not observed in rodents given 15 to 45 times the recommended human sucralfate dose. However, because animal studies are not always predictive of human response, sucralfate should be used during pregnancy only if clearly needed (data on file).

The Committee on FDA-Related Matters of the American College of Gastroenterology published their summary of the use of gastrointestinal drugs during pregnancy and lactation.[36] This committee considered sucralfate to be a drug in which the potential benefit probably outweighs the potential risk in any trimester of pregnancy.

There is a single published report[37] describing the use of sucralfate in pregnant patients. In this study, sucralfate relieved symptoms of pyrosis with minimal maternal adverse effects (one case of diarrhea was reported). However, possible effects of sucralfate on the fetus were not mentioned in this report.

Use in Lactating Women

The excretion of sucralfate into breast milk has not been investigated.

The Committee on FDA-Related Matters of the American College of Gastroenterology concluded that sucralfate appeared to be safe for use in nursing mothers because the drug is minimally absorbed from the gastrointestinal tract.[36]

Conclusion

The remarkable safety record of sucralfate has been established during 20 years of worldwide clinical use. In short- and long-term double-blind studies, the incidence and severity of side effects were similar in the sucralfate and placebo treatments. Because it is minimally absorbed, the most common side effects that occur during sucralfate therapy are gastrointestinal in nature and include constipation, diarrhea, nausea, and indigestion. Its nonsystemic side effect profile may offer potential advantage in special populations such as geriatric patients, and pregnant or lactating women. Sucralfate should be used with caution in ulcer patients with end-stage renal disease, however, because the small percentage of absorbed aluminum may accumulate, especially in patients receiving other sources of aluminum or during prolonged administration.

References

1. Hollander D: Efficacy of sucralfate for duodenal ulcers: A multicenter, double-blind trial. *J Clin Gastroenterol* **3**(suppl 2)**:**153–157, 1981. References 1 through 3 are clinical trials evaluating the efficacy and safety of Carafate tablets in patients with duodenal ulcers.
2. McHardy GG: A multicenter, double-blind trial of sucralfate and placebo in duodenal ulcer. *J Clin Gastroenterol* **3**(suppl 2)**:**147–152, 1981.
3. Behar J, Roufail W, Thomas E, *et al*: Efficacy of sucralfate in the prevention of recurrence of duodenal ulcers. *J Clin Gastroenterol* **9**(suppl 1)**:**23–30, 1987.
4. Giesing D, Lanman R, Runser D: Absorption of sucralfate in man. *Gastroenterology* **82**(5 pt 2)**:**1066, 1982 (Abstract). References 4 and 5 provide quantitative amounts of aluminum and sucrose octasulfate absorbed from sucralfate.
5. Haram EM, Weberg R, Berstad A: Urinary excretion of aluminum after ingestion of sucralfate and an aluminum-containing antacid in man. *Scand J Gastroenterol* **22:**615–618, 1987.
6. Alfrey AC: Gastrointestinal absorption of aluminum. *Clin Nephrol* **24**(1)**:**384–387, 1985.
7. Alfrey AC: Aluminum. *Adv Clin Chem* **23:**69–91, 1983. References 7, 9–13 provide background information on aluminum absorption, excretion, and toxicity.
8. Bannwarth B, Gaucher A, Burnel D, *et al*: Longterm sucralfate therapy. *J Rheumatol* **13**(6)**:**1187, 1986 (Letter). This article evaluates aluminum concentrations in bone obtained from sucralfate-treated patients.
9. Alfrey AC: Aluminum metabolism. *Kidney Int* **28**(18)**:**S8–S11, 1986.
10. Kaehny WD, Hegg AP, Alfrey AC: Gastrointestinal absorption of aluminum from aluminum containing antacids. *N Engl J Med* **296**(24)**:**1389–1390, 1977.
11. Wills MR, Savory J: Aluminum and chronic renal failure: Sources, absorption, transport, and toxicity. *Crit Rev Clin Lab* **27**(1)**:**59–107, 1989.
12. McCarthy JT, Milliner DS, Kurtz SB: Interpretation of serum aluminum values in dialysis patients. *Am J Clin Pathol* **86:**629–636, 1986.
13. Brahm M: Serum aluminum in nondialyzed chronic uremic patients before and during treatment with aluminum-containing phosphate-binding gels. *Clin Nephrol* **25:**231–235, 1986.
14. Burgess E: Aluminum toxicity from oral sucralfate therapy. *Nephron* **59**(3)**:**523–524, 1991 (Letter). References 14 through 19 are case reports of aluminum toxicity in sucralfate-treated patients. All six cases involve renal failure patients.
15. Campistol JM, Cases A, Botey A, *et al*: Acute aluminum encephalopathy in an uremic patient. *Nephron* **51**(1)**:**103–106, 1989.
16. Cappelli G, Facchini F, Malberti F, *et al*: Sucralfate as a cause of aluminum overload in patients undergoing hemodialysis. *G Ital Nefrol* **9**(2)**:**101–103, 1992 (Letter) (English translation of Italian).
17. Lederer ED, Gillum DM: Accelerated development of hypercalcemic aluminum associated bone disease in a patient with protracted acute renal failure. *Kidney Int* **35**(1)**:**378, 1989 (Abstract).
18. Min DI, D'Elia JA: Sucralfate-associated aluminum toxicity in a patient with renal failure: Treatment with deferoxamine. *Clin Pharm* **11**(7)**:**636–639, 1992.
19. Withers DJ, Woolf AS, Kingswood JC, *et al*: Encephalopathy in patient taking aluminum-containing agents, including sucralfate. *Lancet* **2**(8664)**:**674, 1989.
20. Hamdy RC: Aluminum toxicity and Alzheimer's disease. *Postgrad Med* **88**(5)**:**239–240, 1990. This article discusses the difference between Alzheimer's disease and aluminum toxicity.
21. Algozzine GJ, Hill G, Scoggins WG, *et al*: Sucralfate bezoar. *N Engl J Med* **309**(22)**:**1387, 1983 (Letter). References 21 through 26 are case reports of bezoars in sucralfate-treated patients.
22. Anderson W: Esophageal medication bezoar in patient receiving enteral feedings and sucralfate. *Am J Gastroenterol* **84**(2)**:**205–206, 1989 (Letter).
23. Carrougher JG, Barrilleaux CN: Esophageal bezoars: The sucralith. *Crit Care Med* **19**(6)**:**837–839, 1991.
24. Hart RS, Levin B, Gholson CF: Esophageal obstruction caused by sucralfate impaction. *Gastrointest Endosc* **35**(5)**:**474–475, 1989 (Letter).

25. Rowbottom SJ, Wilson J, Samuel L, *et al*: Total oesophageal obstruction in association with combined enteral feed and sucralfate therapy. *Anaesth Intensive Care* **21**(3):372–374, 1993.
26. Shueke M, Mihas AA: Esophageal bezoar due to sucralfate. *Endoscopy* **23**(5):305–306, 1991 (Letter).
27. Roxe DM, Mistovich M, Barch DH: Phosphate-binding effects of sucralfate in patients with chronic renal failure. *Am J Kidney Dis* **13**(3):194–199, 1989. References 27 and 28 are clinical studies evaluating the effect of sucralfate on serum phosphate in dialysis patients.
28. Kozak E, Hudnik V, Drinovec J, *et al*: The influence of aluminum hydroxide and sucralfate on serum aluminum levels in chronic dialysis patients, in *Trace Element Analytical Chemistry in Medicine and Biology*. Berlin, Walter de Gruyter & Co, 1987, pp 473–480.
29. Chines A, Pacifici R: Antacid and sucralfate-induced hypophosphatemic osteomalacia: A case report and review of the literature. *Calcif Tissue Int* **47**(5):291–295, 1990. This article is a case report of hypophosphatemia in a patient receiving sucralfate and antacids.
30. Giesing DH, Bighley LD, Iles RL: Effect of food and antacid on binding of sucralfate to normal and ulcerated gastric and duodenal mucosa in rats. *J Clin Gastroenterol* **3**(suppl 2):111–116, 1981. This reference is an animal study evaluating potential interactions between sucralfate and food or antacids.
31. Cannon LA, Heiselman D, Gardner W, *et al*: Prophylaxis of upper gastrointestinal tract bleeding in mechanically ventilated patients—A randomized study comparing the efficacy of sucralfate, cimetidine, and antacids. *Arch Intern Med* **147**:2101–2106, 1987. References 31 and 32 are stress ulcer prophylaxis studies that describe the administration of sucralfate through a nasogastric tube.
32. Driks MR, Craven DE, Celli BR, *et al*: Nosocomial pneumonia in intubated patients given sucralfate as compared with antacids or histamine type 2 blockers. *N Engl J Med* **317**:1376–1382, 1987.
33. Lamy PP, Kitler ME: Gastric erosions in the elderly: Increased need for cytoprotection. *Gastroenterol Clin Biol* **9**(12):102–105, 1985. References 33 through 35 discuss geriatric considerations in the medical management of PUD.
34. Miller DK, Burton FR, Burton MS, *et al*: Acute upper gastrointestinal bleeding in elderly persons. *JAGS* **4**:409–422, 1991 (Review).
35. Wade WE: Medical management of peptic ulcer disease in the elderly. *J Geriatr Drug Ther* **3**(2): 23–41, 1988.
36. Lewis JH, Weingold AB: The use of gastrointestinal drugs during pregnancy and lactation. *Am J Gastroenterol* **80**(11):912–923, 1985. This review provides the recommendations from the American College of Gastroenterology subcomittee on FDA-related activity concerning the use of gastrointestinal drugs in pregnant or lactating women.
37. Ranchet G, Gangemi O, Petrone M: Sucralfate in the treatment of gravidic pyrosis (Italian). *G Ital Ostet Ginecol* **XXII**(1):1–16, 1990 (English translation). This reference is an open-label study evaluating the use of sucralfate to treat heartburn in pregnant women.

22

Sucralfate Drug Interaction Studies

GILLES CAILLÉ and MANON VÉZINA

Introduction

This section reviews the literature on drug interactions with sucralfate. Since sucralfate is poorly absorbed, most of the dose remains in the gastrointestinal tract and the potential exists for sucralfate to affect the absorption of other drugs. Potential mechanisms of these interactions include adsorption, complexation, decreased dissolution resulting from altered pH, and the formation of a physical barrier to absorption.

In a series of studies in humans, sucralfate coadministration was shown not to influence significantly the absorption of acetaminophen, acetylsalicylic acid, chlorpropamide, erythromycin, prednisone, procainamide, roxatidine, theophylline (nonsustained release), and trisalicylate. In contrast, simultaneous administration of sucralfate with amitriptyline, ciprofloxacin, ketoconazole, norfloxacin, phenytoin, sulpride, and theophylline (sustained release) resulted in a statistically significant reduction in the bioavailability of these agents. No significant effect on bioavailability seemed to occur when digoxin or quinidine was administered 2 hr apart. Sucralfate may also be responsible for altered warfarin and cimetidine absorption in man, although recent studies indicated the absence of such an interaction. Ranitidine absorption may be impaired by large doses of sucralfate. Finally, sucralfate coadministration with NSAIDs resulted in a decrease in the rate but not in the extent of absorption of ibuprofen, indomethacin, ketoprofen, and naproxen. Complete bioavailability may be restored by separating the administration of sucralfate from that of the other agents by 2 hr.

These interactions appear to be nonsystemic and to result from the binding of sucralfate to the coadministered drug in the gastrointestinal tract.

GILLES CAILLÉ • Département de Pharmacologie, Faculté de Médecine, Université de Montréal, Montréal, H3C 3J7, Canada. MANON VÉZINA • Département de Pharmacologie, Faculté de Médecine, Université de Montréal, and Centre de Recherche Fernand Seguin, Hôpital Louis-Hippolyte Lafontaine, Montréal, Canada.

Sucralfate: From Basic Science to the Bedside, edited by Daniel Hollander and G. N. J. Tytgat. Plenum Press, New York, 1995.

Sucralfate—What Is It?

Sucralfate, an aluminum salt of sulfated sucrose, is used in treating patients with active peptic duodenal ulcers. Unlike conventional agents which are currently available for the treatment of peptic ulcer disease, sucralfate neither neutralizes acid nor reduces acid production, but acts mainly through binding with proteins at the ulcer crater, with the formation of a barrier to protect the mucosa against the damaging effect of acid and pepsin. In fact, when exposed to the acidic environment of the stomach, some aluminum is removed from the sucrose octasulfate molecules. This leaves a negatively charged substance that binds to positively charged protein molecules on the ulcer craters. This barrier protects the ulcer site by blocking acid diffusion across the mucosal surface and has been shown to absorb pepsin and bile salts.

Binding of sucralfate occurs mainly and preferentially to altered gastrointestinal mucosa. This barrier to diffusion, as well as the binding capabilities of sucralfate, have led to the hypothesis that altered absorption may occur when other medications are administered concurrently. Potential mechanisms of these interactions include adsorption, complexation, decreased dissolution related to altered pH, and the formation of a physical barrier to absorption.

The following section reviews the effect of sucralfate coadministration on the absorption of other drugs. With few exceptions, only data from human subjects are considered.

Which Drugs Interact with Sucralfate?

The results of trials designed to investigate the drugs that interact with sucralfate are listed in Table I. The data are based on studies carried out with sucralfate tablets.

Anti-inflammatory and Analgesic Agents

Sucralfate, a new antiulcer agent, is often prescribed with drugs that irritate the gastrointestinal mucosal lining or that are ulcerogenic. Sucralfate has been shown to be effective in the prevention of gastritis and gastric ulcers secondary to NSAIDs[1–3] and also to protect the gastroduodenal mucosa against aspirin-induced damage[4] and against a variety of experimental irritants[5] when given before the irritant.

This effect is mediated not only via the formation of a protective barrier but also by mucus release, changes in ion transport, and increase of endogenous prostaglandins and mitotic activity.[5,6]

Combined oral therapy, however, requires evaluation of a potential interaction in absorption between sucralfate and the selected drugs.

Salicylates

The effect of sucralfate on salicylates has been investigated in two different studies, neither of which showed any interaction.

In one study, sucralfate 1 g qid for 2 days did not alter any kinetic parameters of a single dose of aspirin 650 mg given to 12 healthy volunteers.[7] Similarly, in another crossover study of 12 volunteers, sucralfate had no effect on the steady-state bioavailability of choline magnesium trisalicylate.[8]

The lack of a pharmacokinetic interaction between sucralfate and aspirin, and the minimal *in vitro* binding of aspirin to sucralfate[9] would not appear to explain the protective effect of the latter against aspirin-induced gastric mucosal damage.

NSAIDs

Ibuprofen. Two studies in volunteers have examined the potential kinetic interaction of sucralfate with ibuprofen without finding any interaction in terms of extent of ibuprofen absorption.

In one study in which each subject ingested a single 400-mg dose of ibuprofen alone or with sucralfate given as 1-g doses qid for 2 days prior to and during the study, sucralfate coadministration reduced the average peak plasma concentrations, C_{max}, and increased the time to peak plasma concentrations by approximately 0.7 hr, but did not affect the ibuprofen bioavailability.[10]

The decrease in rate of absorption was not seen when ingestion was separated by 1 hr. In a randomized crossover study in which nine healthy subjects were given a single oral 600-mg dose of ibuprofen with and without sucralfate 1 g qid for five doses, with the last sucralfate dose 60 min before ibuprofen, sucralfate had no effect on the peak concentration, time to peak, half-life, and AUC of ibuprofen.[11]

The reduced rate of absorption would not be expected to change the responses of the anti-inflammatory agent. However, in the absence of any specific information, a reasonable general approach would be to separate dosing of ibuprofen and sucralfate by several hours.

Ketoprofen, Indomethacin, Naproxen. The disposition kinetics of ketoprofen, indomethacin, or naproxen with and without sucralfate were each studied in a randomized, crossover volunteer trial.[12] In each study, subjects received either ketoprofen 50-mg capsules, indomethacin 50-mg capsules, or naproxen 500-mg tablets alone or with 2 g sucralfate given 30 min before the drug dose.

The data indicate that sucralfate decreases the C_{max} and increases the t_{max} of ketoprofen, indomethacin, and naproxen without affecting their bioavailabilities.

Analgesic Agent—Paracetamol (Acetaminophen)

Coadministration of sucralfate does not alter the acetaminophen absorption in man.[13] In a double-blind crossover study, six healthy subjects ingested a single oral 1-g dose of acetaminophen with and without a single oral 1-g dose of sucralfate. Sucralfate does not affect the bioavailability of acetaminophen as measured by salivary acetaminophen concentrations.

Table I. Effects of Sucralfate on GI Absorption of Single Doses of Other Drugs

Drugs	Effect of sucralfate on other drugs	Potential interaction (mechanism)	Relevant clinical effect	Comments and recommendations	References
Acetaminophen	None	No interaction	None	No special precaution	13
Acetylsalicylic acid	None	No interaction	None	No special precaution	7, 9
Amitriptyline	Yes	↑ elimination and ↓ absorption	Not known	Cautious in combined use	33
Chlorpropamide	Unlikely	Slight ↓ absorption	Minimal	No special precaution	34
Cimetidine	Unlikely	Possibly ↓ absorption in one report	Unlikely	Combined use not recommended	16
	None	3 studies failed to confirm initial report	None		17–19
Ciprofloxacin	Yes	↓ absorption by 30% (chelation–complexation	Possible ↓ antibiotic effect	Combined use should be avoided	25
Digoxin	Yes	↓ absorption by 19% bioavailability unaltered if given 2 hr apart	Not known	Separating doses by at least 2 hr	27, 30
Erythromycin	None	No interaction	None	No special precaution	35
Ibuprofen	Unlikely	↓ rate but not extent of absorption	Unlikely	Separating dosing schedule	10, 11
Indomethacin	Unlikely	↓ rate but not extent of absorption	Unlikely	Separating dosing schedule	12
Ketoconazole	Yes	↓ bioavailability by 21% (unknown)	Not known	Separating doses as much as possible	36

Ketoprofen	Unlikely	↓ rate but not extent of absorption	Unlikely	Separating dosing schedule	12
Naproxen	Unlikely	↓ rate but not extent of absorption	Unlikely	Separating dosing schedule	12
Norfloxacin	Yes	10-fold reduction in absorption (by chelation–complexation)	Potential treatment failure	Coadministration should be avoided	24
Phenytoin	Yes	↓ absorption	Anticonvulsant effect may be reduced	Separating doses by at least 2 hr	37, 38
Prednisone	None	No interaction	None	No special precaution	39
Procainamide	Yes	Slightly ↓ absorption (unknown)	Minimal	Separating dosing schedule	32
Quinidine	Yes	Altered quinidine absorption (case report)	Subtherapeutic levels	Monitor serum levels—or separating doses	27, 31
Ranitidine	Minimal	1 g sucralfate does not affect ranitidine bioavailability; larger doses ↓ absorption by 29% (unknown)	Unlikely	Combined use not recommended	21, 22
Roxatidine	None	No interaction	None	No special precaution	23
Sulpride	Yes	↓ absorption	Not known	Avoid combined use	40
Theophylline	Unlikely	Minimal effect on bioavailability	None	No special precaution	41, 42
Trisalicylate	None	No interaction	None	No special precaution	8
Warfarin	Likely	Possible ↓ absorption in 2 case reports; two clinical studies failed to confirm	Onset of activity may be delayed	Monitor anticoagulant parameters	26–29

H_2-Receptor Antagonists

A further potentially important source of drug interactions is the coadministration of sucralfate with H_2-receptor antagonist agents, in the hope of an additive or synergistic effect.

Cimetidine

In vitro and animal studies indicate that cimetidine is not likely to inhibit binding of sucralfate to ulcerated tissue.[14,15] With the doses used, cimetidine does not reduce the binding of sucralfate to ulcerated mucosa in animals. Although preliminary work in humans has shown altered cimetidine absorption in the presence of sucralfate,[16] three recent studies failed to confirm the initial report.[17–19] In healthy subjects who received a 1-g sucralfate tablet qid for 2 days prior to and with the cimetidine dose, sucralfate coadministration had no statistically significant effect on the rate or extent of cimetidine absorption.[17] This lack of kinetic interaction is supported by an absence of a pharmacodynamic interaction in patients receiving sucralfate together with cimetidine. In fact, in a double-blind, 2-week study of 61 patients with duodenal ulcer, sucralfate, cimetidine, and a combination of the two were equally effective in ulcer healing, indicating that the drugs do not antagonize each other.[20]

However, since no advantage of combination over single-dose therapy would be found, concurrent use of sucralfate and cimetidine is not recommended.

Ranitidine

Sucralfate appears to have no effect on absorption of another H_2-receptor antagonist, ranitidine. Volunteer studies have confirmed *in vitro* work that ranitidine binds to a small extent (~ 10%) to sucralfate in the gastrointestinal fluids. Pharmacokinetic studies in six volunteers resulted in no differences in absorption or elimination parameters of ranitidine when 150 mg was given alone and when it was given concurrently with 1 g of sucralfate.[21] However, large doses of sucralfate (2 g) reduced the bioavailability of ranitidine 150 mg by 29%.[22]

The clinical importance of these findings has not been established, but it is not likely to be great. However, because of the lack of evidence that the combination is more efficacious than either drug alone, the combined use of sucralfate and ranitidine is not recommended.

Roxatidine

The effect of multiple doses of sucralfate (1 g qid for 3 days) on the pharmacokinetics of a single oral dose of 150 mg roxatidine acetate has been evaluated in 18 healthy male volunteers.[23] No significant difference was observed in pharmacokinetic parameters when roxatidine was given alone and in combination with sucralfate.

Quinolones—A Possible Interaction with Sucralfate

The administration of sucralfate markedly reduces the serum and urine concentrations of norfloxacin[24] and the serum concentrations of ciprofloxacin.[25]

In a randomized, crossover study, norfloxacin 400 mg was administered either alone, or with the fifth dose of sucralfate 1 g qid, or 2 hr following the fifth dose of sucralfate.[24] The relative bioavailabilities were 1.8% when norfloxacin was taken with sucralfate and 56.6% when it was taken 2 hr after sucralfate. The mean 12-hr urine norfloxacin concentration was 119 mg/liter following norfloxacin alone, 6.8 mg/liter when sucralfate was coadministered, and 63 mg/liter when sucralfate was given 2 hr before norfloxacin dosing.

Similarly, administration of a 1-g dose of sucralfate 6 and 2 hr prior to administration of ciprofloxacin 750 mg resulted in a 30% reduction in bioavailability in 12 healthy male volunteers.[25]

The reduced bioavailability seen with quinolones was attributed to chelation complexes of quinolones by the aluminum contained in sucralfate, thereby affecting the absorption of quinolones. This reduction may result in treatment failure. Thus, quinolone–sucralfate coadministration should be avoided.

Anticoagulant Therapy

There have been two case reports indicating that sucralfate coadministration resulted in a reduction of serum warfarin concentrations and prothrombin times (PT). When sucralfate was discontinued, warfarin concentrations increased as did PT.[26,27] While the exact mechanism of this interaction is not known, it is likely to be related to altered warfarin absorption.

However, other works[28,29] in stable warfarin-treated patients reported no significant effect of 14 days of sucralfate coadministration on prothrombin activity or plasma warfarin levels. In view of the theoretical hazard, it is recommended that care should be taken when administering sucralfate with anticoagulants since the onset of hypoprothrombinemia may be delayed.

Antiarrhythmic Agents

Digoxin/Sustained Release Quinidine

A case is reported of a 71-year-old woman who displayed altered absorption of digoxin, quinidine sulfate, and warfarin sodium after being given sucralfate.[27] The administration of sucralfate resulted in subtherapeutic serum concentrations of digoxin and quinidine, and also reduced the patient's PT. Discontinuation of sucralfate increased PT and reestablished therapeutic concentrations of digoxin, quinidine, and warfarin. Patients receiving sucralfate concurrently with digoxin, quinidine, and warfarin should be monitored frequently with regard to serum drug concentration and disease symptomatology.

Digoxin

Recently, in a clinical study of 12 normal subjects who received either 0.75 mg digoxin alone, or concurrently with sucralfate (1 g qid for 2 days) or 2 hr before sucralfate, coadministration of these compounds resulted in a decrease (but not significant) in the AUC (19%) and urinary excretion of digoxin (12%).[30] These differences were not seen when ingestion was separated by 2 hr. No differences were seen in the disposition parameters of digoxin.

The mechanism for the reduced bioavailability is not established. Until more is known about this interaction, it would be prudent to give digoxin and other digitalis glycosides two or more hours before sucralfate.

Quinidine

Similarly the influence of sucralfate on quinidine sulfate absorption has been studied in 14 healthy male volunteers under three conditions: alone, concurrent with sucralfate (1 g qid for 2 days), or 2 hr after sucralfate.[31] The data indicate that co-ingestion of these compounds increased the peak time (41%) and decreased (but not significantly) the C_{max} (12%), AUC (11.5%), and elimination half-life (13%). These differences were not seen when ingestion was separated by 2 hr.

Thus, the administration of sucralfate 2 hr prior to quinidine therapy would not be expected to influence quinidine bioavailability.

Procainamide

Sucralfate appears to have minimal effect on procainamide serum levels. In a study in which four healthy subjects took a single dose of procainamide 250 mg alone or 30 min after a dose of sucralfate, procainamide peak concentration declined about 5% and the area under the concentration–time curve fell by 11%; neither was statistically significant.[32] Neither of these changes would be expected to alter the response to procainamide.

Psychotropic Drugs

Sucralfate may be used in combination with antidepressant drugs since often depressive illness coexists with hyperacidity conditions. Amitriptyline kinetics were studied in six healthy males in a blinded, single-dose, crossover design.[33] The subjects received amitriptyline 75 mg alone or concurrently with 1 g of sucralfate, and there were no significant differences in absorption parameters such as C_{max}, t_{max}, or K_a. However, the data indicate that sucralfate increased the elimination of amitriptyline and decreased its availability. Since sucralfate is minimally absorbed, further work is required to clarify the importance and mechanism of this interaction.

Miscellaneous Agents

Chlorpropamide

A single study in normal subjects indicates that sucralfate has minimal effects on the gastrointestinal absorption of chlorpropamide.[34]

The effect of sucralfate 1 g qid for 3 days on a single oral 250-mg dose of chlorpropamide was studied in 12 healthy male volunteers in a randomized, crossover study. The AUC_{inf} of chlorpropamide was slightly reduced, while its C_{max}, t_{max}, $T_{1/2}$, and $AUC_{0-96\ hours}$ were unchanged. The mechanism for the slight reduction in chlorpropamide bioavailability has not been established. The slight reduction in AUC was regarded by the investigators as having no clinical significance.

Erythromycin Succinate

The pharmacokinetics of 400 mg erythromycin ethylsuccinate were unaltered by concurrent oral administration of 1 g sucralfate in normal volunteers.[35] Thus, combined sucralfate–erythromycin may improve tolerance to erythromycin, although further clinical evidence is required.

Ketoconazole

The coadministration of sucralfate and ketoconazole reduces the plasma concentration of the antifungal agent.[36] The mechanism for reduced absorption is not established. In a study in which each healthy subject received ketoconazole 400 mg alone or with 1 g sucralfate, the bioavailability of ketoconazole was reduced by 21%. The clinical significance of this reduction is not known. Pending further information, doses of ketoconazole and sucralfate should be separated to minimize any interaction.

Phenytoins

Absorption of orally administered phenytoin may be reduced by coadministration with sucralfate.

Two studies[37,38] in normal volunteers have examined the influence of sucralfate on phenytoin absorption. Both demonstrated a significant reduction in bioavailability of phenytoin. In a double-blind, placebo-controlled, crossover study in eight subjects, coadministration of 1 g sucralfate reduced the absorption of 300-mg phenytoin capsules by 20%.[37] In a study involving nine subjects, sucralfate administration decreased the AUC by about 10%.[38] Although small decreases in phenytoin absorption have been observed, this change may be significant in certain patients stabilized on phenytoin. The anticonvulsant effect of phenytoin may be reduced.

In dogs, phenytoin absorption was also decreased by 38% when coadministered with sucralfate; this effect was avoided by separating the administration of these compounds by 2 hr. Therefore, in the absence of a clinical study, doses of sucralfate and phenytoin should be separated by two or more hours.

Prednisone

Sucralfate does not affect the absorption of prednisone. Twelve healthy subjects received 20 mg prednisone under three conditions; alone, concurrently with sucralfate, or 2 hr before the sucralfate dose.[39] Apart from a slight delay of approximately ¾ hr in the t_{max} when sucralfate was given concurrently, no significant difference in the prednisone bioavailability was observed.

Sulpride

The extent of bioavailability of sulpride in humans is reduced by 40% when sucralfate is given concurrently.[40]

Xanthines

Coadministration of sucralfate does not alter the bioavailability of conventional theophylline to a clinically important degree.[41]

Theophylline absorption after a single oral 5 mg/kg dose of non-sustained-release theophylline was evaluated in the absence and presence of sucralfate. Sucralfate was ingested 1 g four times a day for 2 days before the theophylline dose, with the theophylline dose, and 6 hr after the dose. The AUC of theophylline decreased by 5% following sucralfate treatment while its elimination half-life remained unchanged. This slight reduction in AUC is regarded by the investigators as having no clinical significance.

However, one study reported a 40% reduction in theophylline absorption when 1 g sucralfate was given 30 min before the administration of a 350-mg dose of sustained-release theophylline.[42]

Antacids

Because antacids essentially decrease the binding of sucralfate with the gastroduodenal mucosa as a consequence of a change of intragastric pH in animals, antacids should not be taken within half an hour before or after sucralfate intake.

Conclusions: Drug Interactions with Sucralfate

Because of the ability of sucralfate to adsorb charged entities and its affinity to form complexes with proteins, the potential for drug adsorption by sucralfate has been evaluated. These interactions are summarized as follows.

- *No interaction with sucralfate—No special precautions required.*
  Acetaminophen
  Chlorpropamide
  Erythromycin
  Prednisone
  Procainamide
  Roxatidine
  Salicylates (aspirin and trisalicylate)
  Theophylline (nonsustained release)
- *Bioavailability altered—Should be avoided.*
  Amitriptyline
  Quinolones (ciprofloxacin, norfloxacin)
  Sulpride
  Theophylline (sustained release)
- *Bioavailability altered—Caution may be necessary—Effect may be minimized by separating doses by at least 2 hr.*
  Digoxin
  Ketoconazole
  NSAIDs

Phenytoin
Quinidine
Warfarin

- *Altered absorption suspected—Combined use not recommended.*
  H_2-receptor antagonists, cimetidine and ranitidine (a synergistic effect is not evident)
- *Altered binding in animals—Separating doses by one-half hour.*
  Antacids

References

1. Caldwell JR, Roth SH, Wu WC, *et al*: Sucralfate treatment of nonsteroidal anti-inflammatory drug-induced gastrointestinal symptoms and mucosal damage. *Am J Med* **83**(suppl 3b):74–82, 1987. The results of this large randomized, placebo-controlled, double-blind trial indicate that sucralfate partially relieves gastrointestinal symptoms and mucosal damage associated with NSAID therapy.
2. Stern AI, Ward F, Hartley G: Protective effect of sucralfate against aspirin-induced damage to the human gastric mucosa. *Am J Med* **83**(suppl 3b):83–85, 1987. In this small randomized, placebo-controlled study, it was shown that a single oral dose of sucralfate significantly reduced gastric mucosal damage produced by aspirin probably via the stimulation of local prostaglandin production.
3. Lanza F, Peace K, Gustitus L, *et al*: A blinded endoscopic comparative study of misoprostol versus sucralfate and placebo in the prevention of aspirin-induced gastric and duodenal ulceration. *Am J Gastroenterol* **83**:143–146, 1988. The cytoprotective properties of sucralfate against aspirin-induced damage to the gastric and duodenal mucosae were confirmed in this placebo-controlled, double-blind randomized study where healthy volunteers received 1 g of sucralfate or placebo coadministered with 650 mg of aspirin, four times a day for 7 days.
4. Tesler MA, Lim ES: Protection of gastric mucosa by sucralfate from aspirin-induced erosions. *J Clin Gastroenterol* **3**(suppl 2):175–179, 1981. In this randomized placebo-controlled study, complete protection against aspirin-caused damage to the gastric mucosa was achieved in 8 of 12 subjects whereas 3 other subjects had a partial protection.
5. Harrington SJ, Schlegel JF, Code CF: The protective effect of sucralfate on the gastric mucosa of rats. *J Clin Gastroenterol* **3**(suppl 2):129–134, 1981. The effects of sucralfate on the response of the gastric mucosa to ethanol or taurocholic acid were assessed in rats. The results demonstrate that in the presence of sucralfate, the pH of the gastric contents was higher, the disappearance of H^+ was less, and the index of mucosal damage was reduced.
6. Tarnawski A, Hollander D, Krause WJ, *et al*: Effect of sucralfate on normal gastric mucosa, histologic, ultrastructural and functional assessment. *Gastroenterology* **84**:1331, 1983 (Abstract). This animal study found that sucralfate produces in normal gastric mucosa morphological and functional changes which may account for its therapeutic efficacy.
7. Lau AH, Chang CW, Schlesinger PK: Evaluation of a potential drug interaction between sucralfate and aspirin. *Clin Pharmacol Ther* **39**:151–155, 1986. The results of this randomized crossover study (12 volunteers) reveal that the pharmacokinetic parameters of aspirin were not affected by sucralfate either coadministered with aspirin or given qid for 2 days before aspirin.
8. Schneider DK, Gannon RH, Sweeney KR, *et al*: Influence of sucralfate on trisalicylate bioavailability. *J Clin Pharmacol* **31**:377–379, 1991. This study found that sucralfate does not affect the steady-state bioavailability of trisalicylate absorption. No differences were detected in the pharmacokinetic parameters under study (C_{max}, T_{max}, and AUC) when sucralfate was administered with trisalicylate compared with trisalicylate alone.
9. Graham DY, Sackman JW, Giesing DJ, *et al*: *In vitro* adsorption of bile salts and aspirin to sucralfate. *Dig Dis Sci* **29**:402–406, 1984. The *in vitro* adsorption of bile salts or aspirin to sucralfate

was assessed in this study. Aspirin was minimally absorbed by sucralfate, excluding this process as the mechanism of the protective effect.

10. Anaya AL, Mayersohn M, Conrad KA, *et al*: The influence of sucralfate on ibuprofen absorption in healthy adult males. *Biopharm Drug Dispos* **7**:443–451, 1986. In this randomized crossover study on 12 volunteers, sucralfate coadministration with ibuprofen did not alter the extent but did decrease the rate of absorption of the NSAID.
11. Pugh MC, Small RE, Garnett WR, *et al*: Effect of sucralfate on ibuprofen absorption in normal volunteers. *Clin Pharm* **3**:630–633, 1984. In this randomized crossover study on nine volunteers, no decrease in the rate of absorption nor in the extent of absorption was seen when ingestion of sucralfate and ibuprofen was separated by 1 hr.
12. Caillé G, Du Souich P, Gervais P, *et al*: Single dose pharmacokinetics of ketoprofen, indomethacin, and naproxen taken alone or with sucralfate. *Biopharm Drug Dispos* **8**:173–183, 1987. The disposition kinetics of ketoprofen, indomethacin, or naproxen with and without sucralfate were studied in a randomized, crossover volunteer trial. The data indicate that sucralfate decreases the rate but not the extent of absorption of all three drugs.
13. Kamali F, Fry JR, Smart HL, *et al*: A double-blind placebo controlled study to examine effects of sucralfate on paracetamol absorption. *Br J Clin Pharmacol* **19**:113–114, 1985. In this double-blind, placebo-controlled crossover study on six volunteers, the concurrent administration of sucralfate did not affect the bioavailability of acetaminophen.
14. DeChristoforo R: Cimetidine–sucralfate: Drug interaction? *Hosp Pharm* **20**:270, 1985 (Letter). In this letter, the author is concerned about the concurrent use of cimetidine and sucralfate. He addresses the issue in terms of preclinical as well as clinical studies investigating such use of both products.
15. Lacz JP, Drees DT, Browne RK: Effects of antacid therapy on the binding of sucralfate to gastric ulcers in the rat. *Gastroenterology* **84**:1220, 1983 (Abstract). These authors determined in a rat model that the administration of cimetidine in doses that produce a pharmacological response did not affect the binding of sucralfate to acetic acid-induced ulcers.
16. Yoshida Y, *et al*: Effects of concomitant drugs on the blood concentration of a histamine H_2 antagonist (the 3rd report); concomitant or time lag oral administration of cimetidine and sucralfate. *Jpn J Gastroenterol* **84**:1025–1029, 1987. Preliminary work in humans showing altered cimetidine absorption in the presence of sucralfate.
17. D'Angio R, Mayersohn M, Conrad KA, *et al*: Cimetidine absorption in humans during sucralfate coadministration. *Br J Clin Pharmacol* **21**:515–520, 1986. In this randomized crossover study conducted in six healthy male volunteers, coadministration of sucralfate had no significant effect on either the rate or the completeness of cimetidine absorption.
18. Albin H, Vincon G, Lalague MC, *et al*: Effect of sucralfate on the bioavailability of cimetidine. *Eur J Clin Pharmacol* **30**:493–494, 1986. In this randomized crossover interaction study between cimetidine and sucralfate in 12 human volunteers, sucralfate did not reduce the bioavailability of cimetidine.
19. Beck CL, Dietz AJ, Carlson JD, *et al*: Evaluation of potential cimetidine sucralfate interaction. *Clin Pharmacol Ther* **41**:168, 1987 (Abstract). In this randomized blinded crossover trial conducted in eight healthy male volunteers, coadministration of sucralfate had no significant effect on cimetidine's pharmacokinetics.
20. Van Deventer GM, Schneidman D, Walsh JH: Sucralfate and cimetidine as single agents and in combination for treatment of active duodenal ulcers. A double-blind, placebo-controlled trial. *Am J Med* **79**(suppl 2C):39–44, 1985. Double-blind, double-placebo study in 61 duodenal ulcer patients demonstrating a healing rate for combination therapy (cimetidine–sucralfate) higher than for either agent alone.
21. Mullersman G, Gotz VP, Russel WL, *et al*: Lack of clinically significant *in vitro* and *in vivo* interactions between ranitidine and sucralfate. *J Pharm Sci* **75**:995–998, 1986. The influence of coadministration of sucralfate on ranitidine bioavailability was evaluated in an *in vitro* study and in a crossover study in six healthy male volunteers. The *in vitro* results demonstrate a small extent

(≈ 10%) of ranitidine binding to sucralfate paste in the gastrointestinal fluids whereas the pharmacokinetic study showed no diminished ranitidine bioavailability in the presence of sucralfate.
22. Maconochie JG, Thomas M, Michael MF, *et al*: Ranitidine sucralfate interaction study. *Clin Pharmacol Ther* **41**:205, 1987 (Abstract). In a three-period crossover study conducted in 12 healthy male volunteers, coadministration of sucralfate significantly reduced ranitidine's bioavailability.
23. Seibert-Grafe M, Pidgen A: Lack of effect of multiple dose sucralfate on the pharmacokinetics of roxatidine acetate. *Eur J Clin Pharmacol* **40**:637–638, 1991. In an open, randomized, two-way crossover study in 18 healthy male volunteers, roxatidine's pharmacokinetics were not influenced by the coadministration of multiple doses of sucralfate.
24. Parpia SH, Nix DE, Hejmanowski LG, *et al*: Sucralfate reduces the gastrointestinal absorption of norfloxacin. *Antimicrob Agents Chemother* **33**:99–102, 1989. In a three-period, randomized crossover study of eight healthy male volunteers, 2 hr pre- or concurrent administration of multiple doses of sucralfate significantly reduced gastrointestinal absorption of norfloxacin.
25. Nix DE, Watson WA, Handy L, *et al*: The effect of sucralfate pretreatment on the pharmacokinetics of ciprofloxacin. *Pharmacotherapy* **9**:377–380, 1989. The influence of sucralfate pretreatment on the pharmacokinetics of ciprofloxacin was evaluated in a randomized crossover study of 12 healthy male volunteers. The results suggest a decrease in ciprofloxacin's systemic bioavailability on concurrent administration of sucralfate.
26. Mungall D, Talbert RL, Phillips C, *et al*: Sucralfate and warfarin. *Ann Intern Med* **98**:557, 1983 (Letter to the Editor). A case report of a patient in whom sucralfate appeared to hinder warfarin absorption, resulting in a shortened prothrombin time. Prothrombin time returned to normal on discontinuation of sucralfate.
27. Rey AM, Gums JG: Altered absorption of digoxin, sustained-release quinidine and warfarin with sucralfate administration. *DICP Ann Pharmacother* **25**:745–746, 1991. A clinical case of an elderly woman who displayed subtherapeutic serum concentrations of digoxin, quinidine, and reduced prothrombin time when sucralfate was coadministered.
28. Talbert RL, Dalmady-Israel C, Bussey HI, *et al*: Effect of sucralfate on plasma warfarin concentration in patients requiring chronic warfarin therapy. *Drug Intell Clin Pharm* **19**:456–457, 1985 (Abstract). The coadministration of sucralfate to five patients on chronic warfarin therapy did not significantly affect prothrombin time, partial thromboplastin time, or plasma warfarin concentration.
29. Neuvonen PJ, Jaakkola A, Totterman J, *et al*: Clinically significant sucralfate–warfarin interaction is not likely. *Br J Clin Pharmacol* **20**:178–180, 1985 (Letter). In a study of the effect of sucralfate in eight stable warfarin-treated patients, no significant change was found in plasma warfarin concentration or thromboplastin time by the addition of sucralfate.
30. Giesing DJ, Lanman RC, Dimmitt DC, *et al*: Lack of effect of sucralfate on digoxin pharmacokinetics. *Gastroenterology* **84**:1165, 1983 (Abstract). Coadministration of digoxin and sucralfate in 12 normal volunteers resulted in a nonsignificant decrease in the AUC and urinary excretion of digoxin. These differences were not observed when the doses of the two drugs were staggered.
31. Dimmett DC: Unpublished data.
32. Turkistani AAA, Gaber M, Al-Meshal MA, *et al*: Effect of sucralfate on procainamide absorption. *Int J Pharm* **59**:R1–R3, 1990 (Rapid Communication). In this crossover study of four healthy male volunteers, procainamide absorption was not significantly altered by coadministration of sucralfate. Procainamide concentrations were assessed by the volunteer's saliva.
33. Ryan R, Carlson J, Farris F: Effect of sucralfate in the absorption and disposition of amitriptyline in humans. *Fed Proc* **45**(3):205, 1986 (Abstract 299). Blinded crossover study of six healthy male volunteers indicating that sucralfate does not modify the absorption parameters (C_{max}, T_{max}) but does increase the elimination of amitriptyline.
34. Letendre PW, Carlson JD, Seifert RD, *et al*: Effect of sucralfate on the absorption and pharmacokinetics of chlorpropamide. *J Clin Pharmacol* **26**:622–625, 1986. In this two-way randomized, crossover study of 12 healthy male volunteers, pretreatment followed by simultaneous administration of sucralfate had no significant effect on absorption and bioavailability of chlorpropamide.

35. Miller LG, Prichard JG, White CA, *et al*: Effect of concurrent sucralfate administration on the absorption of erythromycin. *J Clin Pharmacol* **30**:39–44, 1990. The possible effect of coadministration of sucralfate on absorption and bioavailability of erythromycin was evaluated in this open label single-dose study of six healthy volunteers. Coadministration of sucralfate did not significantly alter the above-mentioned parameters.
36. Goss TF, Piscitelli SC, Schentag IJ: Evaluation of ketoconazole bioavailability interactions with sucralfate and ranitidine using gastric pH monitoring. *Clin Pharmacol Ther* **49**:128, 1991 (Abstract). The effects of sucralfate and ranitidine on ketoconazole bioavailability were evaluated in this three-period, randomized, crossover study performed in six healthy male volunteers. A significant decrease of ketoconazole bioavailability was reported on coadministration of ranitidine and was related to an elevated gastric pH, whereas the moderate decrease seen with simultaneous sucralfate administration was not linked to an altered gastric pH.
37. Smart HL, Somerville KW, Williams J, *et al*: The effects of sucralfate upon phenytoin absorption in man. *Br J Clin Pharmacol* **20**:238–240, 1985. In this double-blind, placebo-controlled crossover study of eight healthy male volunteers, coadministration of sucralfate significantly reduced phenytoin's absorption.
38. Hall TG, Cuddy PG, Glass CJ, *et al*: Effect of sucralfate on phenytoin bioavailability. *Drug Intell Clin Pharm* **20**:607–611, 1986. The potential effect of coadministration of sucralfate on phenytoin's bioavailability was examined in this open, crossover study of nine healthy male volunteers. Although the results suggest that simultaneous sucralfate administration affects phenytoin's absorption, the difference was not significant.
39. Gambertoglio JG, Romae DR, Yong CL, *et al*: Lack of effect of sucralfate on prednisone bioavailability. *Am J Gastroenterol* **82**:42–45, 1987. Randomized three-way crossover study in 12 healthy volunteers showing that sucralfate does not have a clinically significant effect on the bioavailability of prednisone.
40. Gouda MW, Hikal AH, Babhair SA, *et al*: Effect of sucralfate and antacids on the bioavailability of sulpride in humans. *Int J Pharm* **22**:257–263, 1984. The effect of coadministration of either sucralfate or an antacid on sulpride's bioavailability was determined in this crossover study of six healthy male volunteers. Both sucralfate and the antacid significantly reduced sulpride's oral bioavailability. The bioavailability was also reduced in two volunteers on administration of the two agents 2 hr prior, whereas no significant alteration was seen in one volunteer when the agents were administered 2 hr after sulpride.
41. Cantral KA, Schaaf LJ, Jungnickel PW, *et al*: Effect of sucralfate on theophylline absorption in healthy volunteers. *Clin Pharm* **7**:58–61, 1988. In this two-way, randomized crossover study of eight healthy male volunteers, the rate or completeness of theophylline's absorption was not clinically altered on simultaneous administration of multiple doses of sucralfate.
42. Fleischmann R, Bozler G, Boekstegers P: Bioverfugbarkeit von Theophylline unter Ulkustherapeutika. *Verh Dtsch Ges Inn Med* **90**(II):1876–1879, 1984.

VI

Sucralfate and Therapy of Peptic Disease

23

Therapy of Gastric Ulcer Disease

SHIU KUM LAM

Gastric Ulcer Healing with Sucralfate

Many but not all of the pathophysiological defects in gastric ulcer, including luminal acid and pepsin, duodenogastric reflux, mucus–bicarbonate abnormality, impaired mucosal blood flow, and mucosal defects associated with cigarette smoking and analgesic use, can theoretically be overcome to a significant extent by the gastroprotective actions of sucralfate, which have been detailed in Chapter 17. Because NSAID-associated gastric ulcer represents etiologically a distinct group, present-day therapeutic approach should attempt to separate these ulcers from non-NSAID-related gastric ulcer.

Non-NSAID-Associated Gastric Ulcer

There have been seven placebo-controlled studies and eight comparative studies with H_2-receptor antagonists (Table I), showing that sucralfate 1 g qid is effective for the healing of gastric ulcer, achieving a healing rate of about 79% after 8 weeks, a rate that is similar to that achieved with H_2-receptor antagonists. There are two points worthy of note. First, while a number of earlier studies[1–3,5,7,9] did not report exclusion criteria, most studies either excluded patients taking regular analgesics or asked the patients to stop such medications during the trial. In fact, the combined 8-week healing rate of studies excluding analgesics was 79%, which was close to the corresponding healing rate with H_2-receptor antagonists, which was 82%. Second, in all except three studies,[6,8,13] no attempt was made to exclude or separate prepyloric ulcers from other gastric ulcers. There is evidence that the two types of gastric ulcers are pathophysiologically different. Interestingly, combining the results of the two studies reporting on the efficacy of sucralfate in prepyloric and corpus ulcers shows that the response curves of these two types of ulcers

SHIU KUM LAM • Division of Gastroenterology and Hepatology, Department of Medicine, University of Hong Kong, Queen Mary Hospital, Hong Kong.

Sucralfate: From Basic Science to the Bedside, edited by Daniel Hollander and G. N. J. Tytgat. Plenum Press, New York, 1995.

Table I. Efficacy Studies of Sucralfate in Gastric Ulcer

Reference	Trial duration (weeks)	Sucralfate		Placebo		H_2-receptor antagonists		p value
		No. of patients	Percent healed	No. of patients	Percent healed	No. of patients	Percent healed	
Maybery 1978[1]	4	16	50	12	17			<0.08
Rhodes 1981[2]	4	16	50	15	13			<0.10
Fixa 1981[3]	4	24	71	14	40			<0.05
Orchard 1981[4]	4	13	62	8	25			<0.30
Ishimori 1981[5]	8	67	60	71	42			<0.05
Lam 1985[6]	8	56	84	47	38			<0.01
Brailski 1991[7]	3	26	54	10	10			<0.05
Svedberg 1987[8]	4	68	65			74C	70	
Marks 1980[9]	6	27	63			28C	75	
Pop 1983[10]	6	28	71			25C	83	
Blum 1986[11]	6	66	56			69R	72	
	12	66	82			69R	88	
Kagevi 1987[12]	4	136	65			140C	65	
	8	136	89			140C	91	
Martin 1983[13]	8	12	75			13C	77	
Lahtinen 1983[14]	8	36	80			33C	73	
Herrerias-Gutierrez 1989[15]	8	30	83			30R	86	
Rey 1989[16]	8	101	73			86C	71	
Total	8	438	79	118	40	302	82	All completing 8 weeks
	8	371	82	115	40	302	82	Analgesics excluded
	8	152	85			140	89	Prepyloric ulcers only

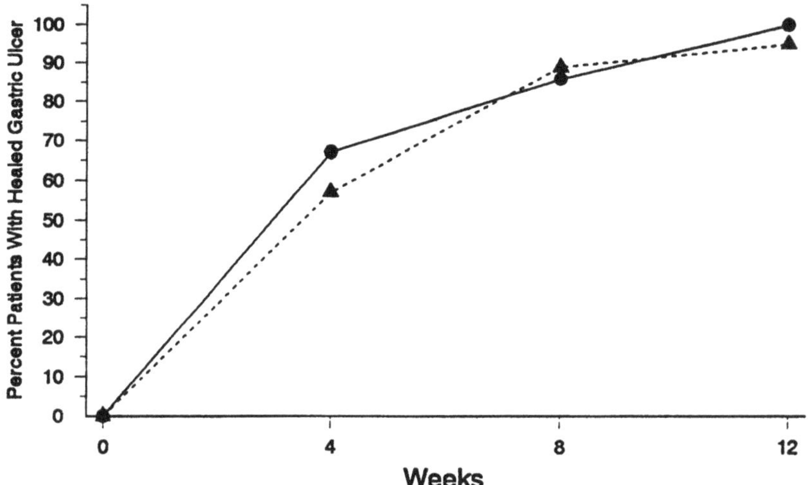

Figure 1. The healing curves of prepyloric (—●—, n = 84) and corpus ulcers (– –▲– –, n = 108) treated by sucralfate completely overlap. This suggests that prepyloric ulcers behave more like gastric ulcer than duodenal ulcer. Both types of ulcers should be treated for at least 8 weeks. Data from Refs. 6 and 12.

completely overlap (Fig. 1). This further supports that the two types of ulcers are closely related pathogenetically, as discussed earlier.

The recommended dosage scheme of sucralfate has been 1 g qid. Recent studies have shown that this can be conveniently changed to 2 g bid with similar efficacy (Table II).

There is some suggestion that if such ulcers are complicated by the need for chronic use of NSAID, such ulcers may be more difficult to heal with conventional treatment. It may be possible to identify some of these ulcers by their association with Helicobacter pylori, in addition to the history of chronic use of NSAID. The role of sucralfate in this situation has not been studied.

NSAID-Associated Gastric Ulcer

It has been debated whether NSAID-associated ulcers respond less well to treatment. In open studies, H_2-receptor antagonists healed 75–100% of gastric ulcers within 12 weeks in arthritic patients who continued to take NSAID during the ulcer therapy. However, a randomized, double-blind study using cimetidine showed that gastric ulcer healing was slower in patients taking NSAID than in those not taking such agents.[20] A recent study on the use of ranitidine in NSAID-associated gastric ulcer showed that the healing rates at 8 and 12 weeks were significantly lower in patients who continued to take NSAID compared with those who stopped these agents,[21] suggesting that the concomitant use of NSAID may lead to more resistant ulcers. However, the results can also be interpreted to indicate that the discontinuation of NSAID in such ulcers is associated with more rapid healing. Similar

Table II. Sucralfate Twice Daily versus Four Times Daily for Gastric Ulcer

		Sucralfate			
		2 g bid		1 g qid	
		n	% healed	*n*	% healed
Asaka 1992	4 wk	24	50	22	35
	8 wk	24	94	22	68
Simjee 1992	8 wk	24	67	17	59
	12 wk	24	92	12	71
		Sucralfate 2 g bid		Cimetidine 400 mg bid	
		n	% healed	*n*	% healed
Hjortrup 1989	4 wk	33	52	31	52
	8 wk		79		81
	12 wk		91		94

to the situation in non-NSAID gastric ulcers, omeprazole heals NSAID-associated gastric ulcers more rapidly than ranitidine.

One center[22,23] examined 14 NSAID-associated gastric ulcers and 51 duodenal ulcers, and observed similar healing rates in sucralfate (70% at 6 weeks)- and ranitidine (69% at 6 weeks)-treated ulcers. Another group[24] studied the endoscopic lesion scores in 26 patients on NSAID who had gastroduodenal lesions ranging from superficial pathologies to actual ulceration, and observed "over 50% improvement" in 71% of patients treated with sucralfate and 33% of patients treated with cimetidine.

There is, therefore, good evidence that NSAID-associated gastric ulcers respond reasonably well to H_2-receptor antagonists, and some hints that sucralfate should do the same. However, at this time, convincing data are not available to support the use of sucralfate in NSAID-associated gastric ulcer.

Prevention of Gastric Ulcer Relapse

Maintenance Treatment

The efficacy of sucralfate in the maintenance treatment of non-NSAID-related gastric ulcer has been well established. There have been at least six placebo-controlled trials[25–30] and three comparative studies with H_2-receptor antagonists,[15,31,32] and the trials are of 6 to 12 months' duration. Figure 2 summarizes the results. The appropriate dosage appears to be 1 g twice daily.

There have been no formal clinical trials on the efficacy of sucralfate, and for that

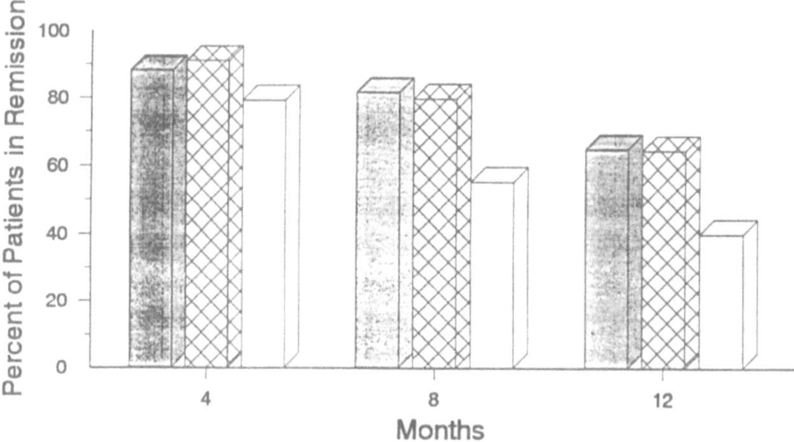

Figure 2. Meta-analysis of six placebo-controlled trials and three comparative studies with H_2-receptor antagonists of the use of sucralfate as maintenance treatment of healed gastric ulcer. (■, sucralfate, $n = 398$; ☒, H_2 antagonists, $n = 217$; □, placebo, $n = 92$). Data from Lam (1992).

matter of any therapeutic agent, in the maintenance treatment of patients with NSAID-induced gastric ulcer.

Eradication of Helicobacter pylori

There are some data to suggest that eradication of *H. pylori* will lead to prolonged remission of a healed gastric ulcer.[33] Eradication of *H. pylori* is usually achieved with triple therapy, consisting of colloidal bismuth or omeprazole and two antibiotics such as amoxicillin and metronidazole. Suppression of *H. pylori* and improvement of antral gastritis by sucralfate has been described.[34] A recent report showed that triple therapy using sucralfate has similar efficacy in *H. pylori* eradication as triple therapy using colloidal bismuth,[35] raising the possibility that "sucralfate triple therapy" might find a role in *H. pylori*-related gastroduodenal ulceration in future. Much more research is needed to define this role before recommendation for clinical use.

Prevention of NSAID-Induced Gastric Ulcer

The development of NSAID-induced gastric ulcer can be prevented by the prophylactic use of misoprostol. One small study examined the use of prophylactic sucralfate in NSAID users ($n = 10$) and did not observe any significant effect in the prevention of gastric mucosal lesions, when compared with misoprostol and placebo.[36] Another randomized, controlled study compared sucralfate 1 g qid and misoprostol 200 μg qid for the prevention of NSAID-induced gastric ulcer, and observed that misoprostol was significantly more effective by about 10 times.[37]

Summary

Many of the pathophysiological defects in gastric ulcer, including luminal acid and pepsin, duodenogastric reflux, mucus–bicarbonate abnormality, impaired mucosal blood flow, and mucosal defects associated with cigarette smoking and analgesic use, can theoretically be overcome to a significant extent by the gastroprotective actions of sucralfate. Seven placebo-controlled and eight comparative studies with H_2-receptor antagonists have shown that sucralfate is effective for the healing of non-NSAID-associated gastric ulcer, achieving a healing rate of about 80% after 8 weeks, a rate that is similar to that achieved with H_2-receptor antagonists. The healing rates of prepyloric ulcers and corpus ulcers by sucralfate appeared identical. Six placebo-controlled studies and three comparative studies with H_2-receptor antagonists have also established the efficacy of sucralfate in the maintenance treatment of non-NSAID-associated gastric ulcer. The approach for prolonging remission by *H. pylori* eradication has not been examined for sucralfate, although triple therapy with sucralfate (and two antibiotics) has been shown to have similar eradication rate as triple therapy with bismuth. Preliminary evidence suggests that sucralfate is as effective as H_2-receptor antagonists in the healing of NSAID-induced gastric ulcer while NSAID is being continued during treatment, although clinical use is not recommendable at this stage. Maintenance treatment of such ulcers in patients who continue to take NSAID has not been studied for any of the known therapeutic agents including sucralfate. Preliminary studies also suggest that sucralfate is not effective for the primary prevention of NSAID-induced gastric ulcer.

References

1. Mayberry JF, Williams RA, Rhodes J, *et al*: A controlled clinical trial of sucralfate in the treatment of gastric ulcer. *Br J Clin Pract* **32:**291–293, 1978. This study used radiological assessment of healing; no exclusion criteria were presented; two patients in each group were on analgesic.
2. Rhodes J, Mayberry JF, Williams FA, *et al*: Clinical trial of sucralfate in the treatment of gastric ulcer, in Caspary WF (ed): *Duodenal Ulcer, Gastric Ulcer: Sucralfate, a New Therapeutic Concept.* Sucralfate Symposium, 11th International Congress of Gastroenterology, Hamburg, June 1980. Munich, Urban & Schwarzenberg, 1981, pp 101–104. This study used radiological assessment and was unable to show any statistically significant advantage with sucralfate.
3. Fixa B, Komarkova O: Aluminum sucrose sulphate (sucralfate) in the treatment of peptic ulcer (double-blind study), in Caspary WF (ed): *Duodenal Ulcer, Gastric Ulcer: Sucralfate, a New Therapeutic Concept*. Sucralfate Symposium, 11th International Congress of Gastroenterology, Hamburg, June 1980. Munich, Urban & Schwarzenberg, 1981, pp 80–84. This placebo-controlled study showed that sucralfate healed gastric ulcer significantly better than placebo.
4. Orchard R, Elliot C: A double-blind placebo-controlled study of sucralfate in the treatment of gastric and duodenal ulcer, in Caspary WF (ed): *Duodenal Ulcer, Gastric Ulcer: Sucralfate, a New Therapeutic Concept*. Sucralfate Symposium, 11th International Congress of Gastroenterology, Hamburg, June 1980. Munich, Urban & Schwarzenberg, 1981, pp 85–88. Because only a total of 21 patients were evaluated, this study showed only a trend in favor of sucralfate.
5. Ishimori A, Arakawa H: A placebo-controlled, double-blind trial using sucralfate for the treatment of peptic ulcer: A multicenter Japanese study, in Caspary WF (ed): *Duodenal Ulcer, Gastric Ulcer: Sucralfate, a New Therapeutic Concept*. Sucralfate Symposium, 11th International Congress of

Gastroenterology, Hamburg, June 1980. Munich, Urban & Schwarzenberg, 1981, pp 93–100. This large-scale study involving close to 140 patients showed significant healing efficacy with sucralfate.

6. Lam SK, Lau WY, Lai CL, *et al*: Efficacy of sucralfate in corpus, prepyloric, and duodenal-ulcer associated gastric ulcers. A double-blind, placebo-controlled study. *Am J Med* **79**(2C):24–31, 1985. This large study stratified patients into the three types of gastric ulcers specified in the title before randomizing the patients into active or placebo treatment, and showed that sucralfate had significant healing efficacy in corpus and prepyloric ulcers but not duodenal ulcer associated gastric ulcers. In this study, concomitant medical diseases were excluded, and 6% of patients were on regular analgesics.
7. Brailski KH, Mendizova A, Matov V, *et al*: Treatment of peptic ulcer with sucralfate. *Klin Med (Moscow)* **69**:78–80, 1991. This placebo-controlled study showed that sucralfate had significant efficacy in the healing of gastric ulcer.
8. Svedberg LE, Carling L, Glise H, *et al*: Short-term treatment of prepyloric ulcer. Comparison of sucralfate and cimetidine. *Dig Dis Sci* **32**:225–231, 1987. This study showed that sucralfate had similar efficacy as cimetidine. In this study, analgesics were stopped, and concomitant medical diseases were excluded.
9. Marks IN, Wright JP, Denyer M, *et al*: Comparison of sucralfate with cimetidine in the short-term treatment of chronic peptic ulcers. *S Afr Med J* **57**:567–573, 1980. This study showed that sucralfate had similar efficacy as cimetidine. Analgesics were stopped during treatment.
10. Pop P, Nikkels RE, Thys O, *et al*: Comparison of sucralfate and cimetidine in the treatment of duodenal and gastric ulcers. A multicenter study. *Scand J Gastroenterol* **83**(suppl):43–47, 1983. This study showed that sucralfate had similar efficacy as cimetidine in the healing of gastric and duodenal ulcers. Bleeding ulcers and analgesic users were excluded.
11. Blum AL, Bode JC, Domschke W, *et al*: Therapy of stomach ulcer with sucralfate and ranitidine: A multicenter double-blind study. *Dtsch Med Wochenschr* **111**:1910–1915, 1986. This study showed that sucralfate had similar efficacy as ranitidine in the healing of gastric ulcer. Concomitant medical illness excluded and analgesics stopped.
12. Kagevi I, Anker-Hansen O, Carling L, *et al*: Swedish multicenter study on prepyloric and gastric ulcer. *Scand J Gastroenterol* **22**(suppl 127):67–76, 1987. This study showed that sucralfate had similar efficacy as cimetidine in the healing of gastric ulcer. Concomitant medical diseases excluded and analgesics stopped.
13. Martin F, Farley A, Gagnon M, *et al*: Short-term treatment with sucralfate or cimetidine in gastric ulcer. *Scand J Gastroenterol* **83**(suppl):37–41, 1983. This study showed that sucralfate had similar efficacy as cimetidine in the healing of gastric ulcer. Drug-induced ulcer, prepyloric ulcer, and duodenal ulcer were excluded.
14. Lahtinen J, Aukee S, Mietinen P, *et al*: Sucralfate and cimetidine for gastric ulcer. *Scand J Gastroenterol* **83**(suppl):49–51, 1983. This study showed that sucralfate had similar efficacy as cimetidine in the healing of gastric ulcer. Analgesic users were excluded.
15. Herrerias-Gutierrez JM, Pardo L, Segu JL: Sucralfate vs ranitidine in the treatment of gastric ulcer: Randomized clinical results in short-term and maintenance therapy. *Am J Med* **86**(suppl 6A):94–97, 1989. This study showed that sucralfate had similar efficacy as ranitidine in the healing of gastric ulcer. Concomitant medical illness, duodenal ulcer, and analgesics were excluded.
16. Rey JF, Legras B, Verdier A, *et al*: Comparative study of sucralfate versus cimetidine in the treatment of acute gastroduodenal ulcer. Randomized trial with 667 patients. *Am J Med* **86**(6A):116–121, 1989. This study showed that sucralfate had similar efficacy as cimetidine in the healing of gastric ulcer. Concomitant medical illness, duodenal ulcer, and analgesic users were excluded.
17. Asaka M, Takeda H, Saito M, *et al*: Clinical efficacy of sucralfate in the treatment of gastric ulcer. *Am J Med* **91**(2A):71S–73S, 1992. This study showed that sucralfate twice daily had similar healing efficacy as sucralfate four times daily in the healing of gastric ulcer.
18. Simjee AE, Pettengell KE, Spitaels JM: Comparative study of sucralfate 2 grams bid versus sucralfate 1 g four times per day in the treatment of benign gastric ulcers in outpatients. *Am J Med*

91(2A):68S–70S, 1992. This study showed that sucralfate twice daily had similar healing efficacy as sucralfate four times daily in the healing of gastric ulcer.

19. Hjortrup A, Svendsen LB, Hoffmenn J, *et al*: Two daily doses of sucralfate and cimetidine in the treatment of gastric ulcer: A comparative randomized study. *Am J Med* **86**(suppl 6A):113–115, 1989. This study showed that sucralfate twice daily had similar healing efficacy as sucralfate four times daily in the healing of gastric ulcer.
20. O'Laughlin JC, Silvoso GR, Ivey KJ: Resistance to medical therapy of gastric ulcers in rheumatic disease patients taking aspirin. *Dig Dis Sci* **27**:976–980, 1982. This randomized, double-blind study using cimetidine showed that gastric ulcer healing was slower in patients taking NSAID than in those not taking such agents.
21. Lancaster-Smith MJ, Jaderberg ME, Jackson DA: Ranitidine in the treatment of non-steroidal anti-inflammatory drug associated gastric and duodenal ulcers. *Gut* **32**:252–255, 1991. This randomized, controlled study using ranitidine in NSAID-associated gastric ulcer showed that the healing rates were significantly lower in patients who continued to take NSAID compared with those who stopped these agents.
22. Malchow-Moller A: Treatment of peptic ulcer induced by non-steroidal anti-inflammatory drugs. *Scand J Gastroenterol* **22**(suppl 127):87–91, 1987. This study examined 14 NSAID-associated gastric ulcer but also 51 duodenal ulcers, and observed similar healing rates in sucralfate- and ranitidine-treated ulcers.
23. Manniche C, Malchow-Moller A, Andersen JR, *et al*: Randomised study of the influence of non-steroidal anti-inflammatory drugs on the treatment of peptic ulcer in patients with rheumatic disease. *Gut* **28**:226–229, 1987. Same study as above but reported in a different journal.
24. Shepherd HA, Fine D, Hillier K, *et al*: Effect of sucralfate and cimetidine on rheumatoid patients with active gastroduodenal lesions who are taking nonsteroidal anti-inflammatory drugs. A pilot study. *Am J Med* **86**(suppl 6A):49–54, 1989. This study examined endoscopic lesion scores in subjects taking NSAID, and observed apparently better response to sucralfate than to cimetidine.
25. Classen M, Bethge H, Brunner G, *et al*: Effect of sucralfate on peptic ulcer recurrence: A controlled double-blind multicenter study. *Scand J Gastroenterol* **18**(suppl):61–68, 1983. This placebo-controlled study examined the efficacy of sucralfate 1 g bid in 77 patients with healed gastric ulcer (and also 174 patients with healed duodenal ulcer), and observed significant prophylactic benefit in duodenal ulcer but not in gastric ulcer in 6 months.
26. Miyake T: Endoscopic evaluation of the effect of sucralfate therapy and other clinical parameters on the recurrence rate of gastric ulcers. *Dig Dis Sci* **25**:1–7, 1980. This randomized controlled study observed better prophylaxis against ulcer recurrence in patients treated with sucralfate than with placebo in 167 patients ($p < 0.06$) over 6 months. The study also observed the remission after stopping maintenance sucralfate for 12 months.
27. Libeskind M: Maintenance treatment of patients with healed peptic ulcer with sucralfate, placebo and cimetidine. *Scand J Gastroenterol* **18**(suppl 83):69–70, 1983. This studied compared sucralfate, its placebo, and cimetidine as maintenance treatment in patients with healed gastric ulcer, and observed 70% remission at 12 months for sucralfate, 50% for cimetidine, and 27% for placebo.
28. Marks IN: Maintenance therapy with sucralfate reduces rate of gastric ulcer recurrence. *Am J Med* **79**(suppl 2C):32–35, 1985. This double-blind placebo-controlled study showed significant prophylaxis with sucralfate maintenance for 6 months.
29. Marks IN, Girdwood AH, Wright JP, *et al*: Nocturnal dosage regimen of sucralfate in maintenance treatment of gastric ulcer. *Am J Med* **83**(suppl 3B):95–98, 1987. This study showed that maintenance treatment with bedtime dose of sucralfate 2 g for 6 months was significantly better than placebo.
30. Blum AL: Sucralfate in the treatment and prevention of gastric ulcer: Multicentre double blind placebo controlled study. *Gut* **31**:825–830, 1990. This randomized, placebo-controlled study showed that short-term healing in 160 patients with gastric ulcer was similar with sucralfate or ranitidine, and that long-term maintenance treatment for 6 months in 105 patients with healed gastric ulcer was significantly better with sucralfate than with placebo.

31. Takemoto T, Kimura K, Okita K, *et al*: Efficacy of sucralfate in the prevention of recurrence of peptic ulcer—double blind multicenter study with cimetidine. *Scand J Gastroenterol* **22**(suppl 140):49–60, 1987. This double-blind comparative study of 127 patients with gastric ulcers and 103 patients with duodenal ulcer showed that after initial healing, maintenance treatment for 12 months with sucralfate had significantly less recurrence than with cimetidine.
32. Takemoto T, Namiki M, Ishikawa M, *et al*: Ranitidine and sucralfate as maintenance therapy for gastric ulcer disease: Endoscopic control and assessment of scarring. *Gut* **30**:1692–1697, 1989. This study compared ranitidine 150 mg nocte and sucralfate 1 g tds for the prevention of gastric ulcer relapse, and observed that relapse was significantly lower at 9 and 12 months.
33. Tatsuta M, Ishikawa H, Iishi H, *et al*: Reduction of gastric recurrence after suppression of Helicobacter pylori by cefixime. *Gut* **31**:973–976, 1990. This study showed that cimetidine 800 mg daily for 12 weeks plus cefixime 100 mg daily for 2 weeks suppressed *H. pylori*, and the suppression was associated with significantly less ulcer recurrence.
34. Hui WM, Lam SK, Ho J, *et al*: The effect of sucralfate and cimetidine on duodenal ulcer associated antral gastritis and campylobacter pylori. *Am J Med* **86**(6A):60–65, 1989. This randomized study showed that the antral gastritis associated with duodenal ulcer improved and that the density of *H. pylori* decreased significantly more with sucralfate than with cimetidine treatment. The study also showed that ulcer relapse at 12 months was significantly less with sucralfate although this was not related to bacterial density.
35. Louw JA, Zak J, Lucke W, *et al*: Triple therapy with sucralfate is as effective as triple therapy containing bismuth in eradicating Helicobacter pylori and reducing duodenal ulcer relapse rates. *Scand J Gastroenterol* **27**(suppl 191):28–31, 1992. This study showed in 40 duodenal ulcer patients that *H. pylori* eradication rates were similar with triple therapy using sucralfate plus metronidazole and tetracycline compared with triple therapy with colloidal bismuth plus the same antibiotics.
36. Lanza F, Peace K, Gustitus L, *et al*: A blinded endoscopic comparative study of misoprostol versus sucralfate and placebo in the prevention of aspirin-induced gastric and duodenal ulceration. *Am J Gastroenterol* **83**:143–146, 1988. This study showed that misoprostol was significantly better than sucralfate and placebo for the prevention of endoscopic mucosal lesions in the stomach, whereas in the duodenum, the prophylactic effect of misoprostol was not different from that of sucralfate, although it was still significantly better than placebo.
37. Agrawal NM, Roth S, Graham DY, *et al*: Misoprostol compared with sucralfate in the prevention of nonsteroidal anti-inflammatory drug-induced gastric ulcer: A randomized, controlled trial. *Ann Intern Med* **115**:195–200, 1991. In this single-blind study, misoprostol (200 μg qid) was significantly better than sucralfate (1 g qid) in the prevention of NSAID-induced gastric ulcer.

24

Therapy of Active Duodenal Ulcers

FRANCOIS MARTIN

Introduction

In 1977, cimetidine had just been released in Canada for the treatment of duodenal ulcers. In view of this powerful acid-suppressing drug, Schwarz's time-honored dictum "No acid, no ulcer" never seemed more appropriate! The high healing rates of active duodenal ulcers, combined with the rapid relief of ulcer symptoms obtained by treating patients with cimetidine over a short period of 6 to 8 weeks, largely explain the rapid, universal acceptance of this new therapeutic breakthrough for peptic ulcer patients.

It was against this background that sucralfate was introduced to some clinical researchers, to test the potential antiulcer capacity of this other new agent, synthesized and already available in Japan since 1971. Reportedly, after its early use for the treatment of peptic ulcer disease in Japan, the preliminary clinical studies seemed to confirm the superiority of the agent over a placebo. In addition, the agent was judged to be extremely safe, as a result of its original nonsystemic mode of action.

The proposed mechanisms of action of sucralfate for the treatment of peptic ulcer were based on the suggestion that, although the drug had little or no effect on intragastric acidity, yet it had a clear ability to heal ulcers through mucosal protective effects. This sulfated aluminum salt of sucrose, when ingested orally, was said to create a physico-chemical gel in an acidic milieu. This gel would then adhere and coat the gastric and duodenal mucosa. Because of its negative electric charge, the molecule would be attracted to the positively charged proteinaceous content of inflammatory exudates; ulcers and their exudative fibrinous base would therefore become the perfect substrate for this original molecule. This "Band-Aid" barrier created at the ulcer base could prevent the acid

---

FRANCOIS MARTIN • Division of Gastroenterology, Hopital Saint-Luc, and University of Montreal, Montreal H2X 3J4, Canada.

Sucralfate: From Basic Science to the Bedside, edited by Daniel Hollander and G. N. J. Tytgat. Plenum Press, New York, 1995.

back diffusion and create an acid-free milieu favoring the natural healing of the ulcer. In addition, the capacity for sucralfate to adsorb bile salts as well as pepsin and pepsinogens, and to create innocuous complexes with these aggressive factors, thus completing the proposed mechanisms of action for the new molecule sucralfate.

Gastroduodenal mucosal-protection mechanisms were subsequently studied in the next 10 years, and this original, rather naive "Band-Aid" effect proposed to explain the healing capacity of sucralfate has progressed toward a much better understanding of these mechanisms, largely from the work of Tarnawski *et al.*[22]

Duodenal Ulcer Healing with Sucralfate

Early Placebo-Controlled Trials

The efficacy and safety of sucralfate in duodenal ulcer therapy were first assessed in three short-term, randomized, double-blind, placebo-controlled trials in which endoscopy was used. These trials were conducted almost simultaneously by the late M. Moshal and colleagues in South Africa and G. McHardy and D. Hollander in the United States.[1–3] A total of 328 patients were evaluated for efficacy in these trials. The healing rates for sucralfate ranged from 75 to 92% versus 44 to 64% for placebo. In each of these studies, sucralfate was shown to be superior to placebo. Few adverse experiences were reported.

This clinically confirmed therapeutic capacity for sucralfate in the short-term treatment of duodenal ulcer was somewhat unexpected in view of the poorly understood mechanism of action of this new agent at that time. This confirmed performance implied, almost heretically, that ulcer could heal rapidly without acid-suppression! The future of sucralfate as an efficient, alternate therapeutic modality for peptic ulceration based on a "mucosal protection" capacity had just begun.

Concomitantly, the widespread acceptance of the new H_2-receptor antagonist (H_2-RA), cimetidine, as the major treatment modality for peptic ulcer had reached such a level of confidence that certain discussions centered on the ethical questions surrounding placebo-controlled duodenal ulcer studies in light of the accepted benefits and wide use of antacids and cimetidine therapy. With these ethical questions around, it was only more difficult for the clinical researchers to plan the needed studies to define the exact therapeutic profile of sucralfate, at least for the treatment of peptic ulcer disease.

These previous considerations should help the younger reader to picture the unique context of thinking that prevailed in the early 1980s, regarding peptic ulcer therapy. It is only because a small number of clinical researchers from several countries around the world accepted to pursue the exploration of the therapeutic capacities of sucralfate, that we can today really appreciate how many important pieces of knowledge on peptic ulcer disease and also on mucosal injury and repair would have escaped us forever without their dedicated work.

Between 1980 and 1989, ten studies were published in which the healing capacity of sucralfate was consistently superior to placebo in 878 duodenal ulcer patients reported; indeed the mean percent healing rate in these ten studies was 75.4% for sucralfate and 48.1% for placebo[1–10] (Table I).

Table I. Placebo-Controlled Studies of Sucralfate in Duodenal Ulcer

		Sucralfate		Placebo		
Year	Authors	*n*	% healed	*n*	% healed	$p <$
1980	Elliot and Orchard[4]	16	69%	17	41%	0.02
1980	Moshal *et al.*[3]	30	60%	29	24%	0.01
1981	Lathinen *et al.*[5]	16	93%	16	31%	0.01
1981	Fixa and Komarkova[6]	69	80%	55	60%	0.05
1981	McHardy[2]	109	75%	107	64%	0.04
1981	Orchard and Elliot[7]	16	80%	17	41%	0.05
1983	Hollander[1]	24	92%	31	58%	0.01
1983	Sung *et al.*[8]	33	72%	32	25%	0.02
1984	Elsborg *et al.*[9]	17	82%	18	39%	0.01
1989	Martin[10]	114	51%	112	34%	0.02

Comparative Trials

In June of 1980, more clinical studies were presented that consistently confirmed the therapeutic capacity of sucralfate in the treatment of peptic ulcer disease. Among the reported studies, two were somewhat different from the usual controlled therapeutic trials since these studies were designed to compare a new agent, sucralfate, against an already accepted control agent, cimetidine.

Indeed, I. N. Marks in South Africa[11] and Martin in Canada[12] had separately, but concurrently conducted such comparative clinical trials. In the Marks study, 55 patients with an endoscopically proven gastric ulcer and 57 patients with a duodenal ulcer were alternately assigned to sucralfate and cimetidine regimens and a repeat endoscopy was carried out after 6 weeks of therapy. Patients with unhealed ulcers at week 6 underwent endoscopy for a third time after a further 6 weeks of therapy. In the duodenal ulcer group, 24 out of 29 patients on sucralfate had healed at 6 weeks (83%) and the remaining 5 patients had healed after a further 6 weeks of therapy (100%), compared with healing rates of 71% at 6 weeks and 86% at 12 weeks in the cimetidine-treated patients.

On the North American side of the Atlantic, we had designed our double-blind, double-dummy randomized trial to compare the efficacy and safety of sucralfate versus cimetidine in the short-term treatment of duodenal ulcer patients. A total of 62 endoscopically proven duodenal ulcer patients entered the trial and 59 completed the treatment. Healing rates for the two treatment groups after 4 and 8 weeks were as follows: of the patients who received sucralfate, 24 of 30 (80%) were healed after 4 weeks compared with 22 of 29 (76%) of the patients who received cimetidine. Patients in whom healing was confirmed at 4 weeks did not continue to receive treatment. After 8 weeks the overall healing rate in the sucralfate group was 90% (27 of 30 patients) versus 86.2% (25 of 29 patients) in the cimetidine group. No statistically significant difference could be shown between these two treatments. We, of course, were aware of the likelihood of making a type II error—declaring as "not significantly different" two treatments that were actually different—since the number of patients studied was small.

We believe that these two early comparative studies contributed to convince the gastroenterology community that the new agent, sucralfate, deserved a niche in the limited therapeutic arsenal for peptic ulcer disease of the early 1980s. Sucralfate could also be recommended as an alternate therapeutic agent for the treatment of duodenal disease.

After the 1980 and 1982 publication of these two comparative trials of sucralfate versus cimetidine, eight more studies were published and in these 1501 patients, the pooled average healing rates were 74.5% for sucralfate and 74.6% for cimetidine, confirming the earlier trials. Also, the healing rates for sucralfate in these comparative trials were similar to those observed in the placebo-controlled studies, namely 75.5%[13–20] (Table II). In 1989, the report of a study comparing the efficacy of sucralfate versus ranitidine for the short-term treatment of duodenal ulcer showed an identical healing rate of 74% for the two treatment groups.[21] The consistency in the healing capacity of sucralfate in the short-term treatment of duodenal ulcer has remained untouched throughout the years of testing and is a reflection of the good sound scientific methods of testing applied.

Symptomatic Improvement

Another highly rated feature of cimetidine therapy in peptic ulcer disease was the capacity for the drug to rapidly relieve ulcer symptoms often within days, if not hours. Any other antiulcer agent needed to be equally efficient in rapidly relieving ulcer symptoms to enjoy an equal acceptability by the ulcer patients. Surprisingly, sucralfate lacking any inherent capacity to suppress acid secretion or to neutralize the secreted acid, could nonetheless achieve a comparable symptomatic relief when systemically recorded by patients using a 10-point severity scale.[12]

Table II. Comparative Studies of Sucralfate versus H_2 RAs

		Sucralfate		Cimetidine	
Year	Authors	*n*	% healed	*n*	% healed
1980	Marks *et al.*[11]	29	83%	28	71%
1982	Martin *et al.*[12]	30	80%	29	76%
1982	Guslandi *et al.*[13]	15	67%	15	73%
1983	Hentschel *et al.*[14]	35	91%	37	84%
1983	Pop *et al.*[15]	31	71%	32	75%
1985	Van Deventer *et al.*[16]	20	65%	20	60%
1986	Glise *et al.*[17]	177	71%	194	77%
1987	Lam *et al.*[18]	141	79%	142	76%
1989	Rey *et al.*[19]	246	80%	234	80%
1989	Tovey *et al.*[20]	24	58%	22	64%
				Ranitidine	
1989	Koelz and Halter[21]	42	74%	35	74%

Safety

In these early studies, the highest incidence of any side effects reported by patients taking sucralfate was for mild constipation. Cimetidine therapy was also considered very safe in these early studies; it was only later that serious adverse events were attributed to the cimetidine therapy, and explained, at least for several of these side effects, by a substrate competition at the P-450 level of the liver metabolism of the drug. Comparatively, the safety profile of sucralfate observed in these early studies has remained intact after close to 15 years of therapeutic use around the world, and even today, constipation is the most frequently reported adverse event (2%). The nonsystemic mode of action of sucralfate is obviously not estranged to the fewer side effects reported by patients taking sucralfate.

Advantages of Sucralfate over H_2-Receptor Antagonists

Cigarette Smoking and Ulcer Healing

Several studies have confirmed that cigarette smoking consistently delays healing of duodenal ulcers often by weeks. Lam and colleagues[18] studied this specific issue of smoking and duodenal ulcer healing and showed that sucralfate overcomes the adverse effect of cigarette smoking on the rate of healing. In pooling several studies in which the effect of smoking on ulcer healing was considered, in more than 500 patients tested, 78.4% of smokers and 77.6% of nonsmokers healed on sucralfate.[23] The mucosal protective capacity of sucralfate seems to counteract in some way the ill effect of smoking on ulcer healing. Since clinical studies have shown that the H_2-RAs and even the more recent proton-pump inhibitors do not harbor this property in smokers, sucralfate could be an alternate therapeutic modality for those unfortunate ulcer patients who cannot stop smoking.

Posthealing Remission Length

Some early studies had shown that a longer remission period followed initial treatment with the mucosal protective agent, colloidal bismuth subcitrate, when compared with cimetidine.[25–27] The relapse rate after healing with sucralfate and cimetidine have also been compared in several studies. When the results of these studies are pooled, it can be shown that approximately 50% of patients treated originally with sucralfate are still in remission after 12 months, while only 25% of the patients treated with cimetidine were in remission after 12 months.[24] A recent 1-year follow-up study on 2045 patients confirmed a longer remission by an average of 80 days in the sucralfate-treated patients when compared with the cimetidine-treated patients.[28] The full understanding of this observation escapes us at present; however, I submit that an original work reported by Moshal on the end-point mucosal healing process, assessed by light and electron microscopy, should perhaps be revisited. Indeed, this work suggested that ulcer healing with sucralfate seems to have produced less fibrous tissue at the site of the healed ulcer than was observed in the cimetidine-treated patients.

Conclusion

Certainly for duodenal ulcer disease, sucralfate-induced healing is comparable to that obtained with H_2RAs. The healing efficacy is of the same magnitude in smokers. Sucralfate-induced healing occurs in the absence of interference with the gastric acid secretory potential. Finally the quality of the healed mucosa may be superior to that seen after healing with H_2RAs.

References

1. Hollander D: A multicenter, double-blind trial of sucralfate in duodenal ulcer therapy. *Scand J Gastroenterol* **18**(suppl 83):25–30, 1983.
2. McHardy GG: A multicenter, double-blind trial of sucralfate and placebo in duodenal ulcer. *J Clin Gastroenterol* **3**(suppl 2):147–152, 1981.
3. Moshal MG, Spitaels JM, Kahn F: Sucralfate in the treatment of duodenal ulcers: A double blind endoscopically controlled trial. *S Afr Med J* **57**:742–744, 1980.
4. Elliot C, Orchard R: A double-blind placebo controlled study of sucralfate in the treatment of gastric and duodenal ulcer. *Hepatogastroenterology* **27**(suppl):384, 1980.
5. Lathinen J, Ala-Kaila, Aukae S, *et al*: Sucralfate and antacid in the treatment of gastric and duodenal ulcer. The preliminary report of a multicenter double-blind trial, in Caspary WF (ed): *Duodenal Ulcer, Gastric Ulcer: Sucralfate, a New Therapeutic Concept*. Munich, Urban & Schwarzenberg, 1981, pp 111–115.
6. Fixa B, Komarkova O: Aluminum sucrose sulfate (sucralfate) in the treatment of peptic ulcer (double-blind study), in Caspary WF (ed): *Duodenal Ulcer, Gastric Ulcer: Sucralfate, a New Therapeutic Concept*. Munich, Urban & Schwarzenberg, 1981, pp 80–84.
7. Orchard R, Elliot C: A double-blind placebo-controlled study of sucralfate in the treatment of gastric and duodenal ulcer, in Caspary WF (ed): *Duodenal Ulcer, Gastric Ulcer: Sucralfate, a New Therapeutic Concept*. Munich, Urban & Schwarzenberg, 1981, pp 85–88.
8. Sung JL, Yu JY, Yang TH, *et al*: A placebo-controlled, double-blind study of sucralfate in the short-term treatment of duodenal ulcer. *Scand J Gastroenterol* **19**(suppl 83):21–24, 1983.
9. Elsborg L, Boysen K, Brunsgaard A, *et al*: Sucralfate vs placebo treatment in duodenal and prepyloric ulcer: A clinical endoscopic, double-blind controlled investigation. *Hepatogastroenterology* **31**:269–271, 1984.
10. Martin F: Multicenter study group. Sucralfate suspension 1 g four times per day in the short-term treatment of active duodenal ulcer. *Am J Med* **86**(suppl 6A):104–107, 1989. In Refs. 1 to 10 inclusive, reports are presented on placebo-controlled studies of sucralfate in duodenal ulcers. In these 878 treated patients, the mean % healing rate for sucralfate was 75.4% versus placebo 48.1%. Very few side effects were observed in these studies.
11. Marks IN, Wright JP, Denyer M, *et al*: Comparison of sucralfate and cimetidine in the short-term treatment of chronic peptic ulcers. *S Afr Med J* **57**:567–573, 1980.
12. Martin F, Farley A, Gagnon M, *et al*: Comparison of the healing capacities of sucralfate and cimetidine in the short-term treatment of duodenal ulcer: A double-blind randomized trial. *Gastroenterology* **82**:401–405, 1982.
13. Guslandi M, Bakkarubm E, Tittobello A: Ulcer healing and mucosa stimulation properties of sucralfate: A study comparing sucralfate to cimétidine. *Fortschr Med* **100**:1778–1780, 1982.
14. Hentschel E, Schutze K, Dufek W: Controlled comparison of sucralfate and cimetidine in duodenal ulcer. *Scand J Gastroenterol* **18**(suppl 83):31–35, 1983.
15. Pop P, Nikkers RE, Thye O, *et al*: Comparison of sucralfate and cimetidine in the treatment of duodenal and gastric ulcer. A multicenter study. *Scand J Gastroenterol* **18**(suppl 83):43–47, 1983.

16. Van Deventer GM, Schneidman D, Walsh JH: Sucralfate and cimetidine as single agents and in combination for treatment of active duodenal ulcers: A double-blind placebo-controlled trial. *Am J Med* **79**(suppl 2C):39–41, 1985.
17. Glise H, Carling L, Hallerback B, *et al*: Short term treatment of duodenal ulcer. A comparison of sucralfate and cimetidine. *Scand J Gastroenterol* **21**:313–320, 1986.
18. Lam SK, Hut WM, Lau WY, *et al*: Sucralfate overcomes adverse effect of cigarette smoking on duodenal ulcer healing and prolongs subsequent remission. *Gastroenterology* **92**:1193–1201, 1987.
19. Rey JF, Legras B, Verdier B, *et al*: Comparative study of sucralfate versus cimetidine in the treatment of acute gastroduodenal ulcer: Randomized trial on 667 patients. *Am J Med* **86**(suppl 6A):116–121, 1989.
20. Tovey FI, Husband EM, Yiu YC, *et al*: Comparison of relapse rates and of mucosal abnormalities after healing of duodenal ulceration and after one year's maintenance with cimetidine or sucralfate: A light and electron microscopy study. *Gut* **30**:586–593, 1989. In Refs. 11 to 20 inclusive, reports of comparative trials of sucralfate versus cimetidine in the short-term treatment of duodenal ulcers are presented. In these 1501 treated patients, the pooled average healing rates were 74.5% for sucralfate and 74.6% for cimetidine. Also, the healing rates for sucralfate in these comparative trials were similar to those observed in the placebo-controlled studies, namely 75.5%.
21. Koelz HR, Halter F: Ulcer study group. Sucralfate and ranitidine in the treatment of acute duodenal ulcer: Healing and relapse. *Am J Med* **86**(suppl 6A):98–103, 1989. In this study the comparative efficacy of sucralfate and ranitidine was tested for the short-term treatment of duodenal ulcers, and an identical healing rate of 74% was found in the two treatment groups.
22. Tarnawski A, Hollander D, Gergely H: The mechanism of protective, therapeutic and prophylactic actions of sucralfate. *Scand J Gastroenterol* **22**(suppl 140):7–13, 1987. This article summarizes the gastroduodenal mucosal protection mechanisms by which sucralfate exerts its ulcer healing capacities.
23. Lam SK: Why do ulcers heal with sucralfate? *Scand J Gastroenterol* **25**(suppl 173):6–13, 1990. With several other mechanisms related to the healing capacity of sucralfate, the specific issue of smoking and duodenal ulcer healing is specifically addressed in this article, and the author reports that on more than 500 pooled patients 78.4% of smokers and 77.6% of nonsmokers healed on sucralfate.
24. Lam SK: Treatment of duodenal ulcer with sucralfate. *Scand J Gastroenterol* **26**(suppl 185):22–28, 1991. In this article the author submits evidence to support the advantages of sucralfate over conventional H_2RAs in the short-term treatment of duodenal ulcers and for the increase in the posthealing remission length.
25. Shreeve DR, Klass HJ, Jones PE: Comparison of cimetidine and tripotassium dicitrato bismuthate in healing and relapse of duodenal ulcers. *Digestion* **28**:96–101, 1983.
26. Hamilton I, O'Connor HJ, Wood NC, *et al*: Healing and recurrence of duodenal ulcer after treatment of dicitrato bismuthate (TCB) tablets or cimetidine. *Gut* **27**:105–110, 1986.
27. Martin DF, Hollander D, May SJ, *et al*: Difference in relapse rates of duodenal ulcer after healing with cimetidine or tripotassium dicitrato bismuthate. *Lancet* **1**:7–10, 1981. In Refs. 25 to 27 inclusive, comparative studies are reported where a longer period of remission seems to follow initial treatment with colloidal bismuth when compared with cimetidine; approximately 25% more patients are still in remission after 1 year when initially treated with sucralfate.
28. Domschke S: Longer relapse-free period after acute treatment with sucralfate than after H2-blocker in peptic ulcer patients. 6th International Sucralfate Symposium Abstracts, ADIS Press, 1990, p 28.

25

Prevention of Ulcer Recurrence

HANS R. KOELZ

The Problem of Ulcer Recurrence

Peptic ulcer disease is a recurrent illness. Within the first year after healing of an acute ulceration, at least one further ulcer attack will occur in approximately 70% of patients with duodenal and in approximately 50% of those with gastric ulcers. Every recurrent ulceration bears the risk of medical and economic complications.

Indications for Prophylactic Treatment

Prophylactic treatment is indicated if the ulcer disease has led to complications and/or frequent relapses (Table I).

There are few, if any, indications for first time (primary) prevention of ulcer disease. Rarely, a patient at high risk for peptic ulcer and its complications, e.g., terminal renal failure or treatment with nonsteroidal anti-inflammatory drugs (NSAID) combined with anticoagulation, may be treated prior to the first ulcer attack.

Strategies of Ulcer Prevention

Three major types of measures are available to prevent ulcer recurrence: (1) long-term treatment with antisecretory or protective drugs, (2) surgery, i.e., vagotomy (in duodenal ulcer) or gastric resection (especially in gastric ulcer), and (3) treatment ("eradication") of *Helicobacter pylori* infection. Advantages and disadvantages of the three types of strategies are summarized in Table II.

In addition, the choice of acute treatment influences the rate of recurrence. This has been shown for duodenal ulcers after short-term therapy with sucralfate (see Chapter 19), colloidal bismuth, and in particular after eradication of *H. pylori*. However, the protection

HANS R. KOELZ • Department of Medicine, Triemli Hospital, CH-8063 Zurich, Switzerland.

Sucralfate: From Basic Science to the Bedside, edited by Daniel Hollander and G. N. J. Tytgat. Plenum Press, New York, 1995.

Table I. Indications for Long-Term Prophylactic Treatment in Peptic Ulcer Disease

Absolute
- Zollinger–Ellison syndrome and related states, not cured by surgery
- Previous life-threatening ulcer complications (bleeding, perforation) in patients who had no acid-reducing surgical procedure after the complication

Relative
- Concomitant disease with high risk of ulcer recurrence (e.g., terminal renal failure) or ulcer complications (e.g., anticoagulation)
- Frequent ulcer relapses
- Troublesome relapses (e.g., severe pain or delayed ulcer healing)
- Patient's wish
- Mandatory use of anti-inflammatory drugs

provided by short-term treatment with sucralfate or bismuth is much less effective than any of the three major prophylactic measures mentioned above. Therefore, if recurrent ulcer must be prevented because of previous life-threatening complications, other means are needed.

While changes in life-style (see section Accompanying Measures below) are recommended, they are usually not effective in preventing relapse. An exception to this rule may be a complete cessation of all NSAIDs in gastric ulcer disease.

Table II. Comparison of Measures to Prevent Ulcer Relapse

Characteristic	Long-term drug treatment	Eradication therapy of *H. pylori*	Surgery (vagotomy, gastric resection)
Effective in prevention of duodenal ulcer	Yes	Yes	Yes
Effective in prevention of gastric ulcer	Yes	Yes	Yes
Need for continuous cooperation	Yes	No, if eradication was successful	No
Experience from controlled clinical trials	Large[a]	Limited	Intermediate
Method established	Yes	No	Probably yes
Morbidity related to unwanted side effects of treamtent	Rare	Common	Depends on type of operation[b]
Mortality related to adverse effects of treatment	Not reported	Very rare (allergic reactions, pseudomembranous colitis)	Yes

[a]Especially with H_2-receptor antagonists.

[b]For example, low after proximal gastric vagotomy without drainage procedure, high after gastric resection.

Long-Term Treatment with Antisecretory or Protective Drugs

Long-term drug treatment with H_2-receptor antagonists or sucralfate is the most commonly used form of prophylactic treatment. It provides good protection against relapse but needs continuous cooperation of the patient. This is important in patients with previous ulcer complications, e.g., acute bleeding, because the risk of recurrent complications is increased at least fivefold as compared with patients without previous complication. In addition, ulcer complications represent the first manifestation in a large proportion of an ulcer attack, i.e., they occur without preceding abdominal pain. This also means that an "on-demand" treatment where patients take their medication only in the presence of symptoms often provides no protection against recurrent complications.

Eradication Treatment of Helicobacter Pylori

More than 95% of patients with duodenal ulcer are infected with *H. pylori*. In comparison, only 30 to 50% of subjects without ulcer disease are infected in Western countries. Evidence is accumulating that *H. pylori* eradication prevents ulcer recurrence. In addition, the reinfection rate with *H. pylori* appears to be very low; it amounts to about 0.5 to 1% per year. However, the optimum eradication regimen has not been defined despite several hundred published trials with more than 100 different schemes. In addition, resistance of *H. pylori* to antibiotics has emerged. Furthermore, all current eradication therapies require (albeit for a limited time) good compliance and they are accompanied by a high rate of side effects. And finally, the success rate of the best available therapies varies between 70 and 90% in most studies. Nevertheless, eradication of *H. pylori* can be recommended in patients for whom *Helicobacter*-associated duodenal ulcer disease represents a serious problem, most commonly those with frequent ulcer relapses, those with slow ulcer healing, and those with severe symptoms during attacks. In addition, eradication therapy may be chosen in patients who had ulcer complications although no convincing evidence from controlled studies is available for the usefulness in this situation. Recent studies suggest that similar indications can be applied to patients with *H. pylori*-associated gastric ulcers, provided they are not taking NSAIDs.

Surgery

The need for elective surgery because of therapy-resistant or recurrent ulcers has become extremely rare with modern therapy. The most frequent cause of recurrent ulcer during long-term drug treatment is insufficient compliance. Surreptitious use of NSAIDs should be identified in gastric ulcer disease. If the patient's compliance appears to be reasonable, additional tests should be performed to ascertain that the patient suffers "common" ulcer disease, and other conditions should be excluded. Specifically, malignancy should be ruled out in gastric ulcer by repeat endoscopy and biopsy. In the case of duodenal ulcer, Zollinger–Ellison syndrome, Crohn's disease, and other rare causes should also be excluded.

There is evidence that proximal gastric vagotomy leads to unsatisfactory results with high relapse rates if used in patients with recurrent duodenal ulcer despite prophylactic drug treatment. This is hardly surprising because vagotomy alone reduces gastric acid secretion approximately to the same degree as a reduced dose of an H_2-receptor antagonist, e.g., ranitidine 150 mg daily. Thus, more invasive procedures such as antrectomy combined with vagotomy should probably be chosen in this situation.

Properties of the Ideal Drug for Prophylactic Long-Term Treatment

The properties of the ideal drug are summarized in Table III. No long-term drug treatment has been shown to completely prevent ulcer recurrences. As mentioned above, good compliance is mandatory. Only about 30% of asymptomatic patients take their medication as prescribed. This figure rapidly increases to about 80% as soon as symptoms recur. Therefore, in order to optimize compliance, the regimen of long-term treatment has to be as acceptable for the patient as possible. Acceptability includes simplicity of drug intake, good (or no) smell and taste of the preparation, and lack of side effects. Finally, the drug should be available at an affordable price.

Prophylactic Long-Term Treatment with Sucralfate

Prevention of Ulcer Recurrence

Long-Term Treatment with Sucralfate in Prevention of Duodenal Ulcer Recurrence

Sucralfate has been studied in the prevention of duodenal ulcer recurrence in several randomized controlled trials (Table IV). As compared with placebo or no treatment, sucralfate in the usual daily dose (1 g bid) reduces the recurrence rate by about 50% within the first year of treatment (Fig. 1). The preventive effect is comparable to that of the H_2-receptor antagonists cimetidine (400 mg) or ranitidine (150 mg) at bedtime (Fig. 2). More and larger studies are needed to prove that sucralfate is equally effective as H_2-receptor antagonists and the pump inhibitors such as omeprazole.

Table III. Properties of the Ideal Drug for Maintenance Treatment

1. Proven efficacy in controlled clinical trials
2. Prevents complications
3. Simple mode of administration
4. No serious adverse effects
5. Good (or no) smell and taste
6. Reasonable price

Long-Term Treatment with Sucralfate in Prevention of Gastric Ulcer Recurrence

The results of randomized controlled trials of the prevention of gastric ulcer are summarized in Table V. It is evident from these data that the prophylactic effect of sucralfate is superior to placebo. No significant difference was detected in most studies between the prophylactic effects of sucralfate and cimetidine or ranitidine; only one study revealed a small superiority of ranitidine (150 mg at bedtime) in comparison with sucralfate (1 g tid). Thus, although the best-investigated regimen of sucralfate treatment is 1 g bid, future studies using direct comparisons may prove that a more convenient regimen with 2 g at bedtime is equivalent or that 1 g tid is more effective.

Prevention of Ulcer Complications

Probably the most important aim of long-term treatment is prevention of ulcer complications, in particular bleeding. Although it appears self-evident that a drug capable of preventing recurrent ulcers will also prevent ulcer complications, direct evidence from controlled clinical trials is needed. Sucralfate has not been tested specifically for this, but it should be emphasized that studies demonstrating prevention of ulcer complications by long-term treatment with H_2-receptor antagonists are scarce.

Ease of Administration, Smell and Taste

The standard regimen for prophylactic use of sucralfate for both duodenal and gastric ulcer is 1 g twice daily. Compared with the once-daily intake of H_2-receptor antagonists, this is less convenient and might impair compliance. There is, however, evidence from one study[14] that a simpler regimen with 2 g of sucralfate at bedtime is equally effective in prevention of duodenal ulcer as cimetidine 400 mg (see Table IV).

Sucralfate has almost no smell. If certain patients dislike the taste of the suspension or of the granulate, which is similar to that of some antacids, tasteless tablets can be prescribed.

Adverse Effects

Adverse effects of sucralfate are virtually unknown in otherwise healthy patients. Simultaneous administration of some other drugs (tetracyclines, phenytoin, digoxin, cimetidine, and chenodeoxycholic acid) should be avoided because sucralfate may inhibit their absorption (see Chapter 22).

Costs

Compared with the costs of recurrent ulcers including diagnostic tests, sick leave, and complications, the price of the drug—within a certain frame—is of minor importance. Precise comparison of the costs of sucralfate with other antiulcer drugs is

Table IV. Efficacy of Sucralfate in Prevention of Duodenal Ulcer: Results of Randomized Trials (Minimum of 15 Patients per Treatment Group) Comparing Sucralfate with Placebo, No Treatment, or Other Drugs

Author	Year	Quality[a]	Treatment and daily dose[b]	No. of patients	Cumulative recurrence rate (%)		
					3 to 4 months	6 to 8 months	12 months
Classen	1983	db	SCF 1 g bid	66	9*	21*	—
			Placebo	60	35	50	—
Marks	1985	sb	SCF 1 g at bedtime	19	—	26	47*
			SCF 1 g bid	20	—	20*	32*
			No treatment	17	—	53	81
Behar	1987	db	SCF 1 g bid	30	—	20*	27*
			Placebo	31	—	74	81
Pääkkonen	1989	db	SCF 1 g bid	40	28*	33*	45*
			Placebo	45	49	64	68
Bynum	1989	db	SCF 1 g bid	122	42*	—	—
			Placebo	117	64	—	—
Bolin	1987	db	SCF 1 g bid	24	18	33*	42*
			Placebo	26	38	69	81
Moshal	1983	db	SCF 0.5 g tid + 1 g	17	29	36*	44*
			Placebo	15	53	73	82
Rodrigo	1987	sb	SCF 1 g bid	24	—	33	—
			Cim 400 mg	29	—	45	—

Jean	1985	db[c]	SCF 1 g bid	20	20	20*	38*
			Cim 200 + 400 mg	25	4*	36	49*
			Placebo	24	27	58	70
Hui	1992	sb	SCF 1 g bid	100	—	28*	40*
			Ran 150 mg	100	—	21*	30*
			Cim 400 mg	94	—	27*	44*
			No treatment	103	—	43	61
Masoero	1986	open	SCF 1 g bid	29	38	38	47
			Ran 150 mg	29	10	15	47
Garcia-Paredes	1991	sb	SCF 1 g bid	33	—	9*	31
			Ran 150 mg	29	—	15	35
Marks	1989	db[c]	SCF 2 g at bedtime	36	8*	41*	55*
			Cim 400	32	22*	47	59*
			Placebo	34	41	67	85
Takemoto	1987	db	SCF 1 g bid	35	17	24	—
			Cim 400 mg	32	6	19	—
			SCF + Cim	36	3	22	—
Tovey	1989	sb	SCF 1 g bid	17	—	0	24
			Cim 400 mg	20	—	10	20

[a]db, double-blind; sb, single-blind.
[b]SCF, sucralfate; Ran, ranitidine; Cim, cimetidine.
[c]Cimetidine group not blinded.
*Significantly lower recurrence rate as compared with control treatment ($p < 0.05$).

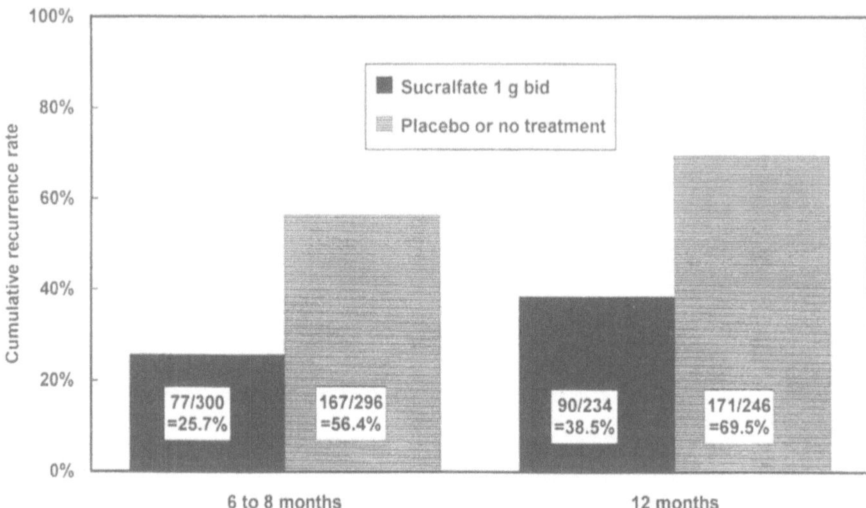

Figure 1. Cumulative recurrence rates of duodenal ulcers during long-term treatment with sucralfate 1 g bid or placebo. The graph represents pooled data from seven randomized studies (Refs. 5, 7, 9, 12, 13, 16, 21).

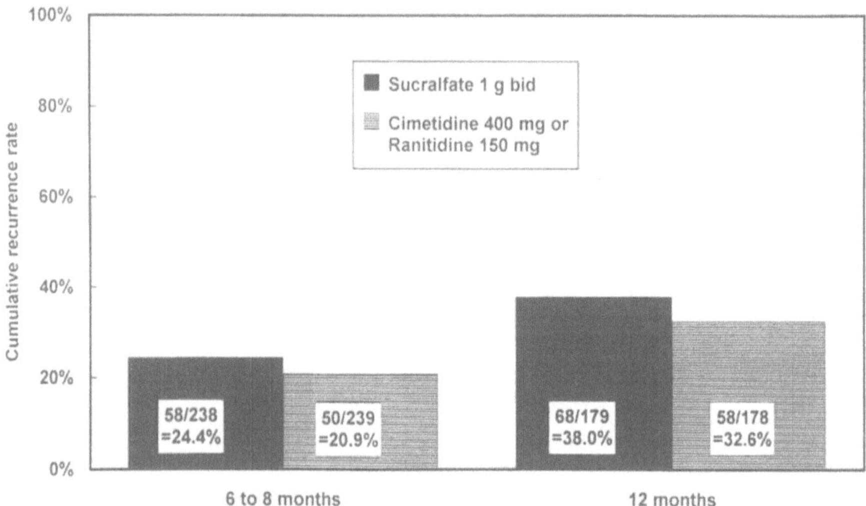

Figure 2. Cumulative recurrence rates of duodenal ulcers during long-term treatment with sucralfate 1 g bid or H_2-receptor antagonist (cimetidine 400 mg or ranitidine 150 mg at bedtime). The graph represents pooled data from six randomized studies (Refs. 10, 12, 18, 22, 23, 25).

Table V. Efficacy of Sucralfate in Prevention of Gastric Ulcer: Results of Randomized Trials (Minimum of 15 Patients per Treatment Group) Comparing Sucralfate with Placebo, No Treatment, or Other Drugs

Author	Year	Quality[a]	Treatment and daily dose[b]	No. of patients	Cumulative recurrence rate (%)		
					3 to 4 months	6 to 8 months	12 months
Blum	1990	db	SCF 1 g bid	49	—	13*	43*
			Placebo	42	—	34	65
Classen	1983	db	SCF 1 g bid	30	—	37	—
			Placebo	25	—	44	—
Herrerias-Gutierrez	1989	open	SCF 1 g bid	21	—	33	44
			Ran 150 mg	18	—	50	50
Marks	1985	db	SCF 1 + 2 g	31	10*	16*	—
			Placebo	30	53	70	—
Marks	1987	db	SCF 2 g at bedtime	29	10	28*	—
			Placebo	27	19	56	—
Miyake	1980	sb	SCF 1 g qid	83	—	7	—
			Antacid	84	—	17	—
Takemoto	1987	sb	SCF 1 g bid	26	—	10	—
			Cim 400 mg	34	—	16	—
			SCF + Cim	38	—	2.4	
Takemoto	1989	db	SCF 1 g tid	175	15	21	30*
			Ran 150 mg	171	9*	15*	21*

[a]db, double-blind; sb, single-blind.
[b]SCF, sucralfate; Ran, ranitidine; Cim, cimetidine.
*Significantly lower recurrence rate as compared with control treatment ($p < 0.05$).

impossible because drug costs vary considerably from country to country. In Switzerland, for example, the daily cost of sucralfate is somewhat lower than that of available H_2-receptor antagonists.

Suitability of Sucralfate for Prophylactic Long-Term Treatment as Compared with Other Drugs

Advantages

Safety is one of the most important aspects of drug treatment, especially in long-term use such as prevention of ulcer recurrence. The almost complete lack of absorption of sucralfate and its (presumably) local action leave little chance for systemic side effects (see Chapter 21). Sucralfate is the treatment modality of choice during pregnancy and lactation. Some authors also believe that preservation of physiological gastric acidity is an advantage of sucralfate as compared with acid-reducing drugs.

Limitations

There is no place for sucralfate in the (rare) Zollinger–Ellison syndrome and other related states of excessive hypersecretion of gastric acid. Also, there are no data to support its use in prevention of NSAID-related gastric ulcer if NSAID treatment will be continued.

Practical Use

Investigations before Treatment

As a general rule, malignant ulcer (especially gastric) should be ruled out by repeat endoscopy with biopsies, and the diagnosis of Zollinger–Ellison syndrome should also be ruled out prior to long-term treatment. Also, complete healing of the acute ulcer should be documented endoscopically. It is very important that a complete history be taken to search for risk factors for ulcer relapse that may be eliminated by changes in life-style (see section Accompanying Measures below).

Duration of Prophylactic Treatment and Surveillance

Current evidence suggests that prophylactic long-term drug treatment should be given for an unlimited time period. Selected patients without major risk factors for relapses or serious complications can be treated for more limited time periods of 1 to 2 years.

Routine endoscopy and other tests are not needed during long-term treatment with sucralfate in asymptomatic patients. However, symptoms suggesting recurrence should lead to prompt investigations directed at identifying ulcer recurrence. Regular visits every few months are recommended in order to reinforce to the patient that compliance is mandatory for effective prevention, although in one study the protective effect of sucralfate—in contrast to acid inhibitors—may act beyond regular intake.[24] This potential benefit is not unexpected considering the preventive action of short-term treatment with sucralfate (see Chapter 19), but it should be confirmed in further studies.

Treatment of "Break-through" Ulcers

An ulcer that recurs during prophylactic long-term treatment is referred to as "break-through" ulcer. If there is no indication of a special situation (e.g., Zollinger–Ellison syndrome or malignancy), these ulcers are treated just like any other ulcer by prescribing an antiulcer drug at full dose followed by prophylactic long-term treatment after healing. The situation is different if the relapse has led to serious complications. In this case, the prophylactic measures must be improved. If the failure was not related to lack of compliance or intake of NSAID that could be avoided, a more effective prophylactic treatment should be chosen. Since there are no data indicating that a higher dose of sucralfate is more effective, an alternate treatment should be given (see Strategies of Ulcer Prevention above).

Accompanying Measures (Table VI)

Smoking should be discouraged because it is a major risk factor not only for delayed healing but also for recurrence of duodenal ulcer. Some authors suggest that smoking might be a less important risk factor during treatment with sucralfate as opposed to acid inhibitors,[4] but these data are not yet completely convincing.

There is no need for the prescription of a strict diet, but individual food intolerances—whether confirmed or not—should be respected. A balanced diet with a normal content of dietary fiber is recommended. While a high intake of fiber does not reduce the risk of relapse, one randomized study indicated that duodenal ulcers recur more readily in patients on a low fiber diet.

Table VI. Accompanying Lifestyle Changes to Prophylactic Long-Term Drug Treatment

Measure	Comment
Stop smoking	Especially important for duodenal ulcer.
Stop excessive intake of alcoholic beverages	Alcoholism may be associated with duodenal ulcer disease. "Hard" alcoholic beverages may directly damage gastric mucosa.
Avoid NSAIDs	NSAIDs are important in the pathogenesis of gastric ulcer, and may provoke bleeding in both gastric and duodenal ulcer. Stop NSAIDs; replace with analgesics (e.g., paracetamol) and/or physical therapy; if not feasible, reduce daily dose as much as possible.
Avoid psychological stress	General importance for ulcer disease disputed, but may be relevant in selected cases.
Use balanced diet, respect individual "intolerances"	There is no special "ulcer diet." Diets with particularly low fiber content may be associated with higher relapse rates of duodenal ulcer.

Summary

As shown in several randomized clinical studies, long-term treatment with sucralfate reduces the risk of both duodenal and gastric ulcer recurrence by approximately 50%. The usual regimen with 1 g sucralfate twice daily is somewhat more complicated than that of H_2-receptor antagonists. However, the excellent safety profile of sucralfate is a strong argument in favor of this nonsystemic treatment that leaves gastric acidity intact. This is particularly important in peptic ulcer disease where drug treatment is often needed for many years, if not indefinitely.

References

1. Bauerfeind P, Blum AL (editors), and 57 co-authors: Ulkusalmanach 1 + 2. Zweite, erweiterte Auflage. Berlin, Springer-Verlag, 1990. This is probably the most comprehensive recent compilation of data on peptic ulcer disease. It includes critical reviews on current topics and an analysis of 1735 original publications. Unfortunately, the 835-page volume is available in German only.
2. Alexander-Williams J: A requiem for vagotomy. Despite the last efforts of surgeons. *Br Med J* **302**:547–548, 1991. In view of the efficacy of current antiulcer drugs and eradication therapy of *H. pylori*, one of the major protagonists of vagotomy for peptic ulcer fails to see any further role for vagotomy in peptic ulcer disease.
3. Lanas A, Sekar MC, Hirschowitz BI: Objective evidence of aspirin use in both ulcer and nonulcer upper and lower gastrointestinal bleeding. *Gastroenterology* **103**:862–869, 1992. Measurement of platelet cyclooxygenase activity in gastrointestinal bleeding reveals that 80% of the patients were currently taking aspirin. 21.5% of the patients were not aware of, or did not admit, current aspirin consumption.
4. Koelz HR: Antisecretory versus protective drugs, in Halter F, Garner A, Tytgat GNJ (eds): *Mechanisms of Peptic Ulcer Healing*. Dordrecht, Kluwer Academic Publishers, 1991, pp 231–242. The two major groups of antiulcer drugs are reviewed, in particular also with respect to potential advantages of sucralfate in smokers.
5. Behar J, Roufail W, Thomas E, *et al*: Efficacy of sucralfate in the prevention of recurrence of duodenal ulcers. *J Clin Gastroenterol* **9**(suppl 1):23–30, 1987. Placebo-controlled, double-blind randomized study in duodenal ulcer patients demonstrating clear superiority of sucralfate.
6. Blum AL, Bethge H, Bode JC, *et al*: Sucralfate in the treatment and prevention of gastric ulcer: Multicentre double blind placebo controlled study. *Gut* **31**:825–830, 1990. This study confirms the efficacy of sucralfate in gastric ulcers. Patients who have never taken NSAIDs had a higher recurrence rate than those who had but had stopped at entry of the study.
7. Bolin TD, Davis AE, Duncombe VM, *et al*: The role of maintenance sucralfate in prevention of duodenal ulcer recurrence. *Am J Med* **83**(suppl 3B):91–94, 1987. Double-blind, placebo-controlled, randomized study in prevention of duodenal ulcer with sucralfate 1 g twice daily.
8. Bynum TE: Sucralfate 1 g twice a day prevents duodenal ulcer recurrence (abstract). *Gastroenterology* **94**:A56, 1988. Preliminary results of a double-blind, randomized, placebo-controlled study with sucralfate in prevention of duodenal ulcer. The duration of treatment was limited to 3 months.
9. Classen M, Bethge H, Brunner G, *et al*: Effect of sucralfate on peptic ulcer recurrence: A controlled double-blind multicenter study. *Scand J Gastroenterol* **18**(suppl 83):61–68, 1983. Prophylactic treatment of patients with duodenal or gastric ulcers with sucralfate 1 g twice daily or placebo for 6 months. Sucralfate prevented recurrence of duodenal ulcers, but a significant difference was not found in gastric ulcers.

10. Garcia-Paredes J, Diaz Rubio M, Llenas F, *et al*: Comparison of sucralfate and ranitidine in the treatment of duodenal ulcers. *Am J Med* **91**(suppl 2A):64S–67S, 1991. Single-blind comparison of sucralfate 1 g twice daily and ranitidine 150 mg daily for up to 12 months in duodenal ulcer disease. The relapse rates were significantly lower in sucralfate-treated patients after 6 months.
11. Herrerias-Gutierrez JM, Pardo L, Segu JL: Sucralfate versus ranitidine in the treatment of gastric ulcer. Randomized clinical results in short-term and maintenance therapy. *Am J Med* **86**(suppl 6A):94–97, 1989. Randomized, but open, prophylactic treatment of patients with gastric ulcers showing no significant differences. The low number of patients precludes firm conclusions.
12. Hui WM, Lam SK, Lok AS, *et al*: Maintenance therapy for duodenal ulcer: A randomized controlled comparison of seven forms of treatment. *Am J Med* **92**:265–274, 1992. Large randomized trial on the preventive effect of several different regimens of prophylactic long-term drug treatment. The "single-blind" design is a serious drawback.
13. Jean F, Bannefond A, Gislon J, *et al*: Traitement d'entretien de la maladie ulcéreuse. Etude multicentrique comparative du sucralfate, de la cimétidine et placébo. *Rev Med Interne* **6**:321–326, 1985. Randomized trial with three small groups of patients. Therefore, and because cimetidine treatment was not blinded, clinically relevant differences between sucralfate and cimetidine cannot be excluded on the basis of this study.
14. Marks IN, Girdwood AH, Newton KA, *et al*: A maintenance regimen of sucralfate 2 g at night for reduced relapse rate in duodenal ulcer disease. A one-year follow-up study. *Am J Med* **86**(suppl 6A):136–140, 1989. Convenient dose of sucralfate (2 g at bedtime). Patients who had acute treatment with or including sucralfate had a lower recurrence rate at 6 months.
15. Marks IN, Girdwood AH, Wright JP, *et al*: Nocturnal dosage regimen of sucralfate in maintenance treatment of gastric ulcer. *Am J Med* **83**(suppl 3B):95–98, 1987. This is the only randomized study available showing a reduction of the relapse rate of gastric ulcers with prophylactic sucralfate treatment using a regimen of 2 g at bedtime.
16. Marks IN, Girdwood AH: Recurrence of duodenal ulceration in patients on maintenance sucralfate. *S Afr Med J* **67**:626–628, 1985. Comparison of sucralfate 1 g twice daily, 1 g at bedtime, and no treatment in prevention of duodenal ulcer. The marginal efficacy of the lower dose of sucralfate does not support its use.
17. Marks IN, Wright JP, Girdwood AH, *et al*: Maintenance therapy with sucralfate reduces rate of gastric ulcer recurrence. *Am J Med* **79**(suppl 2C):32–35, 1985. Double-blind, randomized, placebo-controlled trial. Prophylactic treatment with sucralfate 1 g in the morning and 2 g at bedtime prevents approximately 50% of gastric ulcer relapses.
18. Masoero G, Rocchia F, Rossanino A, *et al*: Comparison of ranitidine and sucralfate in the long-term treatment of duodenal ulcer. *J Clin Gastroenterol* **8**:624–627, 1986. Randomized open trial comparing sucralfate 1 g twice daily and ranitidine 150 mg. Relapse rates at 12 months were identical, but tended to lower earlier with ranitidine treatment.
19. Miyake T, Ariyoshi J, Suzaki T, *et al*: Endoscopic evaluation of the effect of sucralfate therapy and other clinical parameters on the recurrence rate of gastric ulcers. *Dig Dis Sci* **25**:1–7, 1980. Single-blind, placebo-controlled, randomized trial of sucralfate 1 g four times daily and an antacid. No significant difference in relapses of gastric ulcer was found in a relatively large study population.
20. Moshal MG, Spitaels MM, Manion GL: Double-blind placebo-controlled evaluation of one year therapy with sucralfate in healed duodenal ulcer. *Scand J Gastroenterol* **18**(suppl 83):57–59, 1983. Double-blind trial comparing placebo and sucralfate in an unusual dose (three times 0.5 g and 1 g at bedtime).
21. Pääkkonen M, Aukee S, Janatuinen E, *et al*: Sucralfate as maintenance treatment for the prevention of duodenal ulcer recurrence. *Am J Med* **86**(suppl 6A):133–135, 1989. Double-blind placebo-controlled trial in patients with healed duodenal and pyloric (about 25%) ulcers showing superiority of sucralfate.
22. Rodrigo L, Berenger J, Hinojasa J, *et al*: Sucralfate and cimetidine as maintenance treatment in the prevention of duodenal ulcer recurrence. *Am J Med* **85**(suppl 3B):99–104, 1987. Single-blind

randomized study comparing sucralfate 1 g twice daily and cimetidine 400 mg for 6 months, with a follow-up for additional 6 months without therapy. No significant differences were observed.

23. Takemoto T, Kimura K, Okita K: Efficacy of sucralfate in the prevention of recurrence of peptic ulcer—Double-blind multicenter study with cimetidine. *Scand J Gastroenterol* **22**(suppl 140): 49–60, 1987. Double-blind randomized trial in prevention of recurrent duodenal and gastric ulcers with three regimens: Sucralfate 1 g twice daily versus cimetidine 400 mg versus combination therapy. No significant differences were found.
24. Takemoto T, Namiki M, Ishikawa M, *et al*: Ranitidine and sucralfate as maintenance therapy for gastric ulcer disease: Endoscopic control and assessment of scarring. *Gut* **30**:1692–1697, 1989. Large double-blind randomized study demonstrating superiority of ranitidine (150 mg) against sucralfate (1 g thrice daily) in gastric ulcer prevention.
25. Tovey FI, Husband EM, Yiu YC, *et al*: Comparison of relapse rates and of mucosal abnormalities after healing of duodenal ulceration and after one year's maintenance with cimetidine or sucralfate: A light and electron microscopy study. *Gut* **30**:586–593, 1989. Single-blind randomized trial in a small population without significant differences in relapse rates.

26

Therapy of Esophagitis

ROY CHARLES ORLANDO

Introduction

Reflux esophagitis is a chronic disorder characterized by the symptoms of heartburn and regurgitation. Heartburn is extremely common in the United States, reportedly experienced by approximately 1/3 of the population on a monthly basis and by approximately 1/12 of the population on a daily basis. In addition to heartburn and other symptoms, reflux esophagitis has importance because it results in injury to the esophageal tissues ranging from inflammation to ulceration and healing of these lesions occasionally produces such undesirable complications as stricture formation and the development of the premalignant columnar-lined (Barrett's) esophagus.

Although the etiology of reflux esophagitis remains poorly understood, the current view is that the major pathogenetic process involves prolonged contact of the esophageal lining with the highly acidic (and refluxed) gastric content. In this respect reflux esophagitis has much in common with acid–peptic disease of the duodenum, a disease in which the drug sucralfate has been shown to have considerable therapeutic benefit. Chemically, sucralfate is the basic salt of the antacid compound, aluminum hydroxide, and the highly sulfated disaccharide, sucrose octasulfate, and in this form it is insoluble in water. On contact of sucralfate with an acidic medium, however, the molecule polymerizes by the formation of multiple intermolecular and intramolecular hydrogen bonds to form a white viscid material that adheres tenaciously to (positive charged) proteins present in areas of ulcerated mucosa as well as on the surface of healthy tissue. In the presence of excess acid, sucralfate undergoes further changes in that a neutralization reaction occurs that releases aluminum ions and the polymer dissolves releasing the water-soluble sucrose octasulfate. Notably, it is the conversion of sucralfate from insoluble particle to one or more of its active components on contact with acid that appears responsible for its beneficial effects in acid–peptic disease.

In addition to the beneficial effects of sucralfate previously observed in duodenal ulcer disease, its potential for benefit to patients with reflux esophagitis is supported by

---

ROY CHARLES ORLANDO • Tulane University School of Medicine, New Orleans, Louisiana 70112.

Sucralfate: From Basic Science to the Bedside, edited by Daniel Hollander and G. N. J. Tytgat. Plenum Press, New York, 1995.

studies in experimental animals (discussed in greater detail in Chapter 20). To summarize, these studies showed that sucralfate provided significant protection against damage to esophageal epithelium exposed to either acid or acid plus pepsin and that its protective mechanism was complex involving, among others, its ability to bind pepsin, buffer acid, polymerize and generate the water-soluble molecule, sucrose octasulfate (see Chapter 20). In this chapter, the results of the clinical trials in which sucralfate has been used for the treatment of reflux esophagitis are reviewed and this is followed by a discussion that attempts to explain the apparent discrepancy between the dramatic results using sucralfate experimentally (animal models) and the inconsistent findings in clinical trials.

Therapy of Esophagitis

Drug therapy of reflux esophagitis generally involves the following approaches: (a) a reduction in the potency of the noxious material in the refluxate, e.g., by reducing luminal acidity through buffering or inhibition of gastric acid secretion and/or by reducing the concentration of pepsin (and perhaps bile salts), or (b) an enhancement of one of the three esophageal defenses, specifically: (1) the antireflux barriers, e.g., raising lower esophageal sphincter pressure; (2) the acid clearance mechanisms consisting of peristalsis and gravity for volume clearance and salivary and esophageal submucosal gland secretion of bicarbonate ions for intraluminal buffering; and (3) tissue resistance, a group of mucosal structure/functions posed to minimize damage during contact with acid–pepsin or other noxious luminal agents. Notably, sucralfate has actions, discussed above and in Chapter 20, that fall into both of the above categories and so initial optimism regarding its efficacy in reflux esophagitis was predictably high.

Clinical Trials

Clinical trials have been performed comparing the efficacy of sucralfate either to placebo or to an agent presumed effective in the treatment of reflux esophagitis, e.g., the H_2-receptor antagonists, cimetidine and ranitidine, and Gaviscon, an alginate/antacid combination. The results of these trials in terms of symptom (heartburn) relief and/or macroscopic lesion healing (endoscopically documented) are summarized in Table I. In all trials, sucralfate, which is manufactured as tablets, was administered, after crushing, as a suspension. Notably, there were no serious side effects reported from sucralfate in the doses prescribed, and constipation proved to be the most troublesome of the minor side effects. Rarely bezoar formation has been reported as a risk of sucralfate ingestion and the drug's ability to bind other chemicals makes it necessary to avoid taking other medication within 2 hr of sucralfate.

Sucralfate versus Alternative Therapy

At least seven clinical trials have been reported in adult patients in which sucralfate has been compared to monotherapy with another agent, five with an H_2 antagonist[1–5] and

Table I. Clinical Trials of Sucralfate in Reflux Esophagitis

Trial	Rx/No.[a]	Dose	Duration	% patients: Symptoms improved	% patients: Lesions healed
		Sucralfate versus placebo			
Weiss 1983	S, $n = 22$	1 g qid	12 weeks	100	72*
	P, $n = 25$			77	40
Williams 1987	S, $n = 31$	1 g qid	8 weeks	45	36
	P, $n = 37$			24	35
Carling 1988	S, $n = 69$	1 g qid	12 weeks	70	54
	P, $n = 69$			48	41
		Sucralfate versus alternative therapy: H_2 antagonist			
Hameeteman 1987	S, $n = 19$	1 g qid	8 weeks	53	31
	C, $n = 21$	400 mg qid		67	14
Simon 1987	S, $n = 22$	1 g qid	8 weeks	27	64
	R, $n = 19$	150 mg bid		21	68
Elsborg 1991	S, $n = 32$	1 g qid	12 weeks	50	62
	C, $n = 28$	400 mg bid		50	59
Ros 1991	S, $n = 21$	1 g qid	8 weeks	19	48
	C, $n = 20$	400 mg qid		20	55
Bremmer 1991	S, $n = 43$	6 g/day	8 weeks	35	47
	R, $n = 55$	150 mg bid		33	31
		Sucralfate versus alternative therapy: Gaviscon (alginate–antacid)			
Laitinen 1985	S, $n = 36$	1 g qid	6 weeks	70	53
	G, $n = 32$	2 g qid		66	34
Evreux 1987	S, $n = 23$	1 g qid	6 weeks	68	62
	G, $n = 22$	5 g qid		63	64

[a]S, sucralfate; P, placebo; C, cimetidine; R, ranitidine; G, Gaviscon; No., number of patients in group.
*$p < 0.05$ sucralfate versus placebo or alternative therapy.

two with the alginate–antacid combination, Gaviscon.[6,7] The results of these trials are summarized in Table I. Three of the five studies using an H_2 antagonist for comparison to sucralfate, used cimetidine and two used ranitidine. In essentially all of the studies, the data show equal efficacy in the treatment of reflux disease with sucralfate compared to that of the alternative drug in terms of both symptom relief and lesion healing. Additional studies have been carried out in an attempt to extend the profile of patients for which sucralfate may have benefit. In this respect, Pace *et al.* tested its ability to improve patients with grades I–IV (Savary classification) who had initially failed a course of an H_2RA; however, sucralfate failed to heal these refractory subjects.[8] Similarly, the ability of a combination of sucralfate with an H_2RA (cimetidine) has been tested to determine if it would achieve superior effects in patients with reflux esophagitis, but in the two trials performed thus far as exemplified by that of Schotborgh *et al.*,[9] a beneficial effect on lesion healing has been marginal. Further in the same study sucralfate, 2 g qid was administered after successful healing of esophagitis to determine if it could prevent relapse, but this too proved unsuccessful.[9] Although these latter studies have been disappointing, the comparative data shown in Table I can be taken to support the equivalence of sucralfate and a standard dose of an H_2RA for the treatment of reflux disease. Yet, it should be remembered that the spectrum of reflux disease is broad and the management of such patients even with H_2RAs has proven less than ideal. For this reason to establish the efficacy of sucralfate in the treatment of reflux disease, comparative trials with a placebo arm are desirable. At present there are three such clinical trials and these are discussed below.

Sucralfate versus Placebo

The results of the clinical trials comparing sucralfate to placebo in the treatment of patients with reflux esophagitis are summarized in Table I. The results, disappointingly, are mixed. For example, in a study by Weiss and colleagues from Germany, 12 weeks of treatment demonstrated sucralfate to be superior to placebo in the healing of reflux-induced lesions (72 versus 40%, $p < 0.05$), and though symptoms were also improved, the results did not reach statistical significance.[10] The reported success with sucralfate by Weiss *et al.* for healing lesions, however, failed to be duplicated in two subsequent studies. One, a short (8 week) trial conducted by Williams *et al.* in the United States, reported no difference between sucralfate and placebo either in symptom relief or in lesion healing; however, the investigators cautioned that their results were inconclusive because randomization had placed all (6) patients with esophageal ulcers into the same therapeutic (sucralfate) group.[11] The third trial was performed in Sweden and Finland and it was by far the largest in terms of numbers with 138 patients participating.[12] In this study sucralfate was, as noted above, found not to be superior to placebo in healing esophageal lesions and although showing significant improvement in symptoms by sucralfate over placebo at 3 weeks, there was no difference either at the 6 or 12 week period. From these trials it is evident that sucralfate's effectiveness in the treatment of reflux disease can best be described as inconsistent and disappointing in view of the striking benefits from its use against acid and acid–peptic injury in animal models. The possible reasons for this discrepancy are discussed below.

Discussion

In the above review, it has been shown that sucralfate is equipotent to the H_2RAs in the treatment of patients with reflux disease, a finding not too difficult to accept given its equipotency to these agents in the treatment of duodenal ulcer disease. Yet, the lack of clear and consistent superiority of sucralfate over that of placebo in the reflux trials presented, prevents the complete acceptance of this drug as being beneficial (any more so than placebo) for this disease. This inconsistency of sucralfate therapy is all the more troubling given animal experimentation in which its potency in protecting esophageal tissues against acid or acid–peptic injury could be clearly documented. The explanation, however, may lie in methodologic differences between the animal experiments and the clinical situation. Most notably, in the animal models, sucralfate, acid, and esophageal epithelium are simultaneously in contact with one another for an extended period of time. For example, in a typical experiment the esophageal lining is exposed to a solution containing HCl or HCl plus sucralfate for 30 min to 1 hr. In these instances, the morphologic and functional protection of the tissue by sucralfate has been clear-cut and indisputable. Unfortunately, in the clinical realm it is difficult to duplicate such prolonged contact between sucralfate, acid, and epithelium. This is so because humans take oral medication intermittently and exclusively in an upright position, and in the upright position, it generally takes only 7 sec for a swallowed bolus, even of sucralfate, to pass from mouth to stomach. Consequently, the contact time between sucralfate and esophageal epithelium is at best brief. Indeed a study has been performed in which 2 g of radiolabeled sucralfate was ingested and by means of a counter, only 5% of the dose was shown to be retained in the human esophagus for more than a few minutes. There are, however, at least two clinical circumstances in which this may not be the case, as for example when the esophagus is either sufficiently acidic to enable sucralfate to adhere to the lining (either by polymerization or by release of its tissue-reactive component, sucrose octasulfate—see Chapter 15) or sufficiently (grossly) diseased such that sucralfate is physically trapped within an exudate or ulcerated region. Under these conditions, contact of the human esophageal epithelium with both acid (from reflux) and drug may parallel those produced by design in the animal models and as a result confer similar protection to the tissue. Ultimately, then, it is the frequency with which such prolonged contact (between acid, drug, and epithelium) occurs that determines whether the outcome is favorable—and this, being variable for a given patient, may account for the highly variable results produced thus far.

Summary

Reflux esophagitis is a chronic disease that results from the prolonged contact of the esophageal epithelium with gastric contents. Among the agents in gastric juice most responsible for esophageal damage are hydrochloric acid and pepsin—the same factors implicated in the pathogenesis of duodenal ulcer disease. Sucralfate, the salt of aluminum hydroxide and sucrose octasulfate, has been clearly documented to be an effective nonsystemic therapy for duodenal ulcer disease. Since the mechanisms by which sucralfate exerts its therapeutic effect in duodenal ulcer disease include formation of a barrier to acid–pepsin by adherence to the ulcer base as well as by binding pepsin and bile salts, it is reasonable to also expect that sucralfate treatment will be of benefit to patients with reflux esophagitis. The results of experimental studies have shown that sucralfate pretreatment significantly reduces the ability of acid or acid–pepsin to damage rabbit and cat esophagi, and a number of clinical trials have shown that it is equivalent in therapeutic efficacy to the H_2RAs. However, sucralfate has not been consistently shown to be superior to placebo either for relief of symptoms or for healing of esophageal lesions. Such clinical inconsistency may be related to the limited contact time between sucralfate, acid, and epithelium.

References

1. Bremmer CG, Marks S, Segal I, *et al*: Reflux esophagitis therapy: Sucralfate versus ranitidine in a double blinded multicentre trial. *Am J Med* **91**(suppl 2A):119–122, 1991.
2. Jorgensen F, Elsborg L: Sucralfate versus cimetidine in the treatment of reflux esophagitis with special reference to the esophageal motor function. *Am J Med* **91**(suppl 2A):114–118, 1991.
3. Ros E, Toledo V, Bordas JM, *et al*: Healing of erosive esophagitis with sucralfate and cimetidine: Influence of pretreatment on lower esophageal sphincter pressure and serum pepsinogen I levels. *Am J Med* **91**(suppl 2A):107–113, 1991.
4. Simon B, Mueller P: Comparison of the effect of sucralfate and ranitidine in reflux esophagitis. *Am J Med* **83**(suppl 3B):43–47, 1987.
5. Hameeteman W, Boomgaard DM vd, Dekker W, *et al*: Sucralfate versus cimetidine in reflux esophagitis. A single blind multicenter study. *J Clin Gastroenterol* **9**:390–384, 1987. These first five articles compare the efficacy of sucralfate to that of an H_2RA.
6. Evreux M: Sucralfate versus alginate/antacid in the treatment of peptic esophagitis. *Am J Med* **83**(suppl 3B):48–50, 1987.
7. Laitinen S, Stahlberg M, Kairaluoma MI, *et al*: Sucralfate and alginate/antacid in reflux esophagitis. *Scand J Gastroenterol* **20**:229–232, 1985. These two articles compare the efficacy of sucralfate to Gaviscon.
8. Pace F, Lazzaroni M, Bianci Porro G: Failure of sucralfate in the treatment of refractory esophagitis versus high dose famotidine. An endoscopic study. *Scand J Gastroenterol* **26**:491–494, 1991. This article demonstrates the inability of sucralfate to heal lesions in patients refractory to an H_2RA.
9. Schotborgh RH, Hameeteman W, Dekker W, *et al*: Combination therapy of sucralfate and cimetidine, compared with sucralfate monotherapy, in patients with peptic reflux esophagitis. *Am J Med* **86**(suppl 6A):77–80, 1989. This article indicates that the combination of sucralfate with an H_2RA offers minimal advantages over sucralfate alone and that sucralfate in low dose is unable to prevent relapse of reflux esophagitis.
10. Weiss W, Brunner H, Buttner GR, *et al*: Therapie der refluxosophagitis mit sucralfat. *Dtsch Med Wochenschr* **108**:1706–1711, 1983.
11. Williams RM, Orlando RC, Bozymski EM, *et al*: Multicenter trial of sucralfate suspension for the treatment of reflux esophagitis. *Am J Med* **83**:61–66, 1987.
12. Carling L, Cronstedt J, Engqvist A, *et al*: Sucralfate versus placebo in reflux esophagitis: A double-blind multicenter study. *Scand J Gastroenterol* **23**:1117–1124, 1988. These three articles compare sucralfate to placebo in the treatment of reflux disease.

27

Sucralfate for NSAID-Induced Gastroduodenal Lesions

G. BIANCHI PORRO and F. SANTALUCIA

Introduction

Nonsteroidal anti-inflammatory drugs (NSAIDs) are widely used in clinical practice. Their analgesic and anti-inflammatory properties make them useful in many common acute and chronic disorders, especially in various rheumatic and musculoskeletal disorders. However, NSAIDs are often associated with side effects of the gastrointestinal system, producing gastrointestinal symptoms and/or mucosal lesions such as erosions and/or ulcers. Possible complications of these lesions are perforation and hemorrhage, which can even lead to death, albeit rarely. If we consider the high frequency of rheumatic disease in the general population, particularly in the elderly and, consequently, the high consumption of these agents, which is bound to rise as the number of elderly people increases, the problem of NSAID-induced gastric lesions takes on particular importance in clinical terms, both for the physician and for the patient.

The practice of discontinuing NSAID therapy when gastroduodenal lesions are detected endoscopically or when upper gastrointestinal symptoms occur is fairly widespread. However, this often leads to recurrence of joint pain with consequent functional limitation, especially in patients with rheumatoid arthritis. In such cases it is preferable to continue anti-inflammatory treatment, adding an antiulcer agent to treat any gastroduodenal lesions already present or to prevent their occurrence.

This chapter examines the mechanisms by which NSAID-induced gastroduodenal damage occurs, focusing on the role of sucralfate in the prevention and treatment of mucosal lesions induced by these drugs.

G. BIANCHI PORRO and F. SANTALUCIA • Gastrointestinal Unit, L. Sacco Hospital, 20157 Milan, Italy.

Sucralfate: From Basic Science to the Bedside, edited by Daniel Hollander and G. N. J. Tytgat. Plenum Press, New York, 1995.

NSAID-Induced Gastropathy

The term *NSAID-induced gastropathy*, first used in the literature by Roth in 1986,[1] indicates the range of clinical and anatomopathological alterations that develop in the gastrointestinal tract as a result of the use of these drugs. About 60% of patients taking NSAIDs complain of digestive symptoms, mainly painful dyspepsia (epigastric distress, heartburn, hunger pain, nausea, vomiting). These symptoms are not always associated with mucosal damage. Indeed, only a small subgroup of symptomatic patients have acute lesions (submucosal hemorrhage and/or erosions); an even smaller number develop chronic lesions (ulcers), and complications (digestive hemorrhage and perforation) are extremely rare (Fig. 1). Thus, there is no correlation between the presence of symptoms and anatomical damage, as it is possible for severe symptoms to be associated with minimal mucosal damage and vice versa.[2]

The natural history of NSAID-induced lesions of the gastroduodenal mucosa is well known, as is the sequence of macro- and microscopic events underlying each of them. An anatomopathological study[3] in which biopsy samples were taken from the gastric fundus and corpus showed that 10 min after a single oral dose of 600 mg of ASA, 25% of the epithelial cells had already undergone microscopic alterations. The events observed were edema, cytoplasmic vacuolation, clumping and margination of nuclear chromatin, preparing the way for focal loss of apical cells. Cell loss increased between 10 and 30 min after the dose and repair mechanisms started within 1 hr of the drug, reducing the proportion of damaged cells to 9.6%; mucosal integrity was completely restored within 6 hr.

The sequence of macroscopic events that take place in the gastroduodenal mucosa after short-term NSAID therapy (up to 2 weeks) has been identified in numerous acute endoscopic studies.[4–10] Oral ASA causes scattered submucosal hemorrhages in the antrum and fundus within 30–60 min. Within 8–24 hr these became mucosal erosions which surprisingly tend to grow fewer as the anti-inflammatory treatment continues. Even more surprising are the modalities of resolution of acute endoscopic lesions after discontinuation of ASA therapy. After only 1 day of treatment the healing time is 8 days, but this time is halved when anti-inflammatory therapy continues for 1 week (gastric adaptation phenomenon).[11]

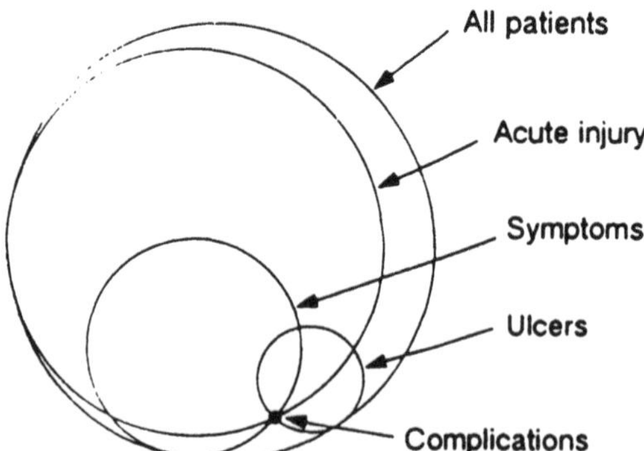

Figure 1. Spectrum of clinical and anatomopathological alterations to be found in NSAID gastropathy.

Although gastric and duodenal ulcers have been reported in healthy volunteers within 24 hr of taking ASA,[5,7,12] the association between ulcers and anti-inflammatory therapy is more evident for long-term treatment (more than 2 weeks).

No studies on long-term NSAID therapy in healthy volunteers are reported in the literature, whereas many such studies have been conducted on patients with rheumatic disease.[13–15] In this group of patients, the incidence of gastric ulcer is lower than that of erosions (15–20 and 40–50%, respectively). Moreover, about two-thirds of patients with gastric ulcer also have erosions. The incidence of duodenal lesions is markedly lower, being about 5% for ulcers and 15% for erosions. Again, adaptation of the mucosa to NSAID-induced damage is seen, resulting in a lower incidence of gastric and duodenal ulcers after 3 months of anti-inflammatory therapy.

The mucosal damage is dose-related, as shown by various experimental and epidemiological findings, and the risk of gastrointestinal bleeding seems to be greater if the daily ASA intake is over 2.4 g.[16]

The damaging effect of ASA is related both to the drug's direct irritant action[3] and to weakening of the defense mechanisms of the gastric wall[17] (dual assault theory) (Fig. 2). In the presence of HCl, ASA is trapped inside the gastric wall cells where it interferes with ATPase-dependent metabolic processes, increasing membrane permeability. The result-

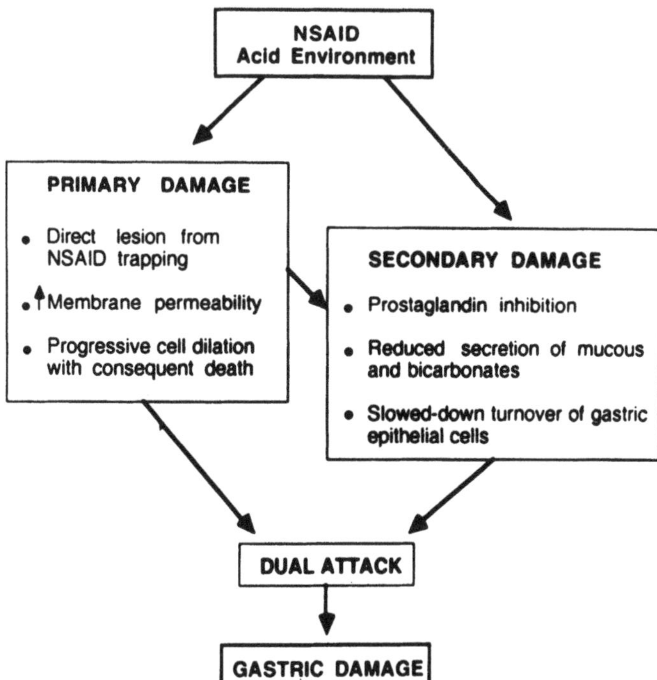

Figure 2. Diagram illustrating the pathogenic mechanisms of NSAID-induced gastroduodenal mucosa damage. Dual attach theory.

ing intracellular accumulation of Na, anions, and H_2O causes progressive dilation through an osmotic effect that culminates in cell death (direct irritant action of the drug).[3] Other mechanisms also contribute to the mucosal damage. ASA reduces mucus secretion and bicarbonate secretion,[17] inhibits prostaglandin synthesis in the gastric mucosa,[18] and interferes with gastric epithelial cell turnover[3] (weakening of defense mechanisms).

The mechanisms by which NSAIDs other than ASA cause mucosal damage are not yet fully understood, but it is likely that they do not differ from those of ASA.[19] In addition, particular pharmacokinetic characteristics of some of these drugs may enhance the damaging effect. For NSAIDs that undergo enterohepatic recycling, repeated exposure of the duodenal and gastric mucosa to the drug (in the presence of duodeno-gastric reflux), even when it has been absorbed, contributes to perpetuation of the damage.[19]

Sucralfate and NSAID Gastropathy

NSAID gastropathy is a distinct clinical entity, with various characteristics that differentiate it from classical peptic ulcer disease (Table I) and call for a different therapeutic approach. NSAID-induced gastroduodenal mucosal damage is not acid-related but is mainly the result of alteration of the defense mechanisms of the gastric wall. The observation of reduced levels of prostaglandins, which are known to have a cytoprotective action, as a result of blocking of the arachidonic acid cascade through inhibition of cyclooxygenase enzymes by NSAIDs, provides the rationale for use of a cytoprotective drug such as sucralfate in the treatment and prevention of gastroduodenal lesions caused by such drugs.

In an acid environment, the aluminum salts contained in the molecule form a gel with a high affinity for the damaged epithelium, and bind substances with an irritant action on the gastric wall, such as biliary acids and pepsin. Sucralfate also increases the defenses of the gastric mucosa: it stimulates secretion of prostaglandin E_2[20] and bicarbonate,[21] increases mucosal blood flow,[22] and binds and transports epidermal growth factor (EGF) to the ulcerated areas.[23]

Acute Studies

Few data are available in the literature on the cytoprotective effects of sucralfate during acute NSAID administration (Table II). Stern *et al.*[24] showed that endoscopically

Table I. Characteristics of NSAID Gastropathy and Peptic Ulcer Disease

	NSAID gastropathy	Peptic disease
Location	Mainly gastric (antral or prepyloric)	Mainly duodenal
Etiology	Connected to taking of NSAIDs	Multifactorial
Pathogenesis	Alteration of the defense mechanisms of gastric wall	Acid-correlated

Table II. Prevention of NSAID-Induced Gastroduodenal Damage with Sucralfate (Short-Term Studies)

Author	Subjects	NSAID	Dosage	Control	Result
Stern *et al.* (1987)	Volunteers	ASA	1.2 g	90 min	Improvement in gastroduodenal endoscopic score
Konturek *et al.* (1987)	Volunteers	ASA	2.5 g	2 days	Reduction in gastric bleeding, evaluated by gastric lavage technique
Tesler and Lim (1981)	Volunteers	ASA	3.6 g	5 days	Protective effect of sucralfate on gastric mucosa
Lanza *et al.* (1990)	Volunteers	Naproxene	1 g	1 week	Noneffectiveness of sucralfate in reducing NSAID-induced gastroduodenal damage
Malchow-Møller and Ranløv (1987)	Volunteers	ASA	1 g	1 week	Noneffectiveness of sucralfate in reducing bleeding, evaluated with ^{51}Cr technique
Aabakken *et al.* (1989)	Volunteers	Naproxene	1 g	1 week	Protective effect of sucralfate on gastric and duodenal mucosa
Wu and Castell (1984)	Volunteers	ASA	2.6 g	1 week	Protective effect of sucralfate limited to duodenal mucosa
Stern *et al.* (1989)	Volunteers	ASA	3.6 g	2 weeks	Noneffectiveness of sucralfate in preventing NSAID-induced gastric mucosal damage

ascertained ASA-induced damage was significantly reduced when sucralfate was given 30 min before the anti-inflammatory drug. The same study also demonstrated that this protective action of sucralfate is abolished by pretreatment with indomethacin, thus confirming the key role of endogenous prostaglandins in the drug's mechanism of action. Konturek *et al.*[25] showed that sucralfate at the dose of 1 g qid for 4 days is able to reduce gastric microhemorrhages in volunteers examined prior to any treatment or after 2.5 g/day of ASA for 2 days. These data, obtained by the gastric lavage method, are in agreement with the improvement in endoscopic score observed by Stern and indicate that the reduction in gastric microhemorrhages is associated with healing of the mucosal damage.

Tesler and Lim[26] confirmed sucralfate's protective effect on gastric mucosa during NSAID therapy. Eight out of twelve patients taking the cytoprotective drug at a dosage of 4 g/day together with ASA 900 mg qid for 5 days proved to be without gastric lesions.

Lanza *et al.*[27] reported results in disagreement with those described above. Four groups of 20 volunteers with endoscopically normal gastroduodenal mucosa were treated for 1 week with naproxen 500 mg bid + cimetidine (300 or 400 mg bid), sucralfate (1 g qid) or placebo. Neither the H_2 antagonist nor the cytoprotective agent significantly reduced NSAID-induced gastroduodenal damage. A Danish study[28] led to similar conclusions. Sixteen patients were treated for 1 week with ASA and sucralfate and then, after a 2-week washout period, with ASA and placebo. Sucralfate failed to reduce fecal blood loss, measured by the ^{51}Cr-labeled erythrocyte method. In the study by Aabakken *et al.*,[29] 16 patients receiving naproxen 500 mg bid were treated concurrently with sucralfate 2 g bid for 1 week, followed by a 3-week washout period, and then by placebo for a further week. Mucosal gastroduodenal damage was assessed endoscopically; alterations of the distal intestine were investigated using the ^{51}Cr-labeled EDTA absorption method. The results showed that sucralfate had a protective effect on the gastric and duodenal mucosa but not on the mucosa distal to the bulb.

A previous study in which a similar protocol had been used,[30] however, came to a different conclusion. Wu and Castell combined treatment with ASA 650 mg qid and sucralfate 1 g/day for 1 week in ten volunteers and, after a 2-week washout period, with placebo for another week. Sucralfate proved effective in protecting only duodenal mucosa from damage caused by ASA. To the contrary, no protective effect was shown concerning gastric mucosa.

Lack of protection of gastric mucosa was also confirmed in the case where acute treatment with NSAIDs was prolonged to 2 weeks. Stern *et al.*[31] treated 19 normal subjects taking ASA 900 mg qid for 14 days with sucralfate 4 g/day, according to a crossover, double-blind trial, with placebo control. The average endoscopic score in sucralfate-treated patients was not statistically different from those taking placebo (2.84 ± 0.27 versus 2.68 ± 0.23, $p > 0.05$ respectively).

These differences are probably explained by the fact that in the various studies sucralfate was used at different dosages, in different formulations, and with different administration times from those of NSAIDs.

Long-Term Studies

Prevention

Only a small number of studies have been carried out on sucralfate coadministered with NSAIDs in the long term (Table III). In one of these, Caldwell *et al.*[32] studied 143 patients with upper gastrointestinal symptoms and NSAID-induced gastric mucosal damage. For 6 months half of the patients were treated with sucralfate 2–4 g/day and half with placebo, the anti-inflammatory therapy remaining unchanged. Coadministration of the cytoprotective agent with NSAIDs proved effective in relieving pain and reducing mucosal damage during follow-up, achieving better compliance to the anti-inflammatory therapy, otherwise interrupted or only used long-term. A pilot study by Shepherd *et al.*[33] confirmed these results. Twenty-six patients with rheumatoid arthritis, under continuous NSAID therapy for at least 3 months and with superficial gastric and duodenal mucosal lesions, received sucralfate 1 g qid or cimetidine 400 mg bid with the anti-inflammatory treatment. Both drugs produced an improvement in the gastroduodenal score. Unlike cimetidine, sucralfate also stimulated prostaglandin E_2 synthesis in the gastric antrum and corpus but not in the duodenum. Prostaglandin E_2 levels in biopsy samples taken after 6 weeks of therapy were significantly higher than in samples taken on entry into the study.

Despite this evidence that protective mechanisms are enhanced only in the gastric wall by sucralfate, there has been no evidence that there are fewer gastric ulcers in patients undergoing treatment with NSAIDs together with sucralfate.

Table III. Prevention of NSAID-Induced Gastroduodenal Damage with Sucralfate (Long-Term Studies)

Author	Disease	NSAID	Control	Result
Caldwell *et al.* (1987)	Various rheumatic pathologies	Naproxen, piroxicam, diflunisal, aspirin, salsalate, ibuprofen, sulindac, others	6 months	Effectiveness of sucralfate in reducing both pain and mucosal damage caused by NSAIDs
Shepherd *et al.* (1989)	Rheumatoid arthritis	Piroxicam, indomethacin, ketoprofen, fenprofen, fenbufen, benorylate, flurbiprofen, diclofenac	6 weeks	Improvement in endoscopic gastroduodenal score
Agrawal *et al.* (1991)	Rheumatoid arthritis	Ibuprofen, piroxicam, naproxen	4–8–12 weeks	Noneffectiveness of sucralfate in reducing NSAID-induced gastric ulcers

In the study by Agrawal *et al.*,[34] 352 patients with rheumatoid arthritis were treated for at least 3 months with NSAIDs. The patients who were free of gastric ulceration were treated with misoprostol 200 μg qid or sucralfate 1 g qid concurrently with the anti-inflammatory treatment and endoscopic examinations were carried out at 4, 8, and 12 weeks. The proportion of patients who developed gastric ulcers was 1.6% in the misoprostol group and 16% in the sucralfate group ($p < 0.001$). Thus, compared with misoprostol, sucralfate does not appear to prevent NSAID-induced gastric ulcerations.

Therapy

Surprisingly, although sucralfate appears to be ineffective in preventing the development of NSAID-induced gastric ulcer, it proved to be effective in the treatment of ulcers in patients continuing anti-inflammatory treatment (Table IV). This was shown in a Danish study[35] which was carried out in the Copenhagen area. Manniche and colleagues enrolled 67 patients suffering from rheumatoid arthritis, osteoarthritis, or other rheumatic pathologies (degenerative lumbo-discopathy, spondylosis, psoriatic arthritis) being treated with NSAIDs and having documented ulcerations (14 with gastric ulcer, 51 with duodenal ulcer, 2 with combined gastric and duodenal ulcers). Only half continued NSAID therapy but all were randomized to receive ranitidine 150 mg bid or sucralfate 1 g qid. The treatment groups were, therefore, the following: (1) ranitidine + NSAIDs, (2) sucralfate + NSAIDs, (3) only ranitidine, (4) only sucralfate. Endoscopic controls were carried out every 3 weeks, up to a total of 9 weeks. There was no statistically significant difference between the group continuing treatment with NSAIDs and that in which the anti-inflammatory treatment was interrupted, both as regards healing percentage (77 versus 91%, respectively) and average time for this (5.0 versus 4.6 weeks, respectively). In the group continuing treatment with NSAIDs, the healing percentage and the average time of healing in patients treated with sucralfate overlapped that achieved in patients treated with

Table IV. Treatment of NSAID-Induced Ulcers with Sucralfate

Author	Disease	NSAID	Comparison drug	Control	Result
Manniche *et al.* (1987)	Various rheumatic pathologies	ASA, azapropazone, diclofenac, fenbufen, fenprofen, ibuprofen, indomethacin, ketoprofen, naproxen, piroxicam, sulindac	Ranitidine 150 mg BID	3–6–9 weeks	No significant statistical difference between sucralfate and ranitidine in inducing recovery from NSAIDs
Bianchi Porro *et al.* (1990)	Rheumatoid arthritis or osteoarthritis	Diclofenac, naproxen, ketoprofen, piroxicam, sulindac, indomethacin	Omeprazole 20 mg o.m.	4–8 weeks	Noneffectiveness of sucralfate in inducing NSAID ulcer recovery at 4 weeks Sucralfate overlaps omeprazole statistically at 8 weeks in inducing healing of lesions

ranitidine. These data suggest that the presence of ulcer in patients being treated with NSAIDs does not demand the interruption of the anti-inflammatory treatment, as both the H_2 antagonist and sucralfate were shown to be equally effective in such situations.

Bianchi Porro *et al.*[36] studied 30 patients with NSAID-induced ulcer (17 with gastric ulcer, 10 with duodenal ulcer, 3 with gastric and duodenal ulcer). The patients continued on the same anti-inflammatory therapy and were treated with omeprazole 20 mg o.m. ($n = 15$) or sucralfate 1 g qid ($n = 15$) for a period of 4–8 weeks. Omeprazole was proved to be statistically superior to sucralfate in healing ulcers (100 versus 64.2%, $p < 0.05$) at 4 weeks. No significant statistical difference was found at 8 weeks between the two drugs (100 versus 76.9%, $p = 0.1$, respectively).

Conclusions and Recommendations

The above data do not permit definitive conclusions as to the possible role of sucralfate in the prevention or treatment of NSAID-induced mucosal damage.

For this purpose, the following are required:

- Further studies, involving well-defined groups of rheumatic patients, in order to identify precise categories of patients at risk for the development of NSAID-induced gastroduodenal lesions.
- Cohort studies into categories at risk.
- Studies having as their end-point not so much prevention or treatment of innocent superficial mucosal lesions (submucosal hemorrhages and erosions) but the prevention of more severe complications of NSAID-induced gastropathy (digestive hemorrhage and perforation) which may constitute the only real if fairly rare danger for patients undergoing anti-inflammatory therapy.

Based on present knowledge, when approaching a patient candidate for acute treatment with NSAIDs and affected at the same time with upper gastroenterological problems, the following observations and recommendations may be useful:

- Obtain a good history in order to identify possible patients at risk with preexisting ulcer history.
- Differentiate between NSAID gastropathy and peptic ulcer disease, both of which can complicate chronic rheumatic pathology and anti-inflammatory treatment.

  NSAID gastropathy is associated with: mucosal hyperemia, submucosal hemorrhages or erosions. Clear ulceration, which is often asymptomatic and rarely causes complications, may be present at the prepyloric area and may be superficial.

  The second, classical peptic ulcer disease depends on individual predisposition where the addition of NSAIDs modifies the course of the disease. The ulcer is most frequently found in the gastric corpus, is deeper, often asymptomatic because of the analgesic effect of NSAIDs (so-called masking effect), and may be complicated with hemorrhage and/or perforation.
- Given the relative rarity of NSAID gastropathy complications, and present incomplete knowledge as to their prevention, there seems no justification for an indis-

criminate use of prophylactic drugs, except in patients with documented risk factors.

- It is possible today to treat NSAID-induced ulcers without interrupting anti-inflammatory therapy, with clear benefit to the patient.

References

1. Roth SH: Nonsteroidal anti-inflammatory drug gastropathy. *Arch Intern Med* **146**:1075–1076, 1986. Definition of gastrointestinal mucosal damage resulting from NSAID use.
2. Lanza FL: Endoscopic studies of gastric and duodenal injury after the use of ibuprofen, aspirin and other non-steroid anti-inflammatory agents. *Am J Med* **77**(suppl 1A):19–24, 1984. Demonstration of dose-dependent upper gastrointestinal mucosal injury induced by acetylsalicylic acid and other NSAIDs.
3. Baskin WN, Ivey KJ, Krause WJ, *et al*: Aspirin induced ultrastructural changes in human gastric mucosa. *Ann Intern Med* **85**:299–303, 1976. Description of ASA-induced microscopic alterations in gastric epithelial cells.
4. O'Laughlin JC, Hoftiezer JW, Ivey KJ: Effects of aspirin on the human stomach in normals: Endoscopic comparison of damage produced one hour, 24 hours, and 2 weeks after administration. *Scand J Gastroenterol* **16**(suppl 67):211–214, 1981. Acute aspirin administration appears to cause predominantly petechial hemorrhage in the fundus and antrum, while longer-term administration causes antral and duodenal erosions.
5. Hoftiezer JW, O'Laughlin JC, Ivey KJ: Effects of 24 hours of aspirin, Bufferin, paracetamol and placebo on normal human gastroduodenal mucosa. *Gut* **23**:692–697, 1982. Short-term use of both unbuffered and buffered aspirin causes upper gastrointestinal damage.
6. Hoftiezer JW, Silvoso GR, Burkis M, *et al*: Comparison of the effects of regular and enteric-coated aspirin on gastroduodenal mucosa in man. *Lancet* **2**:609–612, 1980. Regular aspirin causes a greater amount of gastroduodenal mucosal damage than does enteric-coated aspirin.
7. Lanza FL, Royer GL, Nelson RS, *et al*: Effects of ibuprofen, indomethacin, aspirin, naproxen and placebo on the gastric mucosa of normal volunteers. *Dig Dis Sci* **24**:823–828, 1979. Description of endoscopic changes induced by NSAIDs on upper gastrointestinal tract and their correlation with gastrointestinal complaints.
8. Lanza FL, Royer GL, Nelson RS: Endoscopic evaluation of the effects of aspirin, buffered aspirin, and enteric coated aspirin on gastric and duodenal mucosa. *N Engl J Med* **303**:136–138, 1980. Buffered aspirin offers little protection to gastric and duodenal mucosa, while enteric-coated formulation is less damaging.
9. Graham DY, Smith JL: Effects of aspirin and aspirin–acetaminophen combination on the gastric mucosa in normal subjects. *Gastroenterology* **88**:1922–1925, 1985. Coadministration of acetaminophen with aspirin does not protect from mucosal injury induced by ASA.
10. Graham DY, Smith JL, Holmes GI, *et al*: Nonsteroidal anti-inflammatory effect of sulindac sulfoxide and sulfide on gastric mucosa. *Clin Pharmacol Ther* **38**:65–70, 1985. Evaluation of gastric mucosal damage induced by two different formulations of sulindac.
11. Graham DY, Smith JL, Dobbs SM: Gastric adaptations occurs with aspirin administration in man. *Dig Dis Sci* **28**:1–6, 1983. Gastric mucosal adaptation may occur after continuous aspirin administration and is associated with reduced damage and an accelerated healing process.
12. Eliakim R, Ophir M, Rachmilewitz D: Duodenal mucosal injury with non-steroidal anti-inflammatory drugs. *J Clin Gastroenterol* **9**:395–399, 1987. Description of the effects of various NSAIDs on duodenal mucosa.
13. Caruso I, Bianchi Porro G: Gastroscopic evaluation of anti-inflammatory agents. *Br Med J* **280**:75–78, 1980. Importance of gastroscopy in assessing gastric tolerance of chronic NSAID therapy.

14. Silvoso GR, Ivey KJ, Butt JH, *et al*: Incidence of gastric lesions in patients with rheumatic disease on chronic aspirin therapy. *Ann Intern Med* **91**:517–520, 1979. Endoscopic evaluation of the incidence and characteristics of gastric lesions using long-term ASA.
15. Lockard OO, Ivey KJ, Butt JH, *et al*: The prevalence of duodenal lesions in patients with rheumatic disease on chronic aspirin therapy. *Gastrointest Endosc* **26**:5–7, 1980. Patients on chronic ASA have a high prevalence of duodenal lesions, even though they lack upper gastrointestinal symptoms.
16. Miller R, Jick H: Acute toxicity of aspirin in hospitalized medical patients. *Am J Med Sci* **274**:271–279, 1977. An analysis of the systemic side effects occurring on occasional or regular use of ASA.
17. Garner A: Effects of acetylsalicylate on alkalization, acid secretion and electrogenic properties in the isolated gastric mucosa. *Acta Physiol Scand* **99**:281–291, 1977. Description of ASA action on secretive and electric activities of gastric mucosa.
18. Cohen MM, Clark L, Armstrong L, *et al*: Reduction of aspirin-induced fecal blood loss with low-dose misoprostol tablets in man. *Dig Dis Sci* **30**:605–611, 1985. This study suggests that oral misoprostol reduces aspirin-induced gastrointestinal bleeding even when administered simultaneously and at a dose below its threshold for significant acid inhibition.
19. Rainsford KD: Anti-inflammatory drugs and the gastrointestinal mucosa. *Gastroenterol Clin Biol* **9**(2bis):98–101, 1985. Description of mechanisms of NSAID-induced gastric mucosal damage.
20. Hollander D, Tarnawski A, Gergely H, *et al*: Sucralfate protection of the gastric mucosa against ethanol-induced injury: A prostaglandin-mediated process? *Scand J Gastroenterol* **19**(suppl 101):97–102, 1984. Prostaglandins mediate the protective action of sucralfate against ethanol-induced necrosis.
21. Crampton JR, Gibbons LC, Rees W: Effects of sucralfate on gastroduodenal bicarbonate secretion and prostaglandin E2 metabolism. *Am J Med* **83**(suppl 3B):14–18, 1987. Sucralfate stimulates bicarbonate secretion by gastric and duodenal mucosa and prostaglandin E2 formation by mucosal homogenates.
22. Tarnawski A, Hollander D, Stachura J, *et al*: Effect of sucralfate in the normal human gastric mucosa. Endoscopic, histological and ultrastructural assessment. *Scand J Gastroenterol* **22**(suppl 127):111–123, 1987. Macroscopic and microscopic examination of the gastric mucosa in direct contact with sucralfate.
23. Nexo E, Poulsen SS: Does epidermal growth factor play a role in the action of sucralfate? *Scand J Gastroenterol* **22**(suppl 127):45–49, 1987. Epidermal growth factor is attached to sucralfate at acid pH and accelerates gastric ulcer healing.
24. Stern AI, Ward F, Hartley G: Protective effect of sucralfate against aspirin-induced damage to the human gastric mucosa. *Am J Med* **83**(suppl 3B):83–85, 1987. The protective action of sucralfate on the gastric mucosa of humans may be related to stimulation of endogenous prostaglandins.
25. Konturek SJ, Kwiecien N, Obtulowicz W, *et al*: Gastroprotection by sucralfate against acetylsalicylic acid in humans. Role of endogenous prostaglandins. *Scand J Gastroenterol* **22**(suppl 140):19–22, 1987. Sucralfate is significantly better than placebo in preventing gastroduodenal lesions induced by aspirin.
26. Tesler MA, Lim ES: Protection of gastric mucosa by sucralfate from aspirin-induced erosions. *J Clin Gastroenterol* **3**(suppl 2):175–179, 1981. The authors concluded that sucralfate provided complete or partial gastric mucosal protection from the gastrotoxic effects of 3.6 g aspirin when compared with placebo.
27. Lanza FL, Graham DY, Davis RE, *et al*: Endoscopic comparison of cimetidine and sucralfate for prevention of naproxen-induced acute gastroduodenal injury. Effect of scoring method. *Dig Dis Sci* **35**:1494–1499, 1990. This study indicates that H_2-receptor antagonists are not effective in preventing gastric erosions and ulcers; more importantly, the authors raise doubts about the scoring system that has been widely used in studying this problem.
28. Malchow-Møller A, Ranløv PJ: Does sucralfate reduce acetylsalicylic-acid-induced gastric mucosal bleeding? *Scand J Gastroenterol* **22**:550–552, 1987. Sucralfate did not prevent gastric microbleeding induced by administration of aspirin 1.0 g for 1 week.

29. Aabakken L, Larsen S, Osnes M: Sucralfate for prevention of naproxen-induced mucosal lesions in the proximal and distal gastrointestinal tract. *Scand J Rheumatol* **18**:361–368, 1989. Sucralfate shows a mild protective effect on gastroduodenal lesions induced by naproxen.
30. Wu WC, Castell DO: Does sucralfate protect against aspirin-induced mucosal lesions? Yes and no! *Gastroenterology* **86**:A1303, 1984. Sucralfate may be effective against the development of duodenal, but not gastric lesions induced by aspirin.
31. Stern AI, Ward F, Sievert W: Lack of gastric mucosal protection by sucralfate during long-term aspirin ingestion in humans. *Am J Med* **86**(suppl 6A):66–69, 1989. Sucralfate 4 g daily lacks a mucosal protective capacity in human subjects ingesting large doses of aspirin over a 2-week period.
32. Caldwell JR, Roth SH, Wu WC, *et al*: Sucralfate treatment of nonsteroidal anti-inflammatory drug-induced gastrointestinal symptoms and mucosal damage. *Am J Med* **83**(suppl 3B):74–82, 1987. Sucralfate positively influences dyspeptic symptoms but not gastric or duodenal lesions from NSAIDs.
33. Shepherd HA, Fine D, Hillier K, *et al*: Effect of sucralfate and cimetidine on rheumatoid patients with active gastroduodenal lesions who are taking nonsteroidal anti-inflammatory drugs. A pilot study. *Am J Med* **86**(suppl 6A):49–54, 1989. Sucralfate and cimetidine administration resulted in improved gastroduodenal scores in patients with rheumatoid arthritis continuing with NSAID therapy.
34. Agrawal NM, Roth S, Graham DY, *et al*: Misoprostol compared with sucralfate in the prevention of nonsteroidal anti-inflammatory drug-induced gastric ulcer. A randomized, controlled trial. *Ann Intern Med* **115**:195–200, 1991. Misoprostol is better than sucralfate in long-term (up to 12 weeks) prevention.
35. Manniche C, Malchow-Møller A, Anderson JR, *et al*: Randomized study of the influence of nonsteroidal anti-inflammatory drugs on the treatment of peptic ulcer in patients with rheumatic disease. *Gut* **28**:226–229, 1987. In this study, 77% of gastroduodenal ulcers were healed with ranitidine 150 mg twice daily or sucralfate 1 g four times daily despite continued NSAID use.
36. Bianchi Porro G, Santalucia F, Petrillo M: Omeprazole versus sucralfate in the treatment of NSAID-induced gastric and duodenal ulcer. *Gut* **31**:A1175, 1990. Omeprazole is better than sucralfate in treatment of gastric and duodenal ulcers in patients taking NSAIDs.

VII

The Preventive Use of Sucralfate

28

Sucralfate for Prevention of Acute Gastrointestinal Bleeding

ROBERT S. BRESALIER

Introduction

Patients admitted to critical care units (ICUs) develop a spectrum of gastroduodenal mucosal lesions related to severe *physiologic stress*. *Stress-related gastrointestinal bleeding* from such lesions has been reported in 8 to 33% of patients admitted to ICUs who do not receive prophylactic therapy, but the incidence of severe or clinically significant bleeding is less than 6% and appears to have decreased during the past decade. Routine prophylaxis against stress-related bleeding is commonplace in ICUs worldwide, representing a substantial cost to patients and use of resources. Sucralfate, primarily in suspension form, has been used extensively as prophylaxis against acute upper gastrointestinal hemorrhage in critically ill patients. This chapter will review the rationale for such therapy, and compare its efficacy with other types of treatment. Other uses of sucralfate for prevention of gastrointestinal bleeding will also be briefly discussed.

Stress-Related Upper Gastrointestinal Bleeding

Clinical Description

Acute gastric or duodenal lesions commonly occur in patients admitted to ICUs. Originally described in patients with thermal injury and multiple trauma, such lesions also arise in those with a variety of other underlying conditions, including hypotension, sepsis, renal failure, severe respiratory insufficiency, head injuries, transplant procedures, and hepatic failure.

ROBERT S. BRESALIER • Departments of Medicine, Henry Ford Health Sciences Center and the University of Michigan School of Medicine, Detroit, Michigan 48202.

Sucralfate: From Basic Science to the Bedside, edited by Daniel Hollander and G. N. J. Tytgat. Plenum Press, New York, 1995.

Injury in these settings is represented by a spectrum of lesions ranging from multiple superficial erosions or ulcerations of the mucosa to true ulcers extending through the muscularis mucosae. Stress-related lesions most commonly occur in the proximal stomach, but may be found throughout the stomach and duodenum (usually in conjunction with proximal lesions). Endoscopic examination of critically ill patients suggests an evolution of mucosal changes, beginning with areas of focal pallor, then hyperemia in the proximal stomach. Shallow red-based petechial lesions follow, which evolve to deeper erosions with surrounding edema. This process may spread distally, to involve the body and antrum. Experimental evidence suggests that these stages may correspond pathophysiologically to periods of hypotension and vasoconstriction, followed by reperfusion and damage related to multiple injurious factors (see next section).

Similar lesions arise in experimental animals subjected to hemorrhagic shock or endotoxin-induced shock, restraint, cold stress, immersion stress, and exertion stress. In these models animals develop multiple acute superficial erosions in the corpus (the glandular acid-secreting portion) of the stomach, closely resembling stress-related lesions in man.

Sucralfate's many potential mechanisms of action (described elsewhere in this volume) provide the rationale for its use for the prevention of bleeding from stress-related lesions.

Pathophysiology of Stress-Related Mucosal Damage and the Potential Role of Sucralfate in Prevention

A large body of clinical and experimental evidence suggests that *stress- related gastroduodenal damage* is the result of complex interactions involving both injurious factors and alteration in mechanisms which normally maintain an intact mucosa (Fig. 1).[1–4] Review of the mechanisms of action of sucralfate suggests several ways in which sucralfate may protect the gastroduodenal mucosa from stress-related damage, or ameliorate the severity of stress-related lesions.

Gastric Luminal Factors: Pepsin, Bile, Acid

Small amounts of luminal pepsin are necessary for mucosal damage in some animal models of stress ulceration, and pepsin inhibitors may prevent damage related to experimental hemorrhagic shock. The antipeptic activity of sucralfate may therefore potentially affect this process. It has been suggested that alterations in gastric motility associated with stress may promote gastroduodenal reflux of bile, resulting in bile-induced breakdown of the gastric mucosal barrier. The ability of sucralfate to adsorb bile acids (Chapter 6) or stimulate surface-active phospholipid could help prevent this type of damage as well. While roles for bile acids and pepsin in promoting stress-induced damage have been suggested by some experimental models, their roles in promoting such damage in man remain circumstantial.

The presence of acid and hydrogen ions (H^+) in the gastric lumen is a prerequisite for the development of stress-related mucosal ulceration, and provides justification for the clinical use of antacids, and H_2-receptor antagonists (H_2RAs) for the prophylaxis of these

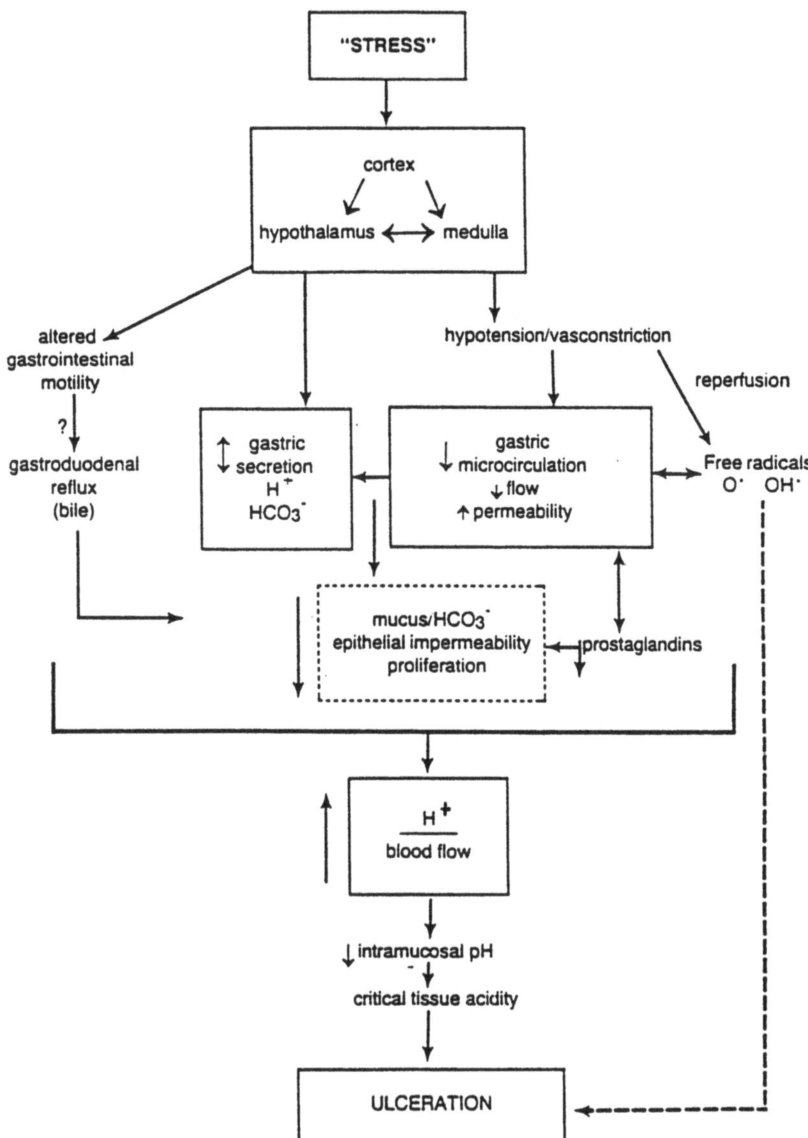

Figure 1. Proposed mechanisms for development of stress-related mucosal damage. The specific relationships depicted are largely based on experimental findings, and remain somewhat speculative. Reproduced with permission from the *Journal of Clinical Gastroenterology* **13**:535–543, 1991.

lesions. Nonetheless, luminal hyperacidity (characteristic in the setting of head trauma, sepsis, and cold-restraint animal models of stress) is not a universal finding in many clinical situations associated with stress ulceration. Hypotension associated with stress ulceration and concomitant decreases in regional gastric blood flow may actually lead to decreased gastric acid secretion. This may have a negative effect since gastric mucosa stimulated to secrete acid may in fact be more resistant to damage than in its basal secretory state. Thus, drugs such as H_2RAs that decrease gastric acid secretion (or gastric mucosal blood flow) may potentially affect mechanisms involved in protecting the gastric mucosa. Blocking secretion of acid and bicarbonate could increase the susceptibility of the mucosal epithelium to acidification and damage. These remain theoretical considerations, however, and substantial evidence exists demonstrating decreased stress-related bleeding with the prophylactic use of drugs that neutralize acid or affect its secretion.

A potential role for sucralfate in treating gastric mucosal damage was originally considered because of its ability to bind to the mucosal surface. While unproven, sucralfate could help prevent stress-related bleeding by binding to early mucosal lesions and acting as a barrier to injurious luminal factors, thus preventing their evolution to more-advanced lesions.

Alterations in Intramucosal pH

Alterations in intramucosal pH may occur as the result of backdiffusion of luminal H^+ through paracellular pathways, or due to systemic acidosis. There is substantial evidence to suggest that such acidification of the gastric mucosa plays a major pathogenic role in the development of stress ulceration. During periods of hypotension which may be associated with stress ulceration, subepithelial tissues are susceptible to acidification in the presence of even low concentrations of luminal acid. A combination of mucosal acid, high pCO_2, and low serosal pH ultimately results in cell death and ulceration. Systemic acidosis may also promote mucosal ulceration since experimental stress ulceration may be prevented by the administration of parenteral sodium bicarbonate. Tissue ischemia and hypoxia associated with physiologic stress impair defense mechanisms which normally protect against H^+ backdiffusion and tissue acidification. Several of these defense mechanisms which include the gastric microcirculation, the mucus–bicarbonate layer, epithelial renewal, and the inherent impermeability of surface epithelial cells may be stimulated by sucralfate.

Altered Mucosal Blood Flow and Vascular Damage

Maintenance of blood flow and of an intact *gastric microcirculation* is essential for protection of the gastric mucosa from injury. Transient hypotension and alterations in mucosal blood flow are common in critically ill patients who develop stress-related mucosal damage. Disturbances in the gastric microcirculation, including regional ischemia, are also common in animal models of stress ulceration such as hemorrhagic shock and restraint. Mucosal ischemia and an impaired microcirculation associated with physiologic stress lead to the accumulation of H^+, cell death, and ulceration. Circulatory compromise also leads to decreased secretion of HCO_3^- in the stomach and duodenum, important for the neutralization of H^+ at the epithelial cell surface. The altered secretory state of the gastric mucosa associated with stress further increases its susceptibility to compromise by H^+. In addition, decreased tissue oxygenation associated with hypotension and ischemia leads to aberrant mitochondrial metabolism and a decrease in ATP and high-energy phosphates. Altered protein phosphorylation and loss of ionic gradients contribute to cell death and ulceration.

Microcirculatory disturbances early in the course of stress-related mucosal damage include increased vascular permeability and resultant mucosal edema. Experimental evidence suggests that *oxygen-derived free radicals* such as superoxides form in the gastric mucosa during reperfusion after transient ischemia, leading to vascular damage. Water-immersion stress related to burn injury in experimental animals, for example, leads to the accumulation of anion radicals and a decrease in the free radical scavenger superoxide dismutase. This results in increased vascular permeability and gastric mucosal injury. Such injury may be ameliorated by administration of superoxide dismutase. Increased vascular permeability during stress is also associated with alterations in glutathione and 5-hydroxytryptamine. The low-molecular-weight phospholipid platelet activating factor (PAF) may act as a mediator of plasma leakage and mucosal ulceration associated with septic shock.

Prostaglandins, sulfhydryl (SH) derivatives, and sucralfate may diminish or prevent the early microvascular lesions associated with stress ulceration. This may then lead to maintenance of blood flow, and decreased mucosal damage.

Epithelial Renewal

Rapid epithelial restitution (a process requiring an intact microcirculation) occurs after superficial damage to the gastric mucosa through migration of epithelial cells and epithelial proliferation. Physiologic stress may depress epithelial proliferation by damage to the microcirculation, or by affecting production of mucosal trophic agents such as gastrin, growth hormone, polyamines, and epidermal growth factor. Epidermal growth factor may act in part by increasing polyamine synthesis associated with epithelial proliferation and mucosal growth. Duodenal mucosal damage in the setting of experimental water-immersion stress has also been reported to be ameliorated by luminal administration of polyamines. Sucralfate has been shown to augment the availability of epidermal growth factor to the gastric epithelium,[4] and thus may attenuate the severity of stress-related damage by enhancing epithelial renewal in this manner.

Mucus

A bicarbonate-rich mucus gel overlies the gastric epithelium and helps to neutralize H^+. This unstirred bicarbonate-rich layer helps to maintain the pH at the apical membrane of the epithelial cell near neutrality despite low luminal pH (the standing pH gradient in the mucus layer may be dissipated at a pH below 2.0–2.5). While the role of gastric mucus in cytoprotection *per se* remains controversial, it is likely that loss of the mucus–bicarbonate layer can contribute to backdiffusion of H^+ into an already damaged mucosa. Mucus secretion is decreased in the stomach of experimental animals subjected to restraint stress. Agents such as sucralfate, prostaglandins, and bismuth stimulate mucus secretion and may protect against experimental and clinical stress ulceration, but a direct contributory role for altered gastric mucus in the pathogenesis of stress-related damage remains speculative.

Prostaglandins

Mucosal prostaglandin levels may be decreased in the setting of physiologic stress. While sucralfate may increase mucosal prostaglandin levels and exogenously administered prostaglandins may prevent experimental stress ulceration, this remains circumstantial evidence for a cause-and-effect relationship between altered mucosal prostaglandins and stress-related mucosal damage.

The Central Nervous System and Neuroendocrine System

The role of the central nervous system and neuroendocrine axis in controlling the response to physiologic stress has been examined in a number of animal models. α-Adrenergic stimulation to the stomach in response to stress is mediated via hypothalamovagal pathways. This has subsequent effects on intragastric blood flow and serotonin (5-HT) release. Serotonin may alter regional blood flow by opening arteriovenular shunts and inducing hyperpermeability of capillaries. Certain peptides such as bombesin, calcitonin, corticotropin-releasing factor, neurotensin, and opioids appear to play an ill-defined role in centrally mediated gastric mucosal protection. The autonomic neurotransmitters dopamine, epinephrine, and norepinephrine have been found to promote gastric mucosal resistance. The central amygdala is important in mediating the cytoprotective effects of neurotensin and dopamine. Other substances such as acetylcholine and histamine may make the mucosa more susceptible to damage. Thyrotropin releasing hormone (TRH) plays a role in mediating stress-induced gastric lesions in the cold-restraint model of stress ulceration in the rat. The relevance of these findings to stress ulceration in humans remains to be determined. Sucralfate is a nonabsorbed, nonsystemic drug. While having no direct effect on the central nervous system, it may help ameliorate the resultant effects of neuroendocrine stimulation (e.g., altered blood flow and vascular damage) at the mucosal level.

The Clinical Significance of Stress-Related Bleeding

Early descriptions of stress-related bleeding in burn patients and those subjected to severe trauma suggested that gastric mucosal lesions occurred in the majority of such patients, and that these lesions were often associated with severe life-threatening hemorrhage.[5] These studies reported gastric erosions or ulcers in 85 to 100% of severely ill patients early in their hospital course. More recent endoscopic studies also demonstrated a variety of gastric mucosal changes ranging from nonhemorrhagic erosions and petechial lesions to ulcers in 74 to 82% of critically ill patients early after admission to the ICU. Endoscopic evidence of bleeding from such lesions in the form of mucosal oozing was often noted, and may have translated clinically into transfusion requirements, but severe hemorrhage was uncommon in these studies.

While it is generally accepted that gastric mucosal lesions are commonplace in severely ill patients, clinical experience has also suggested that associated serious hemorrhage is less common in the modern ICU. The actual incidence of clinically important bleeding is, however, difficult to determine. The incidence of bleeding from stress-related lesions has been inferred from numerous studies examining the efficacy of medical prophylaxis, but few include endoscopic evaluation. Thus, the occurrence of bleeding from stress ulceration is often equated with all clinical evidence of bleeding broadly ranging from microscopic (occult blood in the nasogastric aspirate), overt ("coffee grounds" or frank blood in the nasogastric aspirate) to true life-threatening hemorrhage. Alterations in hemoglobin and hematocrit and general transfusion requirements are also often attributed to stress-related lesions. The difficulty in determining the actual incidence of stress-related bleeding is compounded by the heterogeneity of study populations (medical versus surgical ICUs, burn units, cardiac care units, respiratory ICUs, etc.) with varying illness severity as well as study designs. Most studies are small, and often include too few patients to make accurate assessments.

Given these factors, it is not surprising that the reported incidence of stress-related bleeding in nonprophylaxed patients ranges widely from 8 to 33%. In aggregate, studies that compare antacids, H_2RAs, or cytoprotective agents to no treatment or placebo suggest that the overall incidence of stress-related bleeding in untreated ICU patients is approximately 16%. The incidence of serious or life-threatening bleeding is more difficult to estimate, but would appear to be less than 6–7%. This is also suggested by an independent study which determined the incidence of stress-related bleeding in 174 medical ICU patients who did not receive stress ulcer prophylaxis.[6] *Occult bleeding* was defined as multiple nasogastric aspirates positive for occult blood (hemoccult), and *overt bleeding* as "coffee-ground" emesis, hematemesis, or melena. Evidence of bleeding developed overall in 14% of patients, with a 6% incidence of overt bleeding.

The Impact of Medical Prophylaxis on Stress-Related Bleeding and ICU Care

Antacids, H_2RAs, and more recently agents that enhance mucosal defense (sucralfate, prostaglandins) have been used extensively in the ICU setting to prevent bleeding from stress-related lesions. *Medical prophylaxis* designed to prevent such bleeding has, in essence, become "standard of care" in most ICUs. With more than 3 million patients admitted to ICUs in the United States each year, the impact of such treatment in terms of cost is substantial. A reduction in bleeding as the result of medical prophylaxis has been inferred from a variety of heterogeneous studies, but deficiencies in study design and diverse definitions of bleeding make the impact on morbidity and mortality difficult to determine. Gastric acid plays a significant but not exclusive role in the pathogenesis of stress-related mucosal bleeding and efforts aimed at prophylaxis have often concentrated on measures that reduce gastric acidity. Sucralfate prophylaxis has been shown to decrease the incidence of water-immersion stress-induced erosions in experimental animals. With greater knowledge of the multifactorial pathogenesis of stress lesions and of the mechanisms of action of sucralfate, the efficacy of this compound in preventing stress-related bleeding has been evaluated in a number of clinical trials. Studies using antacids and H_2RAs will be briefly reviewed. The efficacy of sucralfate in preventing stress-related bleeding will then be discussed in detail with comparison to these agents.

Requirements for Study

Adequate evaluation of studies that examine the clinical impact of pharmacological prophylaxis against stress-related bleeding requires knowledge of a number of potential variables regarding the patient population examined. The setting is important. Patients admitted to medical ICUs, for example, may not be at similar risk to those hospitalized in surgical ICUs or burn units. Definition of the number and type of risk factors for development of stress-related bleeding is important, since those who are most severely ill are also most likely to develop stress-related bleeding. This has led to the use of the Acute Physiology and Chronic Health Evaluation (APACHE II) scoring system in some recent studies. Factors such as prolonged mechanical ventilatory assistance and the presence of coagulopathy and sepsis should be noted, since these may be strong predictors of bleeding. The nature of bleeding needs to be strictly defined to help determine the clinical significance of prophylaxis. Nasogastric aspirates positive for occult blood are clearly less significant than overt hemorrhage associated with alterations in hemodynamic status. The source of bleeding should be identified endoscopically when possible, since all bleeding in severely ill patients cannot be attributed to stress-related mucosal damage. The impact of prophylaxis on morbidity, mortality, and cost needs to be ascertained. There is little evidence at present that pharmacological prophylaxis has a significant impact on mortality, for example. This has been difficult to demonstrate, since the incidence of clinically important bleeding is low in the modern ICU. Placebo or no-treatment controls are important given this low incidence of bleeding since equivalence of one form of therapy with another does not prove efficacy. The cost of routine prophylaxis of ICU patients is substantial. Some forms of therapy (including administration) cost in excess of $80 per patient per day. Clearly it would be desirable to define those who would most benefit from prophylaxis. No published study of stress ulcer prophylaxis fulfills all of these requirements. This has led to the recent publication of a number of meta-analyses designed to evaluate the literature at large. These analyses themselves do not provide a uniform opinion of what constitutes the best form of prophylaxis.

Antacids and H_2RAs

Both antacids and H_2RAs reduce stress-related GI bleeding. The use of antacids was popularized when the incidence of upper GI bleeding in surgical patients receiving antacid prophylaxis was compared with those receiving no treatment.[7,8] Bleeding occurred in 20 to 25% of patients in the no-treatment control group, but in only 4 to 5% of those receiving antacids. Many patients had trivial degrees of bleeding (guaiac-positive nasogastric aspirates), few developed hemodynamically significant bleeding, and the sources of bleeding were not documented. This set the stage, however, for a decade and a half of the widespread use of stress ulcer prophylaxis with agents that alter gastric pH. Subsequent studies by this group and others suggested a low incidence of overall bleeding in patients receiving antacid prophylaxis (less than 5%) compared with a greater than 20% incidence of bleeding (all forms) in those not receiving prophylaxis. Clinically significant bleeding appears to occur in less than 6% of these control patients.

H_2RAs have superseded antacids for the most part in ICUs because of antacid-related side effects such as diarrhea and hypermagnesemia. Initial studies suggested that H_2RAs administered intravenously in bolus form provided poor control of gastric pH, and were less effective than antacids, but a large body of literature suggests near equivalence of H_2RAs and antacids in preventing overt forms of bleeding ("coffee grounds," red blood in the nasogastric aspirate, hematemesis, melena). Continuous intravenous infusion of H_2RAs provides more reliable and consistent control of gastric pH, and has been used in most recent studies. Two recent multicenter placebo-controlled studies compared the efficacy of continuous infusion (i.v.) cimetidine with placebo for preventing stress-related upper GI hemorrhage. Both studies entered many patients who would ordinarily be considered at low to moderate risk for bleeding including patients not requiring mechanical ventilation. Criteria for bleeding were bright red blood or persistent "coffee ground" material in the nasogastric tube. Sources of bleeding were not documented. In the first study, which enrolled 87 patients, there was a 21% incidence of overt bleeding in the placebo group compared with 2% bleeding in the treatment group. The second study[10] found a 33% incidence of bleeding in the placebo group (22 of 66 patients) and 14% bleeding (9 of 65 patients) in the cimetidine group. While these studies demonstrated a significant advantage for cimetidine over placebo, the incidence of bleeding in the control group was high given their low severity of illness. Bleeding was relatively minor, and mortality could not be attributed to upper GI hemorrhage in any patient in either study.

Recent *meta-analyses* have examined the efficacy of antacids and H_2RAs in preventing stress-related GI bleeding.[11–13] Cook *et al.*[11] examined 42 randomized clinical trials of stress ulcer prophylaxis. They concluded that stress ulcer prophylaxis with either antacids or H_2RAs decreases the incidence of *overt gastrointestinal bleeding* (H_2RAs were favored), but that only H_2RAs reduced clinically important GI hemorrhage (overt bleeding accompanied by hemodynamic changes or a decrease in hemoglobin requiring transfusion). Tryba examined 44 studies that included "macroscopically visible" bleeding in ICU patients. He concluded that both antacids and H_2RAs are significantly superior to untreated controls, with a trend in favor of antacids over H_2RAs.

Alkalinization of gastric contents may predispose to gastric colonization with gram-negative organisms, retrograde oropharyngeal migration, and aspiration leading to nosocomial pneumonia in mechanically ventilated patients. This has raised concern that the use of antacids and H_2RAs as prophylaxis for stress-related bleeding could lead to an increase in hospital-acquired pneumonias. Studies by Driks, Craven, Tryba, and others suggested that *nosocomial pneumonias* were indeed more common in those receiving agents that neutralize or inhibit production of gastric acid compared with sucralfate. This is not a universal finding, however, and recent studies of patients receiving short-term intravenous infusions of H_2RAs have not demonstrated an increased incidence of pneumonia in this group. A meta-analysis by Cook *et al.*[13] also failed to demonstrate that pH-altering drugs increased the incidence of pneumonia in ICU patients compared with placebo or control therapy. This analysis did suggest, however, that there was a 45% reduction in risk of pneumonia in those receiving sucralfate compared with drugs that raise gastric pH. None of the studies that were analyzed addresses the risk of pneumonia with long-term use of any agent in patients requiring prolonged mechanical ventilation.

Methodologic deficiencies and the small sample sizes of existing studies leave the issue of a relationship between stress ulcer prophylaxis and nosocomial pneumonia unresolved. Studies that have examined the effect of selective decontamination of the GI tract on morbidity and mortality have also failed to shed conclusive light on the issue.

Sucralfate

Several studies have compared the efficacy of sucralfate with antacids or H_2RAs for prophylaxis of stress-related bleeding (Table I).[14] Individually each study shows similar or slightly lower rates of stress-related bleeding in those receiving sucralfate compared with antacids or H_2RAs. Two recent meta-analyses compared the published efficacy of various

Table I. Controlled Trials of Sucralfate for the Prevention of Stress-Related Upper Gastrointestinal Bleeding

	Sucralfate[a]			Control		
Study	Setting[b]	No. of Pts.	Overt bleeding[c]	Regimen[d]	No. of Pts.	Overt bleeding
Borrero, 1985	M&S	80	0	Antacid:2 hr	75	0
Mundinger, 1985	S	100	2	Antacid:2 hr	113	2
				Mecindanol	85	3
Tryba, 1985[e]	S	34	0	Antacid:2 hr	33	2
				Cimetidine:2 g	33	2
Borrero, 1986	S	25	1	Antacid:1 hr	25	0
Tryba, 1987	S	50	1	Antacid:2 hr	50	1
Bresalier, 1987	M&S	38	5	Antacid:2 hr	36	7
Cannon, 1987	M&S	19	0	Antacid:2 hr	19	4
				Cimetidine:2 g	21	1
Driks, 1987	M&S	61	2	Antacid, cimetidine, or ranitidine[f]	69	1
Laggner, 1989	M&S	16	3	Ranitidine: 0.3 g	16	9
Ruiz-Santana, 1991[g]	M&S	24	1	Ranitidine: 0.2 g	19	2
				TPN only	30	1

[a]Sucralfate was given as a noncommercial suspension in doses ranging from 4 to 6 g daily.
[b]M, medical intensive care unit patients; S, surgical intensive care unit patients. The studies by Tryba *et al.* were performed in anesthesiology and neurosurgery units.
[c]Blood or persistent coffee grounds per nasogastric tube, hematemesis, melena.
[d]Dosing interval is indicated for antacids and daily dose for H_2-receptor antagonists.
[e]All patients received pirenzipine (50 mg i.v. daily) in addition to other agents.
[f]Doses not uniform.
[g]All patients received total parenteral nutrition in addition to other agents.

agents used to prevent stress-related bleeding. Tryba[12] analyzed those studies that used "macroscopically visible" bleeding as a minimum criterion for failure. He concluded that sucralfate was significantly superior to H_2RAs, and as effective as antacids in preventing stress-related bleeding. Cook *et al.*[11] considered studies that reported overt bleeding (hematemesis, bloody gastric aspirate, melena, or hematochezia) and "clinically important" bleeding (overt bleeding accompanied by hemodynamic changes or transfusion requirement). Analysis of five trials comparing antacids and sucralfate suggested their equivalence in preventing overt bleeding. Data were considered insufficient to determine the effect of sucralfate in comparison with antacids and H_2RAs in preventing clinically important bleeding. None of the studies in question include a comparison of sucralfate with placebo or no medical therapy. One study that compared sucralfate plus total parenteral nutrition (TPN) to TPN alone, did not demonstrate a difference between the two.

We have recently studied 300 patients hospitalized in the medical ICUs at Henry Ford Hospital, a large metropolitan hospital in Detroit, Michigan. Patients entering the ICUs were prospectively randomized to receive a sucralfate suspension (4 g daily), continuous intravenous infusion of cimetidine (1.2 g daily) or no medical prophylaxis. Potentially significant upper GI hemorrhage was considered if there was (1) frank blood or "coffee grounds" in the nasogastric aspirate or hematemesis not cleared by a 1.5-liter lavage, (2) a drop in hematocrit of greater than 3 points in 24 hr accompanied by melena and no evidence of lower GI bleeding, or (3) a drop of hematocrit of 6 points in 48 hr with no evidence of extra-GI or lower GI bleeding. Patients meeting these criteria were then endoscoped to determine the source of bleeding. Thirteen of one hundred and three patients (12.6%) treated with sucralfate, 16 of 98 (16.3%) treated with cimetidine, and 12 of 99 (12.1%) controls met the minimum criteria for endoscopy. Endoscopy was successfully performed in 81% of patients. Five patients (1 control, 2 sucralfate, 2 cimetidine) had upper GI bleeding as a terminal event and were not endoscoped. One control and two cimetidine patients refused endoscopy. Endoscopically proven stress-related mucosal lesions were documented as the source of bleeding in 5 patients receiving sucralfate (4.8%), 5 of 98 receiving cimetidine (5.1%), and 6 of 99 (6.1%) control patients. Total cost of administration of prophylaxis was calculated to be $3200 for sucralfate versus $17,300 for continuous infusion cimetidine per ICU bed per year. This study demonstrates the need for endoscopic documentation of the bleeding source, and placebo or no-treatment controls in examining the efficacy of agents used for prevention of stress-related bleeding. It also suggests that routine prophylaxis of all medical ICU (MICU) patients for stress-related bleeding is not cost-effective. Whether a subgroup of MICU patients will benefit from treatment remains to be determined. The applicability of these findings to patients in other settings (e.g., surgical or trauma patients) is also unknown.

The Use of Sucralfate for Prevention of Other Types of Acute Gastrointestinal Bleeding

The use of sucralfate has been proposed for prevention or treatment of other forms of GI bleeding. Sucralfate has been reported to protect the GI mucosa from aspirin-induced injury in experimental animal models. It is currently unclear whether this drug prevents the development of bleeding from lesions induced by nonsteroidal anti-inflammatory drugs (NSAID) in man. Some studies suggest partial efficacy in preventing endoscopically documented erosions (especially in the duodenum) during acute NSAID use, but the effect of sucralfate on bleeding during chronic administration remains unproven.

Case reports from Japan suggest the use of sucralfate or sucralfate–thrombin sprays for endoscopic treatment of acute upper GI hemorrhage.

Information in the form of small case reports also suggests a potential use for sucralfate enemas in preventing lower GI bleeding in the setting of inflammatory bowel disease, solitary ulcers of the rectum, and radiation-induced colitis. One case report showed a sucralfate lavage to be effective in stopping postpolypectomy hemorrhage. These potential uses, however, must at present be considered anecdotal.

Conclusion

Sucralfate may prevent the development of acute upper GI mucosal damage associated with physiologic stress in critically ill patients by a number of potential mechanisms. These include protection against injurious factors such as pepsin and bile, stimulation of blood flow, mucus and bicarbonate secretion, epithelial renewal, and prevention of vascular damage associated with physiologic stress. Evidence for these mechanisms comes predominantly from animal models of stress ulceration. Clinical studies indicate that sucralfate prevents the development of bleeding from stress-related lesions in patients admitted to critical care units. The effect of sucralfate and other forms of medical therapy on the prevention of clinically important stress-related GI bleeding, however, remains to be determined. Future studies should emphasize the use of placebo controls, stratify for clinical setting and severity of illness, adequately define the source and degree of bleeding, and examine the impact of prophylaxis on morbidity, mortality, and cost.

References

The Pathophysiology of Stress-Related Gastrointestinal Bleeding

1. Bresalier RS: The clinical significance and pathophysiology of stress-related gastric mucosal hemorrhage. *J Clin Gastroenterol* **13**(suppl 2):S35–S43, 1991. Detailed review of the clinical significance and pathophysiology of stress-related mucosal damage. Includes 100 references.
2. Silen W: Experimental models of gastric ulceration and injury. *Am J Physiol* **255**:6395–6402, 1988. Critical review of animal models of stress-induced ulceration.
3. Schiessel R, Feil W, Wenzl E: Mechanisms of stress ulceration and implications for treatment. *Gastroenterol Clin North Am* **19**:101–120, 1990. Review of potential mechanisms of gastroduodenal damage related to physiologic stress, and their implications for treatment. Includes 65 references.
4. Konturek PK, Brzoozowski T, Konturek S, *et al*: Role of epidermal growth factor, prostaglandin and sulfhydryls in stress-induced gastric lesions. *Gastroenterology* **99**:1607–1615, 1990. Suggests a newly recognized role for epidermal growth factor in protection against stress-induced gastric injury.

Natural History and Incidence

5. Czaja MA, McAlhany JC, Pruitt BA: Acute gastroduodenal disease after thermal injury. An endoscopic evaluation of incidence and natural history. *N Engl J Med* **291**:925–929, 1974. Early article describing the endoscopically monitored evolution of stress-related lesions in critically ill patients.
6. Schuster DP, Rowley H, Feinstein S, *et al*: Prospective evaluation of the risk of upper gastrointestinal bleeding after admission to a medical intensive care unit. *Am J Med* **76**:623–630, 1984. Examines the risk of stress-related bleeding in patients not receiving medical prophylaxis. Suggests a low incidence of clinically significant bleeding. Emphasizes importance of prolonged mechanical ventilation and coagulopathy as risk factors.
7. Hastings PR, Skillman JJ, Bushnell LS, *et al*: Antacid titration in the prevention of acute gastrointestinal bleeding. *N Engl J Med* **298**:1041–1045, 1978. Early series that popularized antacid prophylaxis against stress-related bleeding.
8. Zinner MJ, Zuidema GD, Smith PL, *et al*: The prevention of upper gastrointestinal tract bleeding in an intensive care unit. *Surg Gynecol Obstet* **153**:214–220, 1981. Largest and best early series comparing the efficacy of prophylaxis against stress-related bleeding with antacids and bolus i.v. H_2RAs. Includes a no-treatment control group.
9. Schuman RB, Schuster DP, Zuckerman GR: Prophylactic therapy for stress ulcer bleeding: A reappraisal. *Ann Intern Med* **106**:562–567, 1987. Review emphasizes the need to define the source and magnitude of bleeding in evaluating efficacy of stress ulcer prophylaxis.
10. Martin LF, Booth FVM, Karlstadt RG, *et al*: Continuous intravenous cimetidine infusion decreases stress-related upper gastrointestinal hemorrhage without promoting pneumonia. *Crit Care Med* **21**:19–30, 1993. Multicenter placebo-controlled study of continuous i.v. cimetidine for prophylaxis of stress-related bleeding. Accompanying editorial: Schuster DP: Stress ulcer prophylaxis: In whom? With what? *Crit Care Med* **21**:4–6, 1993. Points out important flaws in this and other existing studies of stress ulcer prophylaxis, and need for better study design.
11. Cook DJ, Witt LG, Cook RJ: Stress ulcer prophylaxis in the critically ill: A meta analysis. *Am J Med* 519–527, 1991.
12. Tryba M: Prophylaxis of stress ulcer bleeding. A meta analysis. *J Clin Gastroenterol* **13**(suppl 2):544–555, 1991. Two recent meta-analyses compare the efficacy of antacids, H_2RAs, and sucralfate for prevention of stress-related bleeding. Analysis by Cook examines effect on both "overt" and "clinically important" bleeding. Review by Tryba uses "macroscopic bleeding" as criterion for analysis.
13. Cook DJ, Laine LA, Guyatt GH, *et al*: Nosocomial pneumonia and the role of gastric pH. A meta-analysis. *Chest* **100**:7–13, 1991. Meta-analysis examining the differential effect of agents used for stress-bleeding prophylaxis on nosocomial pneumonia in critically ill patients.

29

Prevention of Respiratory Tract Infections with Sucralfate in Ventilated ICU Patients

MICHAEL TRYBA

Nosocomial Infections of the Respiratory Tract— A Frequent Complication in Ventilated ICU Patients

Nosocomial infections of the respiratory tract are frequent complications in ventilated ICU patients. The reported incidences vary from 10 to 80% depending on the diagnosis, the duration of ventilation, the underlying disease, and the concomitant treatment. Nosocomial pneumonia occurs significantly more frequently in surgical ICU patients compared with medical patients.[1] In surgical patients, pneumonia significantly prolongs the duration of ICU stay by about 10 days. The impact of pneumonia on mortality is conflicting. While in some studies pneumonia had no influence on mortality, other studies reported a significant increase of mortality in patients with pneumonia. Leu and co-workers[2] determined that the "attributable mortality" or mortality directly related to pneumonia was 33%. Nosocomial infections significantly contributed to the morbidity and mortality of ICU patients in another study. In an analysis of more than 3000 patients who died after a traffic accident, about 25% died as a result of pneumonia, increasing to 60% in patients staying more than 28 days and being older than 70 years. Appropriate antibiotic treatment of pneumonia may improve patient survival, in one study from 36% to 72%. However, the use of broad-spectrum antibiotics in patients without infection is potentially harmful, facilitating colonization and superinfection with highly virulent organisms.

From all of these studies it seems that the impact of pneumonia on mortality of ICU patients mainly depends on the underlying disease. Evidence exists that patients with a

MICHAEL TRYBA • Department of Anesthesiology, Intensive Care Medicine and Pain Therapy, University of Bochum Bergmannsheil, Bochum, Germany.

Sucralfate: From Basic Science to the Bedside, edited by Daniel Hollander and G. N. J. Tytgat. Plenum Press, New York, 1995.

good chance of survival will most likely benefit from prevention or treatment of pneumonia in terms of mortality.

Risk Factors of Pneumonia

Nosocomial pneumonia occurs in about 1% of all hospitalized patients and accounts for about 15% of hospital-acquired infections. ICU patients represent a special group of risk with a 5- to 50-fold higher incidence of pneumonia than other hospitalized patients. Mechanical ventilation increases by 21-fold the risk of pneumonia. Within the ventilated patient group, surgical patients are those with the highest risk of nosocomial pneumonia. In trauma patients, prospective studies reported pneumonia frequencies from 30 to 80%. Patients with femoral fractures, with spinal cord injuries, or with chest injuries constitute special groups with a significant increase of the risk of pneumonia. In an analysis of 294 trauma patients, Rodriguez *et al.*[3] observed an overall pneumonia incidence of 44% with head injury, hypotension on admission, emergent intubation, blunt trauma, and an Injury Severity Score > 25 as independent risk factors. Emergency surgery, impaired airway reflexes, ventilation > 24 hr, and neuromuscular disease were significant risk factors of pneumonia in a large analysis of 1475 ICU patients. In patients with severe thoracic trauma or cervical spine lesion, lung contusion, edema, ischemia, mediator release, atelectasis, paralysis of the diaphragm, and retention of tracheobronchial secretion contribute to the extremely high incidence of respiratory tract complications. Furthermore, the incidence of nosocomial pneumonia increases with the duration of mechanical ventilation, reaching a maximum between the days 10 and 20. The risk of pneumonia was increased by repeated intubation, gastric content aspiration, ventilation > 3 days, COPD, and by the use of PEEP. Craven and co-workers[1] analyzed 233 long-term ventilated patients and found that patients with an intracranial pressure monitor (a sign of CNS depression), winter–fall season, changing of the ventilator circuit every 24 hr rather than every 48 hr, and the use of cimetidine were the only independent risk factors for the occurrence of pneumonia.

These analyses make clear that numerous factors (Table I) may influence the actual incidence of pneumonia in ICU patients, not only depending on the patient but also on the treatment regimen. However, certain risk factors can be found in most of the studies: hypotension or shock, emergency procedures, long-term ventilation, and impaired airway reflexes.

Other potential risk factors may be underestimated because of methodological problems; e.g., if all patients receive the same treatment, no effect of this regimen can be observed in a regression analysis. On the other hand, if a special medication (e.g., prophylactic regimen) will be administered only to those patients at increased risk, then even an inverse correlation can be expected, which might lead to the (false) conclusion that the prophylactic regimen even increases the risk.

Mechanisms of Respiratory Tract Colonization

Respiratory tract infections in the ICU patient may occur by three routes: via exogenous infection and via primary or secondary endogenous infections. In exogenous

Table I. Risk Factors of Nosocomial Pneumonia in ICU Patients

Mechanical ventilation	Neuromuscular disease
Aspiration	COPD
Impaired airway reflexes Repeated intubation	Hypotension/shock
Change of ventilator circuit every 24 hr	Acid-suppressing drugs
Surgery	Winter–fall season
Emergency procedure	
Chest injury	
Head injury	
Spinal cord injury	
Femoral fracture	
Blunt trauma	

infections the organism is introduced into the patient from the environment. Endogenous infections are caused by organisms that are carried by the patient in the oropharynx and/or gastrointestinal tract. Primary endogenous infections are caused by organisms already carried by the patient on admission. Microorganisms acquired after admission to the unit are responsible for secondary endogenous infections (Fig. 1).

Until the early 1980s, exogenous infection was believed to be the main causative route of respiratory tract infection. However, all efforts to prevent nosocomial pneumonia in ICU patients by controlling the exogenous environment were unsuccessful. Even the moving of a whole ICU into a new building had no significant effect on the overall pneumonia rate. Therefore, more and more investigations focused on the other route: endogenous infections. It became clear that 80–90% of all respiratory tract infections are caused by endogenous infections. The causative bacteria could be first observed in the oropharynx or nose in 50–70%. Other primary sources of potentially pathogenic bacteria are the rectum, the skin, or the gastrointestinal tract. Theoretically, bacteria from the gastrointestinal tract can colonize the lungs by different routes. Bacteria from the gut can reach the stomach retrograde by duodenogastric reflux, then be regurgitated into the oropharynx and aspirated into the lungs. Another route of endogenous colonization is the translocation of bacteria from the gut, leading to bacteremia and then pneumonia.

Although the existence of all of these colonization routes could be proved experimentally, it was difficult to support these experimental data by clinical results. Therefore, oropharyngeal colonization was long believed to be the major primary source of potentially pathogenic microorganisms, leading to respiratory tract infections in ventilated patients by the aspiration of colonized oropharyngeal fluids. However, results of recent studies obtained during the last 6 years gave new insights into the mechanisms of respiratory tract colonization in these patients and the importance of different organs in the occurrence of respiratory tract infections.

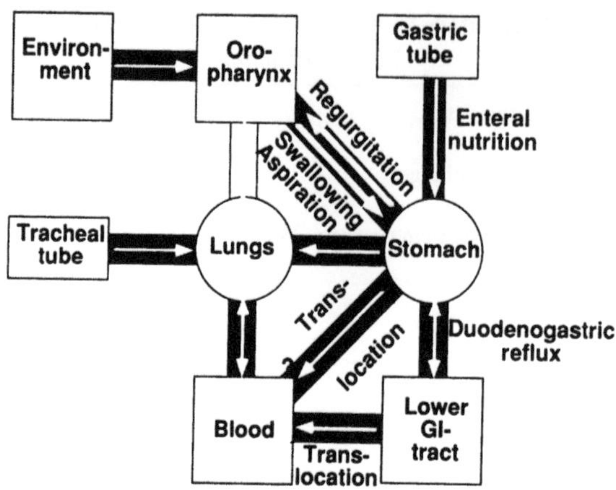

Figure 1. Routes of respiratory tract infection in ventilated patients.

The Stomach—A Pool of Potentially Pathogenic Bacteria?

In healthy humans, gastric bacterial colonization is rare because of the suppressive effect of acid gastric juice. This situation in healthy persons has been confirmed in a number of studies in ICU patients during the last decade. At admission to the ICU, 86% of postoperative ICU patients showed sterile gastric juice. Two days later the gastric juice was colonized in 61% of patients. However, in patients with a gastric juice pH $\geqslant 4$, gastric colonization occurred in 91%. Coliform bacteria $\geqslant 10^5$/ml were isolated only in patients with pH values $\geqslant 4$. In a similar study, 33% of ICU patients with acid-suppressing stress ulcer prophylaxis in whom the pH remained under 4 developed gastric colonization with potential pathogenic bacteria, while this percentage increased to 75% in patients with a pH > 4. Gastric colonization was investigated in 60 ICU patients with antacid or cimetidine prophylaxis.[5] Whereas at pH < 4, gram-negative bacteria were isolated only in rare cases, a significant increase of colonization with gram-negative bacteria relative to increasing gastric pH occurred. These findings were confirmed by Daschner *et al.*[11] in 142 patients undergoing long-term ventilation and in a group of 153 patients. Gastric colonization occurred in all ventilated patients with paralytic ileus, stressing the hypothesis that retrograde colonization may be an important cause of gastric bacterial overgrowth at least in some subgroups of ICU patients. These results clearly show that the risk of gastric bacterial colonization significantly increases in relation to alkaline gastric pH values in ICU patients. Gastric acid secretion is an active process requiring energy-rich phosphates. Because of disturbances of the microcirculation, ICU patients often show reduced gastric acid secretion. Shock and hypotension often leads to spontaneous alkaline gastric juice with pH values > 5.[4] The more severe the underlying disease, the less acid secretion can be observed (gastric exocrine failure). In contrast to healthy men, alkaline gastric pH values are frequently observed in ICU patients. Since the gastric juice loses its barrier function at pH values $\geqslant 4$, gastric gram-negative bacterial overgrowth occurs in the majority of ICU patients within a few days. The pool of bacteria in the stomach must be considered as potentially pathogenic if spread into other organs occurs.

Gastric Colonization—Cause or Consequence of Oropharyngeal and Tracheal Colonization?

Since ICU patients show reduced gastric acid secretion, the questions arise as to whether the increase of gastric colonization is a primary mechanism or whether it reflects only the increased risk of colonization of patients with a severe underlying disease who show reduced acid secretion.

If gastric colonization is only a consequence of oropharyngeal colonization, then it should merely reflect oropharyngeal colonization. However, if gastric colonization occurs at least partly independent from oropharyngeal colonization, then gastric bacterial colonization should be different from oropharyngeal colonization.

Gastric colonization independent of the oropharynx can mainly occur by direct inoculation of bacteria into the stomach, e.g., by administration of colonized enteral nutrition. This route of colonization has been confirmed in a number of investigations.[17] Another source of gastric colonization might be the lower GI tract by retrograde colonization and duodenogastric reflux. After a few hours of drug-induced acid suppression, a significant number of the bacteria in the stomach of ICU patients were typical of the GI tract.[6] This short treatment period is insufficient to induce changes of the oropharyngeal flora. In patients with gastric hypoacidity, the stomach serves as a reservoir of bacteria independent of the oropharynx. In ICU patients a number of studies[8] confirm an enormous increase of the duodenogastric reflux. Recently, Inglis *et al.*[7] proved that in ICU patients the duodenogastric reflux indeed leads to an increase of gastric colonization due to bacteria from the GI tract. In patients with a gastric pH ≥ 4, gastric gram-negative colonization significantly correlated with the detection of bile acids in the gastric juice. The studies leave no doubt that the gastric juice can be colonized independently of the oropharynx (1) by administration of colonized enteral nutrition and (2) by retrograde colonization from the intestine.

The next question is whether (contaminated) gastric juice will be regurgitated into the oropharynx and aspirated into the lungs. Besides numerous indirect investigations that looked at the sequence of colonization, recently a number of studies have directly proven by radiolabeled gastric juice[10] and by detection of glucose in the trachea[9] that microaspiration of gastric juice occurs in 50–90% of mechanically ventilated ICU patients (for further details see Ref. 19).

A significant finding further supporting the hypothesis of gastric colonization as a risk factor of respiratory tract infections was the observation that patients with a gastric pH ≥ 4 showed a higher oropharyngeal and tracheal colonization than those with a low gastric pH. This observation has been confirmed in three prospective randomized studies.[12,13] In ICU patients, enteral nutrition significantly increases gastric pH. Tracheal colonization resulting from gastric bacterial overgrowth in patients on nasogastric enteral feeding has been reported. Recently, Kingston *et al.*[9] showed that enterally fed ventilated patients with positive microaspiration indeed have a significantly higher incidence of pneumonia. While in patients without proof of microaspiration nosocomial pneumonia occurred in 8%, the incidence of pneumonia increased to 100% in patients with positive microaspiration ($p < 0.001$). Investigations in long-term ventilated patients on continuous enteral feeding underline the importance of gastric colonization as a risk factor for the development of pulmonary infections.[16] In patients with a gastric pH intermittently < 3.5

(mean 3.3 ± 0.85), only 9% developed a pneumonia, in contrast to 92% of those with a persistently high gastric pH (mean 6.1 ± 1.05) ($p < 0.0002$). Gastric gram-negative colonization significantly correlated with an alkaline gastric pH. Thurn *et al.*[17] compared two groups of patients with enteral feeding, one group with enteral feeding on bedside versus premixed feeding. In the group with enteral nutrition mixed at the beside there was a high number of organisms in the enteral nutrition relative to premixed. This corresponds with the number of patients who are colonized in the throat and rectum. Sixty percent of the patients showed colonization in the mixed at bedside group, and 20% in the premixed group. Pneumonia occurred in 91% of the patients with colonized gastric juice, and in only 6% of the patients with sterile gastric juice.

In conclusion, gastric colonization partly occurs independent of the oropharynx. Aspiration of colonized gastric juice can be frequently observed in ICU patients with an alkaline gastric pH significantly increasing the risk of nosocomial pneumonia.

The Influence of Stress Ulcer Prophylaxis on Gastric Colonization

Besides the underlying disease, additional risk factors directly increase gastric colonization, e.g., measures that lead to gastric alkalinization (sedation, enteral nutrition, antacids, H_2-antagonists).[11,16,17] The effects of premedication with H_2-antagonists in healthy men have made clear that gastric bacterial colonization with both oropharyngeal and potentially pathogenic bacteria occurs after about 12 hr of acid suppression. Gastric colonization has been demonstrated to occur in 86% of patients pretreated with H_2-antagonists. Forster *et al.*[6] found a sterile gastric juice in 90% of control patients but in only 20/% of patients pretreated with cimetidine. Similar results have been reported by others in patients after premedication with ranitidine and in patients on ulcer therapy with acid-suppressing substances. A study[6] in ICU patients with low gastric pH values (2.5 ± 0.4) at admission may serve as an example of the clinical significance of acid suppression as a risk factor of gastric colonization. A sterile gastric juice was found in 86%. After 24 hr of cimetidine therapy the pH increased to 6.1 ± 0.6 and all gastric juice samples were colonized. Cimetidine was then withdrawn and 12 hr later the gastric juice had a mean pH of 3.1 ± 0.7 with only 21% colonized. This study clearly shows that stress ulcer prophylaxis aiming to increase gastric pH facilitates gastric colonization.

Further studies in ICU patients confirm that the administration of H_2-antagonists or antacids significantly increases gastric gram-negative colonization, compared with regimens like sucralfate without significant influence on gastric pH.[12–14]

Bactericidal Effects of Sucralfate

Early studies of the bacterial colonization of gastric juice during sucralfate therapy revealed that bacterial growth is significantly reduced relative to acid-suppressing medication.[12] This reduction was greater than expected considering the differences in the gastric pH. The question therefore arose whether sucralfate has antibacterial properties in gastric juice independent of the gastric pH.

The antibacterial activity of sucralfate in artificial gastric fluid without proteins was demonstrated by Daschner. We could show in an *in vitro* investigation that this antibacterial effect is also present in human gastric juice at low as well as alkaline gastric juice pH.[18] Apart from gram-negative bacteria, sucralfate was also tested against selected gram-positive cocci for its antibacterial effects. Results of these tests offer support for the hypothesis that the bacterial suppression with sucralfate observed in this study could extend to other bacterial species as well. Further *in vivo* studies in ICU patients with alkaline gastric pH confirmed the antibacterial effect of sucralfate against a number of pathogens. However, in these studies we could show that sucralfate was not equally effective against all bacteria. Furthermore, the *in vivo* dosages necessary to reduce the bacterial concentration by about two log units were above the dosages used up to then for stress ulcer prophylaxis. With dosages of 1 g sucralfate could at best suppress the bacterial growth, therefore this dosage could be considered clinically as "bacteriostatic." On the basis of these investigations we changed our dosage regimen to 3 g sucralfate three times per day. Later, Eddleston *et al.*[13] in a prospective controlled study confirmed the antibacterial effect of sucralfate versus ranitidine. They could show that stress ulcer prophylaxis with sucralfate leads to significantly reduced bacterial growth in patients with low as well as with alkaline gastric pH. However, clinically the effects of sucralfate were more pronounced at alkaline pH values.

To summarize, sucralfate leads to a significant reduction of gastric bacterial overgrowth compared with acid-suppressing drugs. This effect can only partly be explained by differences in the gastric pH. Further *in vitro* and *in vivo* studies have shown that sucralfate has unique dose-related antibacterial effects against a number of pathogens.

Is Sucralfate Effective in Preventing Pulmonary Infections? An Analysis of Prospective Controlled Studies

Numerous prospective studies have investigated the influence of stress ulcer prophylaxis with sucralfate on nosocomial pneumonia in comparison with acid-suppressing drugs such as antacids and/or H_2-antagonists (for further details see Refs. 19 and 20).

In the first randomized study[15] between sucralfate and antacids in ventilated ICU surgical patients without thoracic trauma, we observed a pneumonia rate of 9% with sucralfate therapy, i.e., significantly lower than with antacids where the rate was 34%. In this study an antacid dosage was chosen that guaranteed alkaline gastric pH values. A similar pH-titrated regimen was used in another study by Eddleston *et al.*[13] This study came to the same conclusions as our own study. Long-term ventilated patients titrated to a gastric pH > 4 with ranitidine (+ sodium citrate, if necessary) developed a significantly higher frequency of pulmonary infections (35%) as did patients on sucralfate (9%). Patients on sucralfate who had a pH $\geqslant 4$ showed a pneumonia frequency much higher than those with a low gastric pH.

Driks *et al.*[12] prospectively compared the pneumonia rate with sucralfate to antacids, H_2-antagonists, and a combination of both. Randomization was carried out only between sucralfate and conventional prophylaxis but not between the subgroups within conventional prophylaxis. In the 39 patients treated with antacids there was a pneumonia rate of 23%

and in the patients treated with antacids + H_2-antagonists, 46%, while the pneumonia rate in the small group of 17 patients treated with H_2-antagonists (6%) was on the same order of magnitude as in the 55 patients treated with sucralfate during the whole study period (9%). However, the latter group differed in several respects from the other groups. Patients treated with H_2-antagonists were mainly medical patients, were ventilated for a shorter period of time, and none of the patients had signs of gastrointestinal disease.

Laggner *et al.* investigated 133 tracheal swabs of patients undergoing long-term ventilation, randomly assigned to sucralfate or ranitidine prophylaxis. They found a significantly higher frequency of tracheobronchial colonization with ranitidine than with sucralfate therapy (43.3 versus 18.6%). Seventy-three patients ventilated for at least 48 hr were randomly treated with sucralfate, cimetidine, or antacids and retrospectively analyzed for pneumonia frequency. Twelve percent of patients with sucralfate prophylaxis developed nosocomial pneumonia versus 21% of patients in both groups with acid-suppressing medication. Kappstein *et al.* compared the pneumonia rate in 104 ICU patients undergoing long-term ventilation with sucralfate or H_2-antagonists (cimetidine). In the sucralfate group the pneumonia rate was 29%, in the cimetidine group 46%. In another study 41 patients ventilated for more than 24 hr were analyzed (Garcia-Labattut *et al.*). In the sucralfate group 25% developed pneumonia versus 43% of those treated with cimetidine. A recent study[14] in 244 ventilated surgical patients comparing sucralfate, antacids, and ranitidine showed a significantly lower pneumonia rate in sucralfate-treated patients. This study proved that only secondary pulmonary infections were reduced by sucralfate but not early onset pneumonia. However, the administration of sucralfate is not necessarily associated with a lower pneumonia rate. Colardyn *et al.* retrospectively did not observe a higher frequency of pneumonias in patients treated with cimetidine compared with sucralfate. A similar result has been reported by Ryan *et al.* Both studies differ in some important characteristics from the other studies involving sucralfate. Colardyn *et al.* almost exclusively included medical patients, who already showed signs of infection on admission in about 80%. More than 50% of the patients had been resuscitated prior to the admission with a high likelihood of aspiration. The most relevant difference seems to be, however, that the study period was limited to a maximum of 7 days. Thereafter all patients were switched to ranitidine. Moreover, the patients in both groups had an alkaline gastric juice and therefore no differences could be observed in the bacterial colonization rate between the groups. In Ryan's study both patient groups had a pneumonia rate below 20% and an overall mortality rate of 15%, distinctively lower than in other studies. It seems to be of even greater importance that the cimetidine dosage was only 900 mg/day. In this dosage range no increase of the gastric pH can be expected. Therefore, the gastric bacterial colonization can be expected to be the same in both groups.

Another study comparing sucralfate, antacids, and cimetidine also failed to show any differences in gastric colonization rates between the three groups. The main reason seems to be that the groups did not differ in the gastric pH. Only 6 of 30 sucralfate-treated patients had mean gastric pH values < 4, but also 3 patients in the cimetidine and a further 3 patients in the antacid group. Therefore, it is not surprising that no significant differences in the pneumonia rates could be observed between the three groups. Confirming the study by Eddleston *et al.*[13,19] in those sucralfate-treated patients with a low gastric pH the pneumonia rate was about half of that observed in all other groups.

Taking all these studies together (Fig. 2) it becomes clear that drugs that significantly increase the frequency of gastric pH values above 4 increase the risk of pulmonary infections at least in ventilated ICU patients. However, the studies also show some limitations of sucralfate, and therefore the use of sucralfate does not lead necessarily to a significant reduction of the pneumonia rate.

Potentials and Limitations of Sucralfate for the Prevention of Respiratory Tract Infections in Ventilated Patients

Several factors may influence the gastric pH independently of stress ulcer prophylaxis. Continuous enteral feeding significantly increases gastric pH compared with intermittent feeding,[16] resulting in a corresponding increase of the pneumonia rate. Furthermore, it has to be considered that inactivation of sucralfate might occur if the time interval between sucralfate and enteral nutrition is less than 1 hr. This interaction may also inhibit the bactericidal effect of sucralfate.

Pneumonias resulting from the gastropulmonary route of infection are time-dependent. Godard *et al.* showed that antibiotic decontamination of the stomach was effective in reducing pneumonias only in those patients treated for more than a week. Pneumonias occurred after a mean time of about 9 days. Therefore, it becomes apparent that in patients with a very short duration of treatment, no differences in the rate of pneumonia caused by stress ulcer prophylaxis can be expected.

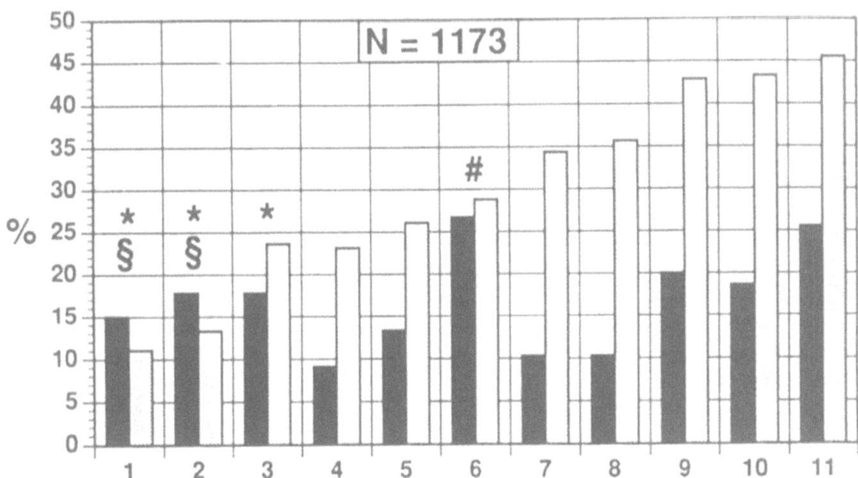

Figure 2. Frequency of nosocomial pneumonia in ICU patients in relation to stress ulcer prophylaxis with sucralfate (■) or antacids/H_2 antagonists (□) (prospective studies through August 1992). *Low-dose H_2 antagonists/antacids; §maximum duration of treatment was 7 days; #no difference in gastric colonization.

In neurosurgical patients the gastro-oropharyngeal reflux is significantly reduced because of the head-up position. Moreover, this patient group in general has no impairment of the gastrointestinal motility. Therefore, no increased risk of a gastropulmonary route of colonization can be expected in neurosurgical patients. On the other hand, patients with cervical spine lesion have a very high incidence of pulmonary infections caused by factors completely independent of microaspiration of gastric content.

A gastropulmonary route of colonization becomes relevant only in patient groups with a high risk of pneumonia.[19] This has been confirmed in our own studies with sucralfate[15] and pirenzepine. Therefore, it seems unlikely that in patient groups with a low pneumonia risk (< 20% with antacids, H_2-antagonists) any significant differences of pneumonia rates related to stress ulcer medication can be observed.

Several criteria must be taken into consideration when evaluating studies on the pneumonia rate under various regimens of stress bleeding prophylaxis. On the basis of these criteria we have developed a risk score that should allow a more detailed evaluation of studies. Furthermore, this risk score should describe those patients who are at the highest risk for the development of respiratory infections related to the gastropulmonary route of colonization (Table II).

In studies where the H_2-blocker or antacid group reached scores above 2, there was an increased risk of pulmonary infections relative to a medication that did not influence the

Table II. Risk Scores Relating to an Increased Risk of Pulmonary Infections via the Gastropulmonary Route of Colonization in Patient Groups Treated with Drugs That Lead to an Alkalinization of Gastric Juice

	Score			
	−2	−1	+1	+2
Patients	Neurosurgical Inhalation trauma Cerv. spinal cord lesion		Mainly surgical	
Ventilation	None	Mean duration ≤2 days	Mean duration >3 days	Mean duration >7 days
Pneumonia rate in groups with H_2RAs/antacids		<20%		
Gastric colonization	No difference			
Study period	Limited to ≤7 days			
Enteral feeding		+		
Stress ulcer prophylaxis	Low-dose H_2RAs (<1 g cim. equiv.) or/and no *increase/difference* in gastric pH >4 in many patients		H_2RAs (≥1.2 g cim. equiv.) Antacids >2 and <6 hourly	Antacids ≤2 hourly
Dose adjustment/ titration of gastric pH			+	

gastric pH (no medication, pirenzepine, sucralfate). On the other hand, if the risk score was below 2, no increased risk could be demonstrated. This result allows definition of those patients who are at an increased risk of pulmonary infections via the gastropulmonary route of colonization.

Reducing the Risk of Pulmonary Infections in Ventilated Patients—A Rational Approach

Physiological barriers such as gastric acidity effectively prevent the occurrence of respiratory infections. However, in ICU patients these barriers are often eliminated. Lying in the bed with a gastric tube significantly increases the risk of regurgitation and aspiration of gastric content. Gastric colonization increases with the severity of the underlying disease as well as with the administration of acid-suppressing drugs or enteral feeding. Gastric colonization is at least partly independent from oropharyngeal colonization. The sources of oropharynx-independent gastric colonization are the lower GI tract relating to the increased duodenogastral reflux observed in ICU patients and administration of nonsterile enteral nutrition.

Nosocomial pneumonia in ventilated patients should no longer be considered an unpreventable misfortune. Different approaches have been proven effective in the prevention of this complication. Since they all aim at different sites of the colonization sequence, they should not be considered competing regimens. They all have their own place in a general prophylactic concept. There is good evidence now that in patients with low gastric pH and without further risk factors, stress ulcer prophylaxis with sucralfate reduces the overall frequency of pneumonia to about 10%, which is in the same range as with selective digestive decontamination. Any drugs that increase gastric pH should be avoided. Sterile enteral nutrition should be administered as early as possible and intermittently with a fasting interval of about 6 hr daily to avoid a continuous elevation of the gastric juice. Gastric pH should be measured at least twice a day, not for stress ulcer prophylaxis but for determining the risk of gastric colonization. In patients with alkaline gastric juice (e.g., spontaneous or related to enteral nutrition), those with a significant risk of pathological oropharyngeal colonization on admission, or patients on immunosuppressive drugs, selective digestive decontamination should be considered as an additional prophylactic measure. However, since sucralfate may bind some antibiotics if administered concurrently, antibiotics should be administered at least 1 hr prior to sucralfate (Table III).

Clinical Experiences with Sucralfate for Stress Ulcer Prophylaxis

After the first papers appeared suggesting sucralfate as an effective alternative for stress ulcer prophylaxis with a reduced risk of nosocomial pneumonia, this substance gained wide popularity throughout the world and in many countries superseded H_2-antagonists and antacids as the drug of choice for stress ulcer prophylaxis.

Repeated questionnaires and multicenter studies from France may serve as an example of how the introduction of sucralfate has changed the routine practice of stress ulcer prophylaxis. Soon after the papers by Driks and our own appeared in 1987, a

Table III. Physiological Measures for the Prevention of Nosocomial Pneumonia in Ventilated Patients

1. Start enteral feeding as early as possible in order to stimulate gastrointestinal motility, bile acid secretion, and IgE secretion.
2. Do not put your patients on continuous enteral feeding. Instead interrupt feeding for 6 h daily. (We stop feeding from midnight to morning.)
3. Let your patient sit in the bed as early as possible even if he is on mechanical ventilation.
4. Avoid any drug that reduces gastric acidity. (If stress ulcer prophylaxis is necessary we use sucralfate 3 × 3 g daily, or pirenzepine i.v. if enteral medication should be avoided.)
5. Measure gastric pH at least once daily after the fasting period (not for stress ulcer prophylaxis but for the evaluation of the risk of respiratory infections). If gastric pH is >4 on two days running, consider additional measures for the prevention of respiratory infections.

questionnaire was done in France. H_2-antagonists were still the most often prescribed drugs for stress ulcer prophylaxis and only 10% of the ICUs used sucralfate. Two years later a similar questionnaire showed a significant change in management. Sucralfate was used in about 50% of the ICUs. In 1992 a French multicenter study in ventilated ICU patients showed that H_2-antagonists were used in only about 10% of the patients and that antacids played no role, while sucralfate was used in almost 80% of the patients who received stress ulcer prophylaxis. This large placebo-controlled multicenter study investigated the effect of selective digestive decontamination (SDD) on the frequency of nosocomial pneumonia. In contrast to almost all other studies published hitherto, SDD was ineffective in the prevention of nosocomial pneumonia, mainly because of the low overall frequency of about 12%. However, the major difference of this study in contrast to others studies dealing with the same topic was that about 90% of the patients did not receive any acid-suppressing drugs. Therefore, this study can be taken as a further proof that the overall frequency of nosocomial pneumonia in ventilated patients will be in the range of 10–15% if acid-suppressing drugs for stress ulcer prophylaxis are avoided.

In our ICUs we have abandoned the use of H_2-antagonists or antacids for stress ulcer prophylaxis since 1987 and have accumulated more than 4000 patients treated with sucralfate three times daily only (3 × 3 g) or pirenzepine without any problems. Although about 60% of these patients were on long-term ventilation, only two patients had to be operated on because of acute upper gastrointestinal bleeding. In one patient with severe burns, stress ulcer prophylaxis was accidentally stopped 3 days prior to the occurrence of macroscopic bleeding from a duodenal ulcer (Forrest la); the other patient had developed an autolytic gastric perforation resulting from a necrotizing pancreatitis. Therefore, none of our patients who received adequate prophylaxis developed severe stress ulcer bleeding.

References

1. Craven DE, Kunches LM, Kilinsky V, *et al*: Risk factors for pneumonia and fatality in patients receiving continuous mechanical ventilation. *Am Rev Respir Dis* **133**:792–796, 1986.

2. Leu HS, Kaiser DL, Mori M, *et al*: Hospital acquired pneumonia: Attributable mortality and morbidity. *Am J Epidemiol* **129**:1258–1267, 1989.
3. Rodriguez JL, Gibbons KJ, Bitzer LG, *et al*: Pneumonia: Incidence, risk factors, and outcome in injured patients. *J Trauma* **31**:907–914, 1991. References 1–3 analyze risk factors of pneumonia in ICU patients.
4. Stannard VA, Hutchinson A, Morris DL, *et al*: Gastric exocrine "failure" in critically ill patients: Incidence and associated features. *Br Med J* **296**:155–156, 1988. Spontaneous alkaline gastric juice frequently occurs in critically ill patients.
5. Du Moulin GC, Paterson DG, Hedley-White J, *et al*: Aspiration of gastric bacteria in antacid-treated patients: A frequent cause of postoperative colonisation of the airway. *Lancet* **1**:242–245, 1982.
6. Forster A, Niethamer T, Suter P, *et al*: Influence de la cimetidine sur la croissance bacterienne dans le liquide gastrique. *Nouv Presse Med* **11**:2281–2283, 1982.
7. Inglis TJJ, Sproat LJ, Sherratt MJ, *et al*: Gastroduodenal dysfunction as a cause of gastric bacterial overgrowth in patients undergoing mechanical ventilation of the lungs. *Br J Anaesth* **68**:499–502, 1992. References 5–7 demonstrate that gastric gram-negative bacterial colonization increases in ICU patients with alkaline gastric pH.
8. Schindlbeck NE, Lippert M, Heinrich C, *et al*: Intragastric bile acid concentrations in critically ill, artificially ventilated patients. *Am J Gastroenterol* **84**:624–628, 1989. Duodenogastric reflux is significantly increased in ICU patients.
9. Kingston GW, Phang PT, Leathley MJ: Increased incidence of nosocomial pneumonia in mechanically ventilated patients with subclinical aspiration. *Am J Surg* **161**:589–592, 1991.
10. Torres A, Serra-Batlles J, Ros E, *et al*: Pulmonary aspiration of gastric contents in patients receiving mechanical ventilation: The effect of body position. *Ann Intern Med* **116**:540–543, 1992. References 9 and 10 show that aspiration of gastric contents frequently occurs in intubated patients and that patients with aspiration have a significant increase in incidence of pneumonia.
11. Daschner F, Reuschenbach K, Pfisterer J, *et al*: Der Einfluß von Streßulcusprophylaxe auf die Häufigkeit einer Beatmungspneumonie. *Anaesthesist* **36**:9–18, 1987.
12. Driks MR, Craven DE, Celli BR, *et al*: Nosocomial pneumonia in intubated patients randomized to sucralfate versus antacids and/or histamine type 2 blockers: The role of gastric colonization. *N Engl J Med* **317**:1376–1382, 1987.
13. Eddleston J, Vohra A, Scott P, *et al*: A comparison of the frequency of stress ulceration and secondary pneumonia in sucralfate- or ranitidine-treated intensive care unit patients. *Crit Care Med* **19**:1491–1496, 1991.
14. Prodhom G, Leuenberger P, Blum AL, *et al*: Effect of stress-ulcer prophylaxis on nosocomial pneumonia in ventilated patients: A randomized comparative study. *31st Intersci Conf Antimicrob Agents Chemother*, Chicago, 1991.
15. Tryba M: The risk of acute stress bleeding and nosocomial pneumonia in ventilated ICU-patients: sucralfate vs antacids. *Am J Med* **83**(3B):117–124, 1987. References 11–15 compare the rate of pneumonia with sucralfate therapy versus antacids, H_2-antagonists for stress ulcer prophylaxis.
16. Lee B, Chang RWS, Jacobs S: Intermittent nasogastric feeding: A simple and effective method to reduce pneumonia among ventilated ICU patients. *Clin Int Care* **1**:100–102, 1990.
17. Thurn J, Crossley K, Gerdts A, *et al*: Enteral hyperalimentation as a source of nosocomial infection. *J Hosp Infect* **15**:203–217, 1990. References 16 and 17 investigate the influence of enteral nutrition on the rate of pneumonia in ICU patients.
18. Tryba M, Mantey-Stiers F: Antibacterial activity of sucralfate in human gastric juice. *Am J Med* **83**(3B):125–127, 1987. Investigation of the antibacterial effect of sucralfate.
19. Tryba M: The gastropulmonary route of infection—Fact or fiction? *Am J Med* **91**(2A):135S–146S, 1991.
20. Tryba M: Sucralfate vs antacids or H2-antagonists for stress ulcer prophylaxis—A metaanalysis on the efficacy and pneumonia rate. *Crit Care Med* **19**:942–949, 1991. References 19 and 20 contain a more detailed list of references dealing with stress ulcer prophylaxis and the risk of pneumonia.

30

Sucralfate in Nonulcer Dyspepsia, Gastritis, and Duodenitis

M. GUSLANDI

Introduction

Nonulcer dyspepsia (NUD) is a generic term used to describe the presence of dyspeptic symptoms in patients unaffected by pancreatic or biliary disorders (i.e., with normal abdominal ultrasound), without endoscopic signs of peptic ulcer disease or reflux esophagitis, and no symptoms clearly suggestive of irritable bowel syndrome.

The prevalence of NUD in the population is high. According to some studies it appears that more than one-third of the general population complains of dyspeptic symptoms within a period of 6 months.

A possible way to classify dyspepsia is to distinguish "organic" forms related to or at least accompanied by inflammatory changes of the gastroduodenal mucosa (gastritis, duodenitis, mucosal erosions) and those where no mucosal abnormalities are detectable ("functional" dyspepsia) where symptoms are presumably related to motor abnormalities (e.g., delayed gastric emptying, duodenogastric reflux) or functional disturbances of the nervous system. Alterations of the gastroduodenal motility can account for up to 30% of patients with functional dyspepsia.

NUD either functional or organic is usually not associated with increased gastric acidity. Instead mucosal defensive factors such as secretion of mucus and bicarbonate appear to be defective in patients with chronic gastritis or gastric erosions.

M. GUSLANDI • Gastroenterology Unit, S. Raffaele Hospital, University of Milan, 20132 Milan, Italy.

Sucralfate: From Basic Science to the Bedside, edited by Daniel Hollander and G. N. J. Tytgat. Plenum Press, New York, 1995.

Sucralfate in Nonulcer Dyspepsia

The therapeutic role of sucralfate in patients with NUD in its broader meaning, including both functional and organic forms, was first evaluated in 1987 in Finland[1] in a double-blind randomized trial versus placebo involving 175 patients. Sucralfate 1 g tid or placebo were given for 4 weeks. The drug was found to be more effective than placebo in inducing symptom relief, the percentages of patients being symptom-free or greatly improved at the end of treatment being 77 and 56%, respectively ($p < 0.01$). The best results were observed in subjects with symptoms of mild to moderate intensity and, oddly enough, without endoscopic or histological evidence of inflammation of the gastric or duodenal mucosa. It must be noted, however, that, as will be discussed below, the duration of therapy (4 weeks) is too short to allow morphological improvement of mucosal alterations, when present, and that a longer course with sucralfate could result in a higher rate of disappearance of symptoms in subjects with mucosal inflammation.

Direct comparisons between sucralfate and other drugs in NUD are few. Rather surprisingly, no studies comparing sucralfate with acid-inhibiting drugs are available.

The only published data come from two double-blind Italian studies where sucralfate was compared to sulglycotide, a gastroprotective drug derived from porcine duodenal mucosa.[2,3] Predictably, the two drugs, endowed with similar modes of action, provided comparable clinical results. After 6 weeks of therapy with either sucralfate 1 g tid or sulglycotide 200 mg tid, symptoms were significantly reduced and endoscopic signs of gastric or duodenal inflammation (when detectable) were abolished by therapy in up to 41% of cases.

Sucralfate in Organic Dyspepsia

Sucralfate and Helicobacter pylori

The association between histological gastritis and *H. pylori* is recognized in a number of studies. Eradication of the microorganism appears to promote improvement of histological features, the effect on symptoms being much less straightforward. Hence, the interest has been strong to ascertain the possible effect on *H. pylori* by drugs employed in the treatment of peptic ulcer and allied gastroduodenal disorders.

The large majority of the studies have ruled out a direct inhibitory effect of sucralfate on the microorganism, although *in vitro* studies suggest that sucralfate can inhibit *H. pylori* hemagglutination and counteract the mucolytic effect of the microorganism on human gastric mucus. It is unclear whether the latter effect is related to the mucus-stimulating properties of sucralfate rather than to a specific antagonistic activity. In fact, sucralfate improves the Na^+/H^+ ion exchange through the mucus gel both in infected and in uninfected stomachs.

On the other hand, histological examination of the mucosa in patients with gastritis treated with sucralfate showed conflicting results with respect to *H. pylori* colonization.

On the whole, sucralfate cannot be considered as an agent able to either clear or eradicate *H. pylori*. The possible therapeutic effects of the drug in chronic gastritis are therefore to be related to different mechanisms.

Sucralfate in Chronic Gastritis

Chronic gastritis is a pathological condition where acid secretion is usually normal, while mucosal defensive factors such as gastric bicarbonate and mucus secretion appear to be defective. Hence, on theoretical grounds, a gastroprotective agent such as sucralfate should represent a first-line therapeutic approach for this condition.

Patients with endoscopic signs of gastritis have been included in various NUD trials, but detailed information on the efficacy of the drug in patients with gastritis can be obtained only in studies specifically designed for that purpose (Table I).

In a double-blind placebo-controlled Danish trial, sucralfate promoted endoscopic and clinical improvement not significantly superior to placebo, the healing rates at 6 and 12 weeks being 43 and 62% with sucralfate and 37 and 62% with placebo.[4]

The inclusion of patients with erosive gastritis and the possible existence of a type-2 error related to the relatively low number of evaluable subjects (30 per group) may

Table I. Morphological Results of Sucralfate Therapy in Gastritis, Duodenitis, and Duodenal Erosions

Ref.	No. of patients	Weeks	Disappearance of gastritis (%) Endoscopic		Histological	
		Gastritis				
Skoubo-Kristensen *et al.* (1989)	60	6	SUC 43			
			PLA 37			
Guslandi *et al.* (1989)[5]	473	8	SUC 56.8*		SUC 39.7*	
			RAN 46.9		RAN 29.5	
Barbara *et al.* (1990)[2]	89	6			SUC 70.8[b]	54.1[c]
					SGC 54.1	40.0
Psilogenis *et al.* (1990)[3]	124	6	SUC 30.2[d]	25.4[c]		
			SGC 26.9	23.0		
		Duodenitis				
Guslandi *et al.* (1990)[7]	30	4	SUC 50			
			PIR 50			
Psilogenis *et al.* (1990)[3]	66	6	SUC 34.4			
			SGC 41.2			
		Duodenal erosions				
Safrany and Schott (1983)[8]	25	4	SUC 100*			
			ANT 62			
Guslandi *et al.* (1989)[9]	30	8	SUC 64.3			
			RIO 57.2			

[a]Abbreviations: SUC, sucralfate; PLA, placebo; SGC, sulglycotide; PIR, pirenzepine; RAN, ranitidine; ANT, antacids; RIO, rioprostil.
[b]Fundus.
[c]Antrum.
[d]Corpus.
*Significantly superior.

possibly explain the discrepancy with the superior results observed in other trials (see below).

In a double-blind Italian study carried out in dyspeptic patients with histological evidence of active gastritis, sucralfate induced a significant regression of inflammatory changes after 6 weeks of therapy.

The present author coordinated a multicenter randomized trial including 500 patients with dyspeptic symptoms and endoscopic features of nonerosive gastritis comparing an 8-week treatment with either sucralfate or ranitidine.[5] Both drugs induced a significant reduction in the endoscopic severity score, sucralfate being significantly more effective ($p < 0.02$) in promoting healing or improvement of endoscopic gastritis. Sucralfate was also superior in promoting normalization of histological features ($p < 0.001$). Dyspeptic symptoms were eliminated in the majority of patients by both drugs which appeared to be equally effective in this respect. However, during the first 4 weeks of therapy the number of patients becoming symptom-free was significantly higher ($p < 0.01$) with ranitidine, confirming the notion that H_2-receptor antagonists relieve symptoms faster than gastroprotective agents.

Scarce information is available on the longer-term outcome of gastritis after successful medical treatment. In a recent study[6] we followed up for 3 months without further therapy 48 patients in whom previous endoscopic signs of chronic gastritis had been eliminated by treatment with either sucralfate 1 g tid or famotidine 40 mg hs. Cumulative endoscopic relapse rates at 3 months were 21.7% in the sucralfate group and 57.1% in the famotidine group ($p = 0.017$). All patients with endoscopic recurrence of gastritis also reported recurrence of dyspeptic symptoms of various degree. Most patients with endoscopic relapse had persisting histological gastritis, but up to 67% of subjects with histological gastritis at the time of initial endoscopic healing did not have subsequent endoscopic or clinical recurrence. Our results not only suggest that gastritis, especially if histologically active, tends to recur quickly after endoscopic healing but also indicate that early relapses are significantly more frequent after treatment with an H_2RA than after sucralfate.

Since both sucralfate and H_2RAs are virtually ineffective against *H. pylori*, it seems reasonable to conclude that healing of gastritis is easier and longer-lasting when mucosal defensive factors are strengthened by the gastroprotective properties of sucralfate.

Sucralfate in Duodenitis

To date only one small study performed by us[7] has investigated the efficacy of sucralfate in the treatment of dyspeptic patients with endoscopic diagnosis of nonerosive duodenitis. In a double-blind trial, 30 patients were treated for 1 month with either sucralfate 2 g bid or pirenzepine (a selective antimuscarinic agent) 50 mg bid. Both drugs significantly reduced the symptom score compared with baseline values. Normalization of the endoscopic aspect of the duodenal mucosa was attained in 50% of cases in both groups.

Reporting the results of a double-blind trial versus sulglycotide in dyspeptic patients, Psilogenis and co-workers[3] provided information on the endoscopic normalization in the subgroup of patients with duodenitis. At 6 weeks, only 34.4% of sucralfate-treated patients and 41.2% of subjects receiving the comparative drug showed healing of endoscopic duodenitis, the difference being statistically not significant.

Sucralfate in Mucosal Erosions

Duodenal Erosions

The cause of chronic erosions of the duodenal bulb (also described as "erosive duodenitis") is still a matter of speculation. Gastric acid secretion is usually within the normal range and the rate of endoscopic healing attained with antisecretory agents such as H_2RAs is comparatively low, especially in comparison with the results obtained in peptic ulcer therapy.

For instance, in a double-blind comparative trial, despite its superior acid-inhibiting effect, ranitidine promoted healing of duodenal erosions in only 39.3% of cases, a modest result, significantly inferior to the 70.4% healing promoted by pirenzepine, an antimuscarinic agent with only mild antisecretory properties. An explanation for these results is perhaps the ability of pirenzepine to increase mucosal blood flow, suggesting a possible involvement of reduced mucosal blood flow in the pathogenesis of erosions.

More recently, measurements performed in our laboratory by means of laser Doppler flowmetry confirmed that in duodenal erosions, local microcirculation is in fact impaired.

The effect of sucralfate on gastric mucosal blood flow in humans is still under evaluation. The results of animal studies, however, suggest that the drug exerts a stimulating effect on gastric mucosal blood flow.

The experience with sucralfate in the treatment of erosive duodenitis is limited. According to a small German trial by Safrany and Schott,[8] sucralfate is significantly more effective than antacids in inducing endoscopic healing.

A comparative study versus rioprostil, a PGE_1 analogue, showed that the two drugs were equally effective in promoting symptom relief. At 8 weeks, complete disappearance of erosions was noted in 64.3% of cases with sucralfate and 75.2% with rioprostil, a difference not statistically significant, but in a further 14.3% of sucralfate-treated patients (versus only 7% of subjects receiving rioprostil) the number of erosions was reduced.[9]

Thus, it must be concluded that in a field where medical treatment in general remains ill-defined, the possible therapeutic role of sucralfate, although promising, needs to be more clearly established.

Gastric Erosions

Information about the therapeutic efficacy of sucralfate in the treatment of dyspeptic patients with antral erosions is very limited.

In 1983 Safrany and Schott reported the results of a very small trial where 22 patients with endoscopic erosive gastritis were treated for 4 weeks with either sucralfate or antacids. Endoscopic healing was obtained in 82 and 90% of cases, respectively.[8]

In an unpublished series of 63 patients with antral erosions recruited by various centers in northern Italy, sucralfate, given for a period of 6 weeks, induced endoscopic normalization in 60% of cases.

Conclusion

Sucralfate appears to be effective in promoting symptom relief in patients with NUD both of organic and of functional origin.

When dyspepsia is associated with mucosal abnormalities, sucralfate can induce normalization of inflammatory or erosive alterations. This appears to be especially true in the treatment of chronic gastritis, where sucralfate, although devoid of substantial effects on *H. pylori*, is capable of inducing healing or marked improvement of both endoscopic and histological inflammation.

In this respect the drug is significantly superior to H_2RAs, healing of gastritis being more frequent and longer-lasting.

Additional data are needed to confirm the possible therapeutic role of sucralfate in dyspeptic patients with duodenitis or gastroduodenal erosions.

References

1. Kairaluoma M, Hentilae R, Alavaikko M, *et al*: Sucralfate versus placebo in the treatment of nonulcer dyspepsia. *Am J Med* **83**(suppl 3B):51–55, 1987. A major study on the use of sucralfate in dyspeptic patients with either organic or functional forms of dyspepsia.
2. Barbara L, Biasco G, Capurso L, *et al*: Effects of sucralfate and sulglycotide treatment on active gastritis and Helicobacter pylori colonization of the gastric mucosa in non-ulcer dyspepsia patients. *Am J Gastroenterol* **85**:1109–1113, 1990. An important study on the effects of sucralfate on histological gastritis and on the (lack of) relation to *H. pylori* infection.
3. Psilogenis M, Nazzari M, Ferrari PA: A multicenter double-blind study of sulglycotide versus sucralfate in nonulcer dyspepsia. *Int J Clin Pharmacol Ther Toxicol* **28**:369–374, 1990. Possibly the only published study where the efficacy of sucralfate in nonulcer dyspepsia has been compared with that of an active drug.
4. Skoubo-Kristensen E, Funch-Jensen P, Kruse A, *et al*: Controlled clinical trial with sucralfate in the treatment of macroscopic gastritis. *Scand J Gastroenterol* **24**:716–720, 1989. The only example of negative results of sucralfate in the treatment of gastritis. A matter of type-2 error?
5. Guslandi M: Comparison of sucralfate and ranitidine in the treatment of chronic nonerosive gastritis. A randomized, multicenter trial. *Am J Med* **86**(suppl 6A):45–48, 1989. The largest trial on the treatment of gastritis with sucralfate and the only one directly comparing the drug with an H_2-receptor antagonist as regards clinical, endoscopic, and histological results.
6. Guslandi M, Ballarin E, Fanti L, *et al*: Follow-up of endoscopic gastritis after healing with sucralfate or an H_2-receptor antagonist. *Scand J Gastroenterol* **27**(suppl 191):25–27, 1992. Probably the first attempt to investigate the outcome of endoscopic gastritis after healing by pharmacological agents.
7. Guslandi M, Molteni V, Dell'Oca M, *et al*: Double-blind trial of pirenzepine versus sucralfate in the treatment of endoscopic duodenitis. *Clin Ther* **12**:26–30, 1990. The only source of information on the potential role of sucralfate in the treatment of duodenitis.
8. Safrany L, Schott B: Vergleich von Sucralfat und Antazida in der Behandlung der unspezifischen erosivhamorrhagischen Duodenitis. *Therapiewoche* **33**:5233–5236, 1983. The first data, although scarce and only preliminary, on the possible use of sucralfate in erosive lesions.
9. Guslandi M, Ballarin E, Tittobello A: Rioprostil in the treatment of duodenal erosions. *Scand J Gastroenterol* **24**(suppl 164):174–177, 1989. The only published comparative study of sucralfate and a prostaglandin analogue in duodenal erosions.

31

Use of Sucralfate in Variceal Sclerotherapy-Induced Ulcerations

W. SCOTT BROOKS, JR.

Introduction

Injection sclerotherapy of esophageal varices has become the standard therapy for patients bleeding from these lesions. Studies have shown this technique to be superior to other nonsurgical therapies and to selective shunt surgery in terms of survival and quality of life. The efficacy of this therapy, though, has been reduced by sclerotherapy-induced ulcerations. Tissue necrosis from the necrotizing chemical injected to sclerose the varices may result in deep ulceration with both arterial and venous bleeding, occasionally with perforation of the esophagus. Sucralfate has been suggested as an agent to assist in healing of these lesions, and reduce ulcer-related bleeding.

Factors in the Pathogenesis of Sclerosis-Related Ulcerations

Injection of sclerosing agents into esophageal varices results in a significant local inflammatory reaction with venous thrombosis and submucosal fibrosis, the latter event being the factor that prevents or deters variceal recurrence. The agents used for sclerotherapy vary considerably in their nature, and little work has been done to define the mechanisms of tissue injury that result from their injection.

W. SCOTT BROOKS, JR. • Piedmont Hospital, Atlanta, Georgia 30309.

Sucralfate: From Basic Science to the Bedside, edited by Daniel Hollander and G. N. J. Tytgat. Plenum Press, New York, 1995.

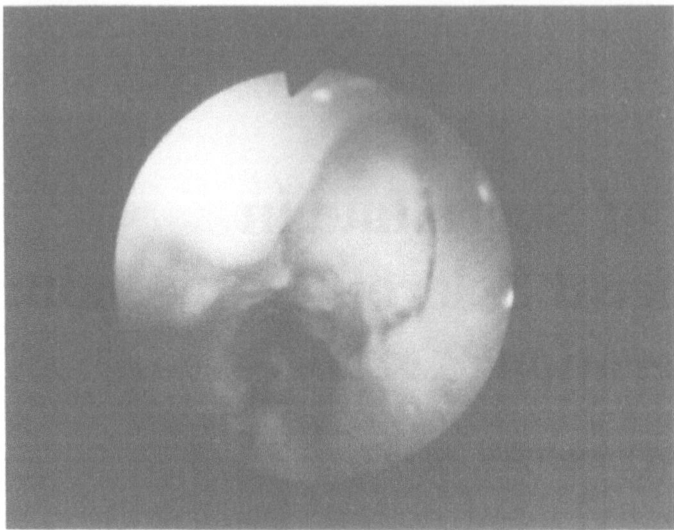

Figure 1. Large postsclerotherapy ulceration. (A color version of this figure can be found in the color insert following p. 6.)

Local activation of the coagulation system and fibrinolysis indicated by an increase in fibrinopeptides has been described with ethanolamine oleate. This sclerosant, *in vitro*, though, actually interferes with coagulation, probably because of the chelating effect of the ethanolamine component on calcium ions. The oleate component, on the other hand, does promote clotting *in vitro*.

The inflammatory reaction produced by all sclerosants no doubt releases tissue factor and Hagemann factor resulting in variceal coagulation. This coagulation is not sufficient to account for the necrosis seen with sclerotherapy-related ulcerations (Fig. 1). Similar variceal clotting and local arteriolar clotting is seen with variceal ligation by banding, but the necrotic response to this therapy is considerably more restricted. Even so, coagulation of submucosal varices has been seen to extend to the stomach following variceal ligation. The arteriolar clotting is likely restricted to the banded tissue, which sloughs after a few days leaving only a limited mucosal defect, but submucosal fibrosis and venous clotting work to prevent further bleeding and variceal recurrence.

Variceal banding results in clearly limited and defined mucosal injury, limited by the small amount of tissue banded, but the results of injection sclerosis are quite variable because of operator-dependent factors. Needle placement, choice of sclerosant, and volume injected vary between operators. Deep ulceration from extensive necrosis may lead to perforation, with the extent of injury being determined by the volume and location of the injection as well as the concentration of the sclerosant.

Sclerosants

A multiplicity of chemical agents have been selected for variceal sclerotherapy. Phenol was used in the late 1930s for the first reported case of injection sclerosis of esophageal varices. In the United States, sodium tetradecyl sulfate and sodium morrhuate are widely used. Ethanolamine oleate use is limited in the United States, no doubt because of its lack of availability initially, pending FDA approval. Ethanolamine is used widely in Great Britain, Europe, and Japan and appears to have a good safety profile. Comparative studies indicate that the use of this agent results in more rapid obliteration of varices with limited tissue injury. Polidocanol is used in Europe as well. Absolute ethanol is used in many areas also, and, additionally, is commonly used for injection to stop peptic ulcer bleeding because of its ability to produce arteriolar coagulation. In animal studies this agent was found to be more ulcerogenic in the esophagus than the other agents tested.[1] No study has compared these agents in terms of complications from the ulcerations that often develop.

Location of Injection

Most sclerotherapists prefer to inject directly into the varix with the intent of producing the inflammatory reaction and the clot in the varix, limiting the exposure of the adjacent tissue. Unfortunately, fluoroscopic studies indicate that as often as not, when the injection is made, the needle is outside the varix. Since the endoscopist is unaware of the location of the needle tip, he may inject significant amounts of the necrotizing agent into the esophageal soft tissues. As noted above, some endoscopists with excellent results prefer submucosal injections adjacent to the varix ("paravariceal"), rather than intravariceal injections. In this instance, though, the agent injected (polidocanol) is relatively nontoxic and can be injected in significant volumes with limited reaction. When ethanolamine oleate is injected intentionally into the submucosa for the purpose of creating submucosal fibrosis, only small volumes are injected. In either circumstance, ulcerations may result.

Acid Reflux

Injection sclerotherapy does have a short-term effect on esophageal motility and the ability of the esophagus to clear an acid load. The ulcerations that are seen following sclerotherapy do not have the typical smooth appearance of peptic esophageal ulcerations, and occur only at the point of prior injection. While the topical effect of acid probably plays no part on the initial development of an ulcer, acid reflux may play a role in delayed healing. Several investigators have shown more rapid healing of these ulcerations with the use of potent acid inhibitory agents, and some use these drugs routinely through the course of sclerotherapy.[2] Potent acid inhibition does not appear to reduce the incidence of bleeding from these lesions, which often occurs early in the postinjection period. In one report, though, omeprazole did heal ulcerations that had not healed with other therapies, including sucralfate, and did eliminate further bleeding from these ulcerations in six of seven cases.[2] This suggests that there may be a subset of patients in whom acid reflux is a major factor in delayed healing.

Patient Factors

Perhaps the most important variable in the development of sclerotherapy-related ulcerations is the status of the patient. Unfortunately, most of the patients at risk for dying from bleeding esophageal varices and for repeated bleeding episodes, those who would potentially benefit the most from sclerotherapy, are the ones at greatest risk for development of injection-related ulceration. Patients classified by Child's classification as Class C by virtue of prolonged prothrombin time, low albumin, elevated bilirubin, malnutrition, hepatic encephalopathy are more likely to develop injection-related ulcerations than those patients with only limited abnormal parameters. After injection sclerotherapy, one out of three patients classified as Child's C will develop deep ulcerations. The reasons for this increased risk are not clear, but it probably relates to tissue factors and nutrition.

Effects on Morbidity of Sclerotherapy-Induced Ulcerations

Reports of ulceration and morbidity from ulcerations have been quite variable. Bleeding following sclerotherapy may be caused either by recurrent variceal bleeding or by bleeding from the injection-related ulceration. Bleeding from these ulcers is often intermittent and may be missed at the time of repeat endoscopy. The true incidence of bleeding from these lesions is not clear. Nor is there any standardization as to the depth of these lesions.

Esophageal perforation has been reported, particularly in the early experience with sclerotherapy. The incidence of perforation in reported series has ranged from 1 to 6% (Table I).[3] Perforation is caused by extensive necrosis from the injected sclerosant, with ulceration extending beyond the muscular layers of the esophagus through the serosa (Fig. 2). Perforation can be assumed to be a direct effect of the sclerosant, as the use of flexible endoscopy apart from sclerotherapy is rarely associated with this complication.

Review of the data in Table I would suggest that concentration of the various sclerosants is an important determining factor in patient outcome. Tetradecyl in 3% concentration was associated with one of the highest perforation rates and perforation-related deaths. This concentration is rarely used now, with concentrations ranging from 0.5 to 1.5% in use currently. The most common concentration in use currently is 1.0%, deriving from Jensen's studies on sclerosant effects.[1] This is often used in combination with alcohol, diluted with saline.

Polidocanol at 3% concentration was also associated with both a high perforation incidence and a high death rate in these patients, with five of six patients dying in the Copenhagen study. This had an overall effect on the efficacy of this study as well. The Copenhagen Sclerotherapy Group reported that no improvement in survival with sclero-

Table I. Perforation following Esophageal Variceal Sclerotherapy[a]

Author	Sclerosant	Pts	Perforation	Deaths
Lewis	5% morrhuate	101	1 (1%)	0
Kjaerjaard	3% polidocanol	61	1 (2%)	0
Huizinga	5% ethanolamine		1 (3%)	1
McGrew	5% morrhuate	40	1 (3%)	1
Korula	1.5% tetradecyl	63	2 (3%)	2
Sarles	1.5% tetradecyl	50	1 (2%)	1
Shenesh	5% ethanolamine	55	2 (4%)	0
Perino	3% tetradecyl	54	3 (6%)	3
Copenhagen	3% polidocanol	93	6 (6%)	5

[a]Adapted from Perino *et al.*[3]

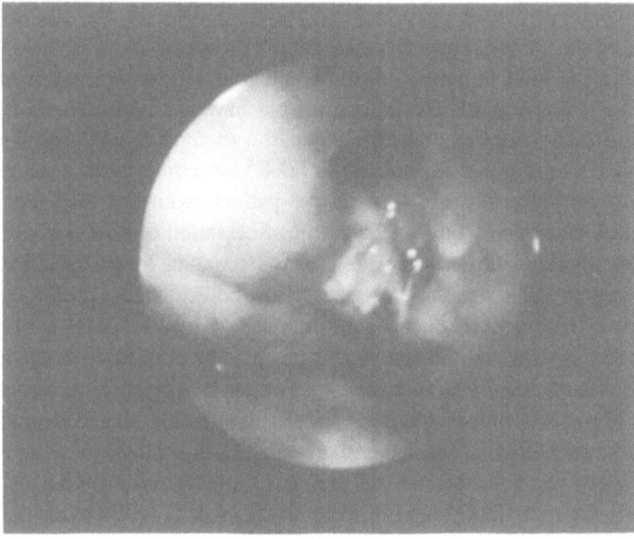

Figure 2. Esophageal perforation following variceal sclerotherapy. (A color version of this figure can be found in the color insert following p. 6.)

therapy was noted compared with medical controls until after the first 45 days, the point at which most of the sclerotherapy complications would have been already manifested. Polidocanol at 1% concentration is most often used today.

Effect of Sucralfate in the Esophagus

Sucralfate has clearly demonstrated benefits in the stomach and duodenum related to many different effects of this agent: cytoprotection, pepsin inhibition, physical barrier, stimulation of mucosal prostaglandins. Benefits in the esophagus have been more difficult to show in the clinical setting of reflux esophagitis, with some studies, but not all, showing significant symptomatic relief and endoscopic healing compared with placebo. The esophageal mucosa, in fact, would appear to respond in a fashion different from the gastric mucosa in some respects. Indomethacin, an agent that inhibits prostaglandins, has been shown to protect the esophagus from radiation injury and acid-related injury in animal studies.

Protection of the esophageal mucosa has been demonstrated with the use of sucralfate, noting a reversal of the decline seen in esophageal mucosal resistance with acid exposure following the administration of sucralfate.[4] These effects were seen both with sucralfate and with its component parts, and do not appear to be prostaglandin-mediated. Other investigators have confirmed this effect of sucralfate protecting the esophageal mucosa from acid exposure independent of a prostaglandin effect.

Use of Sucralfate for Sclerotherapy-Related Ulceration

Because of the unique properties associated with sucralfate, it is not surprising that this agent has been used in patients with complications from variceal injection-related ulcerations, particularly since the lesions do not have the appearance of acid–peptic ulcerations and did not respond particularly to initial attempts at acid control with H_2RAs. Roark published a brief report of such use in 1984.[5] He administered a suspension of 1 g sucralfate in 5 ml glycerol every 4 hr to five patients who had bled repeatedly from injection-related ulcerations. Four of the five had cessation of bleeding within 24 hr.

This report by Roark lead to widespread use of sucralfate for postinjection ulcerations (Fig. 3). The agent was known to have an excellent clinical safety profile, and had been found to have cytoprotective effects in the stomach that were not initially appreciated. Physicians were hopeful that this use would prove to be another such new effect.

This use was studied by Tabibian and co-workers in a prospective randomized trial, randomizing 19 patients with esophageal varices and injection-related ulceration either to treatment with a sucralfate suspension or to placebo, each administered four times a day.[6] Weekly endoscopy was done for a 4-week period. Complete healing of the ulcerations was seen in 7 of 9 in the sucralfate group (78%) but in only 4 of 10 (40%) in the placebo group. The authors concluded, surprisingly, that no beneficial effect had been seen since the difference did not reach statistical significance.

Additionally, the authors noted that the ulcerations in the patients randomized to

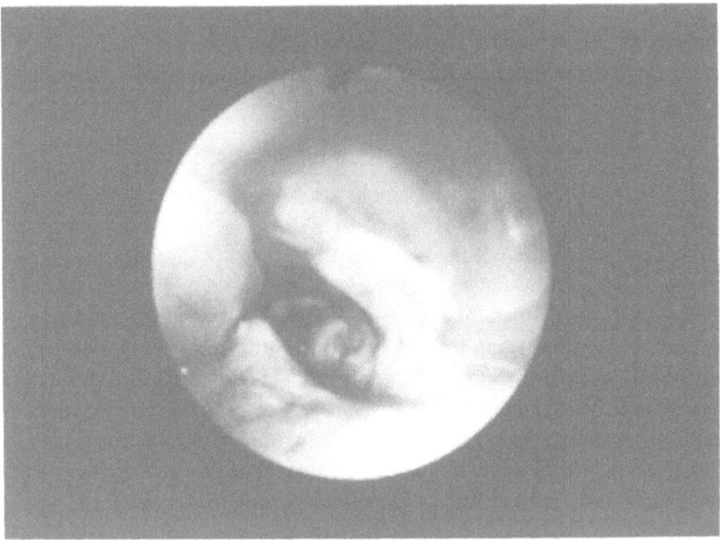

Figure 3. Sucralfate coating of postsclerotherapy esophageal ulcerations. (A color version of this figure can be found in the color insert following p. 6.)

sucralfate were somewhat smaller than those in the control patients, so that any apparent difference might be related to that factor. While a minor difference in ulcer size was apparent in their data, it was also clear that the only patients with ulcerations greater than 2 cm that did in fact heal were those who had been treated with sucralfate. None of the placebo-treated patients with comparable size ulcerations showed healing.

A more correct interpretation of these findings would be that the data suggest a beneficial effect of sucralfate on healing, but that the study was too small to demonstrate this conclusively. In any event, in none of the patients was the clinical course affected by the ulcerations.

A larger study was reported from Paquet's group, with 60 patients randomized prospectively following sclerotherapy with 1% polidocanol to either sucralfate suspensions or placebo.[7] No statistically significant difference was noted between the groups but the observation was made that those randomized to sucralfate had larger ulcerations and appeared to show more rapid healing. In other words, if there had been no drug effect, one might have expected the sucralfate group to have had a slower healing rate, since the ulcers were larger. Such was not the case.

A still larger study was reported by Polson and co-workers from Kings College, with 180 patients being randomized after sclerotherapy.[8] In this study a beneficial effect was seen with sucralfate which was statistically significant. Of interest the effect was more apparent in those patients with well-compensated liver disease, than in the higher-risk group. Bleeding of any sort occurred in only 24% of compensated patients treated with sucralfate, compared with 42% of similar placebo-treated patients ($p < 0.05$). Bleeding thought to be related to the postinjection ulceration occurred in only 10 instances in the sucralfate-treated group compared with 20 in the placebo group ($p < 0.05$). Even so, there was no clear effect on the speed of ulcer healing, and no difference in mortality between the two groups.

Conclusions

Deep ulceration of the esophageal mucosa remains a significant risk of variceal sclerotherapy and a limiting factor in the success of this therapy. Studies would suggest that sucralfate does have a beneficial role in this setting, but the clinical significance is relatively minor. The one study that shows a reduction in bleeding does not show an improvement in healing, and the reduction in bleeding in this study was seen only after the higher-risk patients were removed from analysis. Improvement in survival more logically would follow preventive measures such as reduction in sclerosant concentration or volume, or perhaps use of an alternate technique such as variceal ligation by banding, which has been shown to have fewer complications than sclerotherapy.[9]

References

1. Jensen DM: Sclerosants for injection sclerosis of esophageal varices. *Gastrointest Endosc* **29**:315–317, 1982. One of the few articles comparing sclerosants and mixtures of sclerosants in an animal model. From this article came the popular "Wadsworth solution," a tetradecyl, alcohol, saline mixture.
2. Gimson A, Poison R, Westaby D, *et al*: Omeprazole in the management of intractable esophageal ulceration following injection sclerotherapy. *Gastroenterology* **99**:1829–1831, 1990. Describes results of the use of omeprazole in ten cases with refractory injection-related ulceration. High-dose omeprazole (40 mg/day) healed ulcerations that had been refractory to high dose H_2RAs and sucralfate.
3. Perino LE, Gholson CF, Goff JS: Esophageal perforation after fiberoptic variceal sclerotherapy. *J Clin Gastroenterol* **9**:286–289, 1987. This article reports the authors' experience with this particular complication of sclerotherapy and provides a review of the available literature.
4. Orlando RC: Cytoprotection by sucralfate in acid-exposed esophagus: A review. *Scand J Gastroenterol* **22**(suppl 127):97–100, 1987. A review of animal and clinical studies of the effects of sucralfate on esophageal mucosal protection.
5. Roark G: Treatment of postsclerotherapy esophageal ulcers with sucralfate. *Gastrointest Endosc* **30**:9–10, 1984. The first report of apparent beneficial effects from the use of sucralfate for postinjection ulceration bleeding (an uncontrolled observation—but dramatic results).
6. Tabibian N, Smith JL, Graham DY: Sclerotherapy-associated esophageal ulcers: Lessons from a double-blind, randomized comparison of sucralfate suspension versus placebo. *Gastrointest Endosc* **35**:312–315, 1989. The first randomized trial of sucralfate for injection-related ulceration. No clear effect found despite 78 versus 40% benefit for sucralfate in healing, as numbers were insufficient for significance.
7. Paquet KJ, Koussouris P, Keineth R, *et al*: A comparison of sucralfate with placebo in the treatment of esophageal ulcers following therapeutic endoscopic sclerotherapy of esophageal varices—a prospective randomized trial. *Am J Med* **91**(2A):147S–150S, 1991. A large randomized trial showing faster healing for ulcerations in patients randomized to sucralfate, but no difference in the percent healed, as the patients randomized to sucralfate had significantly larger ulcerations.

8. Polson RJ, Westaby D, Gimson AE, *et al*: Sucralfate for the prevention of early rebleeding following injection sclerotherapy for esophageal varices. *Hepatology* **3**:279–282, 1989. A large randomized trial showing reduced bleeding in the postinjection period, but the benefit was not seen in the decompensated patients, only those with reasonably well-compensated liver disease.
9. Steigmann G, Goff J, Michaletz-Onody P, *et al*: Endoscopic sclerotherapy as compared with endoscopic ligation for bleeding esophageal varices. *N Engl J Med* **326**:1527–1532, 1992. A large randomized cooperative trial showing variceal ligation by endoscopic banding to be superior to variceal injection sclerotherapy with reduced complications and improved survival.

VIII

The Clinical Role of Sucralfate in Peptic Ulcer Therapy—Comparison with H-2 Blockers and Pump Inhibitors: A Projection for the Nineties

32

Future Research into the Mechanisms of Action of Sucralfate

DANIEL HOLLANDER

Sucralfate is a nonabsorbable, nonsystematic agent for the therapy and prevention of peptic ulcer disease. The drug was originally developed in Japan as an agent to deactivate peptic activity. Sucralfate was found to adhere to both ulcerated and normal mucosa with a preference for damaged areas of the gastric mucosa.[1] For these reasons, the original proposals to explain sucralfate's therapeutic efficacy and its mechanisms of action included both pepsin antagonism and surface adhesion which presumably protect ulcerated areas from luminal acid, enzymes and exogenous damaging agents such as NSAIDs, or alcohol.

There is no question that the original thoughts as to the mechanisms of action of sucralfate did explain, in part, the mechanisms by which sucralfate exerts its therapeutic effect. However, it is equally clear that surface adherence and pepsin antagonism are only two of the several known mechanisms by which sucralfate exerts its therapeutic effects. Subsequent research in the United States by Hollander and Tarnawski discovered that sucralfate stimulated the normal gastric mucosa to synthesize protective prostaglandins of the PGE_1 and PGE_2 groups.[2–5]

The discovery that sucralfate stimulates prostaglandin production[2] was important because of the emerging recognition at that time of the great importance of prostaglandins in both maintaining normal gastric and duodenal mucosal integrity as well as accelerating the healing of ulcerated areas.[6–8] Prostaglandins stimulate the production of mucus and bicarbonate at the surface of the gastric mucosa which form an alkaline microclimate. Prostaglandins also stimulate cell proliferation in the gastric glands, augment renewal of the surface epithelium, and increase the resistance of the endothelium of blood vessels to

DANIEL HOLLANDER • Dean's Office, University of Kansas School of Medicine, Kansas City, Kansas 66160-7300.

Sucralfate: From Basic Science to the Bedside, edited by Daniel Hollander and G. N. J. Tytgat. Plenum Press, New York, 1995.

injury by a variety of agents including alcohol and nonsteroidals. By maintaining the integrity of the vasculature of the stomach, prostaglandins improve gastric mucosal resistance to injury and stimulate restitution of the mucosa by ensuring adequate supplies of blood, oxygenation, and nutrients to the gastric mucosa.[6–8] The discovery that sucralfate stimulates production of prostaglandins by the gastroduodenal mucosa was a great step forward because it was the first therapeutic agent which was found to depend on prostaglandin stimulation for its efficacy.[9]

This discovery raised the question of how a nonabsorbable surface-acting compound, such as sucralfate, would act to induce the synthesis of prostaglandins by the stomach and duodenum. Since it had always been assumed that prostaglandins are synthesized predominantly by cells in the lamina propria and not by surface epithelial cells, the ability of surface-acting nonabsorbable sucralfate to stimulate synthesis of prostaglandins could not be readily explained. We will return to this question later in the discussion and discuss research that might clarify this important physiological question.

Subsequent studies of its mechanisms of action suggest that sucralfate may modulate sulfhydryl compounds such as glutathione.[10,11] More recent evidence suggests that sucralfate promotes healing of ulcerations by binding growth factors, such as basic fibroblast growth factor, in the lumen and concentrating them at the site of ulcerations.[12]

Future research on the mechanisms of action of sucralfate should investigate the effects of sucralfate on *Helicobacter pylori*, on reactive forms of oxygen, and on the elaboration of nitric oxide. Perhaps the most interesting area of all would be to study sucralfate's role in the activation of surface receptors which trigger the activities of leukocytes, mast cells, macrophages, and cytokine-dependent immune activities. In the discussion that follows, these areas will be discussed briefly. By necessity, these possibilities are strictly speculative, have very little experimental evidence to support them, and, in fact, may turn out not to be true. However, the intent of what follows is to stimulate new research about sucralfate's mechanisms of action.

A major question which needs to be answered is whether sucralfate penetrates the surface epithelium and enters the lamina propria of the gastroduodenal mucosa. The substitution of sulfated aluminum salts on the sucrose backbone prevents the sucralfate molecule from being hydrolyzed and absorbed through the normal disaccharide pathways. However, we know that there are multiple routes by which large molecules penetrate the surface epithelium. The three major routes of penetration of the mucosa that need to be explored are uptake by the paracellular route, transport through transcellular pinocytosis, and sampling of sucralfate by small intestinal M cells.[13]

Contrary to previous beliefs, recent experimental evidence demonstrates that larger molecules such as lactulose, intact sucrose, inulin, and dextran penetrate the gastrointestinal epithelium through tight junctional paracellular routes. Penetration of such large molecules occurs in amounts that are less than 1% of the administered amounts. However, even small amounts can be significant in instigating reactions and interactions between molecules such as sucralfate and immune components of the lamina propria and submucosa of the gastrointestinal mucosa. Therefore, studies need to be done to ascertain whether 1% or less of ingested sucralfate does indeed penetrate through the tight junctions of the stomach and proximal small intestine and could perhaps reach the basolateral portion of the gastrointestinal epithelial cells. Separate experiments need to explore the question of transcellular penetration of sucralfate into the lamina propria perhaps by pinocytosis.[13]

If sucralfate is shown to be transported into the basolateral space of the surface epithelium and into the lamina propria of the gastroduodenal mucosa, the implications regarding its mechanisms of action could be very significant. Once sucralfate has been transported to the lamina propria, it can have access to mucosal lymphocytes and mast cells which are important in immune reactions, secretion of cytokines, and in defensive and repair mechanisms of the gastrointestinal mucosa. In addition, once having penetrated the surface epithelium, sucralfate could conceivably activate various receptors on the basolateral surface of the gastrointestinal epithelium and on cells within the lamina propria. The cells in the lamina propria that are of particular interest include leukocytes, lymphocytes, mast cells, and macrophages. If sucralfate can reach these cells, it could activate surface receptors on these cells in order to stimulate the secretion of prostaglandins, interleukins, nitrous oxide, and a wide variety of growth factors. Thus, the partial penetration of sucralfate into the lamina propria, if substantiated experimentally, could explain its ability to stimulate the secretion of prostaglandins, growth factors, nitrous oxide, and cytokines which could be involved in a wide host of proliferative, reparative, and defensive functions of the mucosa. Penetration of sucralfate into the lamina propria could also explain the ability of sucralfate to stimulate angiogenesis and to protect blood vessels and capillaries in the lamina propria from injury by luminal factors such as alcohol.

Another area which is quite separate from the ability of sucralfate to penetrate the lamina propria across the gastroduodenal epithelium is the question of stimulation of surface receptors on the luminal side of the gastroduodenal epithelium. At the time of sucralfate's initial development, information was very scanty regarding surface receptors on cells in general and on gastroduodenal epithelial cells in particular. Therefore, the assumption at that time was made that a nonsystemic agent such as sucralfate could not possibly interact with cells except for a physical interaction such as adhesion. Now, more than 20 years later, we have a much greater understanding regarding surface receptors of all cells. We know that all cells possess a wide array of surface receptor molecules which include receptors of immunoglobulin family, the integrins, and specific receptors for hormones, cytokines, and growth factors.[14] We are beginning to learn more about surface receptors on the luminal surface of intestinal epithelial cells and undoubtedly this area will become better developed in the future. Therefore, another potentially productive area for research is the interaction between luminal sucralfate which has not been absorbed and surface receptors on the luminal surface of gastroduodenal epithelial cells. It is quite possible that luminal sucralfate could indeed stimulate a whole host of cellular proliferation, cell renewal, and cell signaling reactions in epithelial cells of the stomach and duodenum without being absorbed. These reactions could explain the ability of sucralfate to stimulate epithelial renewal and restitution and could explain how sucralfate may in fact stimulate production of compounds such as prostaglandins, cytokines, nitric oxide, and growth factors without penetrating the surface epithelium.

Another area of research which needs to be expanded has to do with the potential ability of sucralfate to interact with *H. pylori*. It is not entirely clear whether sucralfate can modify the viability and pathological effects of *H. pylori* nor is it entirely clear whether sucralfate in combination with antibiotics could in some way enhance the eradication of *H. pylori*. This area needs to be investigated since the eradication of *H. pylori* can prevent the recurrence of duodenal ulcerations.[15]

Two other relatively new areas in peptic ulcer disease research need to be investigated as potential mechanisms of action of sucralfate. These two new areas have to do with the injurious effect of oxygen radicals and with the role of nitric oxide as a messenger system within the mucosa. Oxygen radicals are known to be damaging to tissues and cells. Oxygen radicals may play some role in mucosal injury of the stomach and duodenum. Sucralfate needs to be examined as to its potential ability to scavenge oxygen free radicals or inhibit their formation. Whether sucralfate has a direct effect on oxygen free radicals or whether some of the reactions which it stimulates could in some way modify oxygen free radical activity is not known.

The area of nitric oxide as a major mediator of a variety of reactions within the mucosa is new. It will be useful to examine whether sucralfate administration modifies nitric oxide-dependent reactions. Likewise it will be important to know whether any of the reactions which are stimulated by sucralfate such as prostaglandin release may also modify the nitric oxide system. At present, little information exists along these lines but the question nevertheless needs to be investigated.

The last area of research that should be considered is the interaction between sucralfate and the small intestinal and large intestinal epithelium. There are some preliminary studies suggesting that sucralfate may have some activity in controlling inflammatory bowel disease.[16] There are no mechanistic studies that could explain why or how sucralfate may be helpful in inflammatory bowel disease. However, in our discussion, we have indicated that some percentage of sucralfate may penetrate the surface epithelium and could reach the lamina propria of the gastrointestinal mucosa by either paracellular or transcellular routes. This possibility should be investigated in the colonic epithelium. If sucralfate can penetrate the colonic surface epithelium and reach the lamina propria of the colon, it could interact with inflammatory cells such as lymphocytes, leukocytes, neutrophils, mast cells, and macrophages in the colon. Such interaction could perhaps lead to suppression of inflammation and stimulation of restitution of the mucosa and could point to therapeutic possibilities of the use of sucralfate in inflammatory bowel disease. Clearly, this area is highly speculative and needs basic scientific studies to show whether sucralfate can reach the lamina propria of the large bowel and thus perhaps exert a therapeutic effect.

In summary, sucralfate could activate numerous defensive and regenerative mucosal functions by interaction with surface receptors of the epithelium or by absorption through the tight junctions into the lamina propria of the gastrointestinal mucosa. By either route sucralfate could activate several immune, biochemical, or cell stimulatory reactions which could account for its cytoprotective and reparative mechanisms.

References

1. Bighley L, Giesing D: Mechanism of action studies of sucralfate, in Caspary W (ed): *Duodenal Ulcer, Gastric Ulcer: Sucralfate, a New Therapeutic Concept*. Munich, Urban & Schwarzenberg, 1981, pp 3–12. Early thoughts as to the mechanisms of action of sucralfate.

2. Hollander D, Tarnawski A, Gergely H, *et al*: Sucralfate protection of the gastric mucosa against ethanol-induced injury: A prostaglandin-mediated process? *Scan J Gastroenterol* **19**:97–102, 1984.
3. Hollander D, Tarnawski A, Krause WJ, *et al*: The protective effect of sucralfate against alcohol-induced gastric mucosal injury in the rat. Macroscopic, histologic, ultrastructural and functional time sequence analysis. *Gastroenterology* **88**:366–374, 1985.
4. Tarnawski A, Hollander D, Krause WJ, *et al*: Does sucralfate affect the normal gastric mucosa? Histologic, ultrastructural and functional assessment. *Gastroenterology* **90**:893–905, 1986.
5. Tarnawski A, Hollander D, Stachura J, *et al*: Effect of sucralfate on the normal human gastric mucosa. Endoscopic, histological and ultrastructural assessment. *Scand J Gastroenterol* **22**:111–123, 1987. References 2–5 explored the mechanisms of sucralfate interaction with the normal and ulcerated gastric mucosa and sucralfate's cytoprotective mechanisms.
6. Tarnawski A, Hollander D, Stachura J, *et al*: Prostaglandin protection of the gastric mucosa against alcohol injury, a dynamic time related process. The role of the mucosal proliferative zone. *Gastroenterology* **89**:366–374, 1985.
7. Tarnawski A, Stachura J, Gergely H, *et al*: Microvascular endothelium—A major target for alcohol injury of the human gastric mucosa. Histochemical and ultrastructural study. *J Clin Gastroenterol* **10**:53–64, 1988.
8. Tarnawski A, Stachura J, Hollander D, *et al*: Cellular aspects of alcohol-induced injury and prostaglandin protection of the human gastric mucosa. Focus on the mucosal microvessels. *J Clin Gastroenterol* **10**:35–45, 1988. References 6–8 represent some of the key experiments regarding the mechanisms of cytoprotective activity of prostaglandins.
9. Hollander D, Tarnawski A: *Gastric Cytoprotection: A Clinician's Guide*. New York, Plenum Press, 1989. A general review of the concept of cytoprotection, its mechanisms, and its clinical applications. This book is directed at both investigators and clinicians.
10. Szabo S, Brown A: Prevention of ethanol-induced vascular injury and gastric mucosal lesions by sucralfate and its components: Possible role of endogenous sulfhydryls. *Proc Soc Exp Biol Med* **185**:493–497, 1987.
11. Szabo S, Hollander D: Pathways of gastrointestinal protection and repair. *Am J Med* **86**(6A):23–31, 1989.
12. Konturek SJ, Brzozowski T, Bielanski W, *et al*: Epidermal growth factor in the gastroprotective and ulcer-healing actions of sucralfate in rats. *Am J Med* **86**(6A):32–37, 1989. References 10–12 add other mechanisms to the list of mechanisms of action of sucralfate.
13. Hollander D: Permeability in Crohn's disease: Altered barrier functions in healthy relatives? *Gastroenterology* **104**:1848–1851, 1993. A review of the concept of intestinal permeability of larger molecules. Permeability of the gastrointestinal barrier by sucralfate could instigate immunological and reparative reactions in the subepithelial layers and explain some of sucralfate's clinical activity.
14. Hollander D: Integrins: A family of cell surface adhesion receptors—Relevance to intestinal immune defenses. *Eur J Gastroenterol Hepatol* **5**:593–599, 1993. Review of cell surface adhesion molecules of the gastroduodenal mucosa.
15. Thomson ABR: Helicobacter pylori and gastroduodenal pathology. *Can J Gastroenterol* **7**:353–358, 1993. Recent review of the importance of *H. pylori* in ulcer disease.
16. Bianchi Porro G, Hollander D: *Treatment of Digestive Disease with Sucralfate*. New York, Raven Press, 1989. Review of the mechanisms of action of sucralfate with preliminary data on the possible activity of sucralfate in intestinal inflammation.

33

Future Clinical Development of Sucralfate

G. N. J. TYTGAT

Predictions of future clinical applicability of sucralfate are obviously frought with difficulty. Nevertheless, based on the current knowledge of sucralfate's mode of action, one can envisage several clinical disease states where evaluation of its applicability might be considered useful. Such evaluations would be the more desirable the lesser other therapeutic possibilities are available for both symptomatic and objective improvement of these disease states.

At first some clinical conditions will be discussed where there is already some preliminary evidence of potential efficacy. The second part will be devoted to speculation with respect to future potential applicability in as yet unexplored areas. Such speculation is largely based on sucralfate's binding capacity to mucosal surfaces especially when inflamed or denuded and its stimulating action on mucus production and bicarbonate secretion together with its effects on surface phospholipids, prostaglandin synthesis, mucosal blood flow, cell proliferation, and availability of epidermal growth factor.

Prevention and Therapy of Irradiation-Induced Discomfort and Mucosal Damage

Irradiation is often a cornerstone in the management of various malignancies, but patients receiving such cancer therapy are regularly afflicted with a diversity of adverse effects.

Radiation damage is a well-known complication of the therapy of esophageal and pulmonary cancer, cancer of the prostate, urinary bladder, or other malignancies in the pelvis since various parts of the small and/or large intestine are positioned in the field of therapy. Enteropathy during and after irradiation can be seen in almost all patients

G. N. J. TYTGAT • Department of Gastroenterology–Hepatology, Academisch Medical Centre, University of Amsterdam, Amsterdam, The Netherlands.

Sucralfate: From Basic Science to the Bedside, edited by Daniel Hollander and G. N. J. Tytgat. Plenum Press, New York, 1995.

following radiation doses of 40–80 Gy. Proctitis accounts for more than 75% of radiation injuries in the gut. Acute radiation injury is attributed mainly to the sensitivity of the epithelial cells resulting from their short cell cycle time. Late radiation injury is attributed mainly to obliterative damage of the vasculature of the bowel, jeopardizing adequate blood supply.

The postulated mechanisms of action of sucralfate in radiation-induced enteropathy relate to coating and protection of denuded surfaces (Fig. 1), perhaps stimulation of cytoprotective mechanisms and binding of irritating bile salts. Coating of denuded surfaces may provide local protection against various luminal irritants, enzymes and toxic factors, bile salts, food constituents, etc.[1] Especially the binding capacity for bile salts can have an additive effect in preventing discomfort when the terminal ileum is damaged causing cholorrheic diarrhea.[2]

Forty-five patients with ENT malignancies treated with 60–70 Gy in two opposing fields were treated either with 1 g sucralfate suspension qid orally for 5 min or with standard oral hygiene.[3] Minimal or absent oral mucosal inflammation, pain, or dysphagia were found in the majority of the sucralfate-treated patients. Topical efficacy appeared to be less in the hypopharynx presumably because of the shorter dwell time compared with the mouth.

Fifty-one consecutive patients with various gynecological malignancies were treated with sucralfate tablets 2 g qid in a randomized but open study.[4] Pelvic irradiation with the

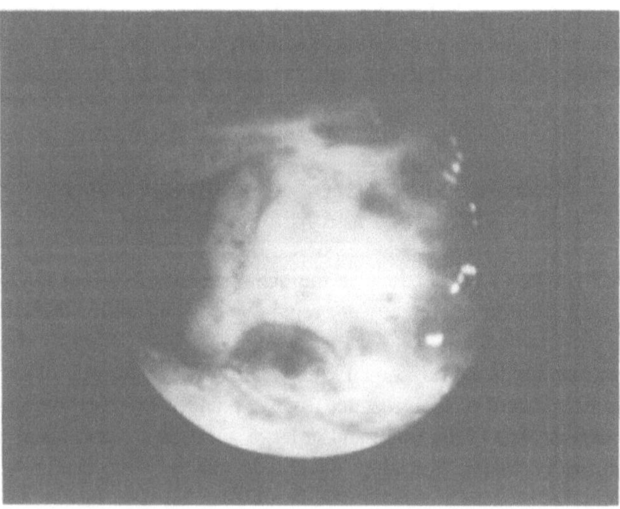

Figure 1. Distal rectal postradiation ulceration, selectively coated with sucralfate suspension (2 g/20 ml). (A color version of this figure can be found in the color insert following p. 6.)

four-field technique was given to all patients with ovarian carcinoma and to patients with more advanced stages of cervical carcinoma. The frequency of diarrhea was almost 50% less in the sucralfate group compared with the controls. The patients receiving sucralfate in general displayed only minor alterations of bowel habits and therefore required less loperamide compared with controls. Symptoms such as nausea, vomiting, and loss of appetite were also reduced in the sucralfate group.

These findings were largely confirmed in a double-blind placebo-controlled study in 70 patients receiving pelvic irradiation with a curative intent for carcinoma of the prostate or urinary bladder without distant metastases.[5] The total pelvic radiation dose in a four-field technique was 62–66 Gy and the total treatment time was 6½ weeks. Sucralfate granules or placebo were dispensed 2 weeks after radiation started and continued for 6 weeks. One dose package of 1 g was to be dissolved in water six times daily. Seven of thirty-four evaluable patients in the placebo group and 18 of 32 patients in the sucralfate group did not develop diarrhea during the observation period. In the others, the frequency of defecation and stool consistency were significantly improved by sucralfate. Fourteen patients in the placebo group and only three in the sucralfate group required symptomatic therapy with loperamide. There was, however, no significant difference in the appearance of blood or mucus in the stool or abdominal cramps between the groups. One year later, the patients in the sucralfate group displayed significantly less problems with bloody mucoid diarrhea. Thus, sucralfate appears to be of benefit in diminishing bowel discomfort during radiotherapy of pelvic malignancies. This study confirms previous uncontrolled observations in patients but is in contradiction with an irradiation-induced proctitis study in the rat.

Eight patients with radiation proctitis were treated with enemas of 10% sucralfate suspension of 2 g in 20 ml water bid for 3 weeks in an open study.[6] These patients were unresponsive to a prior 4-week course of conventional therapy including sulfasalazine and topical steroids. The majority of the patients experienced reduced stool frequency and bleeding stopped in six of them. In addition, all patients showed sigmoidoscopic improvement. These results confirm earlier data in chronic radiation proctitis, where sucralfate suspension was seen to adhere to the injured bleeding mucosal surface.

Commentary

The fact that sucralfate substantially diminished irradiation-induced diarrhea and abdominal discomfort in patients receiving radiotherapy for pelvic carcinoma and most importantly also reduced the late intestinal damage should be of significant interest to clinicians. Whether this beneficial effect is unique for sucralfate or whether similar results may also be obtained with other pharmaceutical regimens requires further study. There is uncertainty with respect to the most optimal way of administering sucralfate. It may perhaps be preferable to have the drug designed as a slow-release preparation for optimal effect in the lower part of the gastrointestinal tract. Also the most optimal composition for topical application with respect to binding quality, dwell time, etc. requires further study. It also remains to be studied whether long-term sucralfate therapy can prevent the late postradiation consequences?

Prevention and Therapy of Chemotherapy-Induced Discomfort and Mucosal Damage

Mucositis is a common and distressful complication of chemotherapy (Fig. 2). Approximately 40% of patients will develop oral complications during cancer chemotherapy depending on the regimen used. In addition, a destroyed epithelial layer favors infectious complications. Patients complain of discomfort, dry mouth, burning sensation, and pain. Severe erythema and ulceration may be seen when stomatitis is severe. Stomatitis usually appears after 4–6 days, reaches a peak intensity around the 10th day, and resolves in another week or two.

The application of 1 g sucralfate during 1 min on the buccal mucosa six times per day in patients treated with cycles of epirubicine after failed cisplatin therapy was evaluated in an open study.[7] There was no evidence of buccal mucositis in 55% of the treatment cycles. Failures were always related to noncompliance or delay in starting therapy.

Mouth-swishing with sucralfate as prophylaxis against chemotherapy-induced stomatitis was evaluated in a double-blind crossover study.[8] Using radioactively labeled sucralfate, the authors found that 20–30% was still adherent to the oral mucosal lining 2.5 hr after mouth-swishing. Forty-five patients receiving cisplatin and continuous infusion with 5-fluorouracil for 5 days were entered in this placebo-controlled study. Among 23 evaluable patients a significant reduction in the objective score of edema, erythema, erosion, and ulceration was seen during treatment with sucralfate. Ten patients did not complete the study since the swishing procedure aggravated chemotherapy-induced

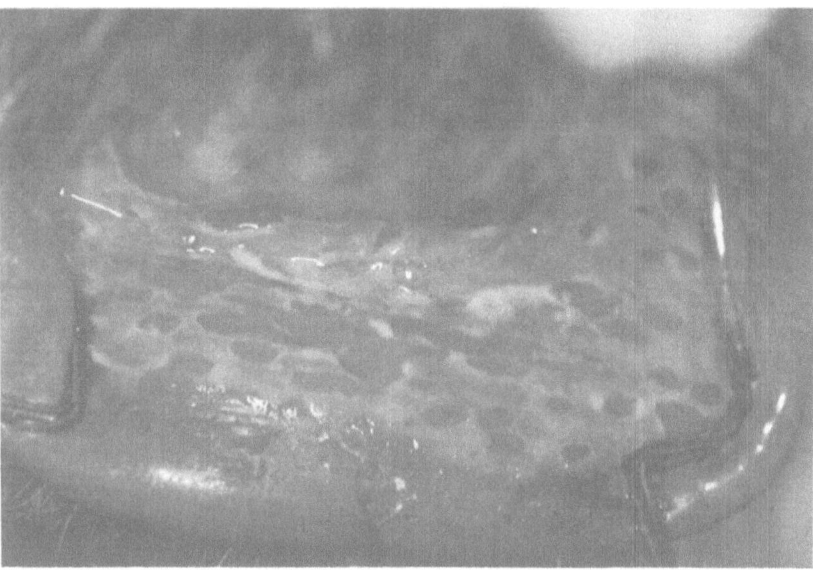

Figure 2. Severe oral chemotherapy-induced mucositis. (A color version of this figure can be found in the color insert following p. 6.)

nausea. According to the authors, the oral medication should have a neutral taste, the solution should not be swallowed, and swishing should not be started until nausea has ceased or is adequately dealt with pharmacologically.

Such results confirm initial pilot studies indicating that patients treated with stomatotoxic chemotherapeutic agents may benefit from oral sucralfate suspension.

The further usefulness of sucralfate was prospectively evaluated in 98 patients with a spectrum of malignancies, treated with chemotherapy.[9] The patients received at least three cycles of chemotherapy with various chemotherapeutic agents. Incidence and severity of heartburn, paleness, nausea, and abdominal cramps were scored. Of the 98 patients, 47 developed such symptoms under chemotherapy. After sucralfate therapy, symptoms improved in 38 (81%) patients. In 8 patients there was transient worsening of heartburn and nausea. Overall improvement was significant for heartburn and nausea. The authors conclude that long-term sucralfate is effective in prophylaxis and treatment of chemotherapy-induced complaints.

In contrast, negative results were reported for 48 children and adolescents with acute nonlymphocytic leukemia treated with sucralfate suspensions or placebo qid during 10 weeks of intensive chemotherapy.[10] Discomfort and severity of mucositis were similar but sucralfate reduced colonization of the alimentary tract with potential pathogens perhaps through interference with adherence to mucosal membranes.

Commentary

Sucralfate suspension may be useful in chemotherapy-induced mucositis. Obviously other measures such as meticulous mouth hygiene are of equal importance in this distressful condition. Coating of the inflamed surface is presumably the dominant aspect of sucralfate's action. It is interesting to note that colonization with pathogenic microorganisms seems to be reduced after coating the inflamed mucosa with sucralfate. Improvement in the composition of the sucralfate suspension or the development of more appropriate forms of dispension (chewing tabs?) may enhance patient acceptability.

Solitary Rectal Ulcer Syndrome

Solitary rectal ulcer syndrome (Fig. 3) is an uncommon condition. The cause is presumably multifactorial (excessive straining at stool, invagination, automanipulation, etc.). Conventional medical therapy with abstinence from straining at stool, high-fiber diet, and enemas or suppositories with mesalazine and/or corticosteroids occasionally fails.

As previous studies had shown that ^{99m}Tc-labeled sucralfate adheres to colonic ulcerations, it was logical to find out whether sucralfate was useful in solitary rectal ulcer syndrome.[11] Topical sucralfate may be administered using either water or propylcellulose as vehicle.

In a first study, six patients were treated with a 10% sucralfate suspension.[12] Gradual healing of the ulcers was obtained in five of the six patients.

In a second study, five patients with solitary rectal ulcer unresponsive to conventional

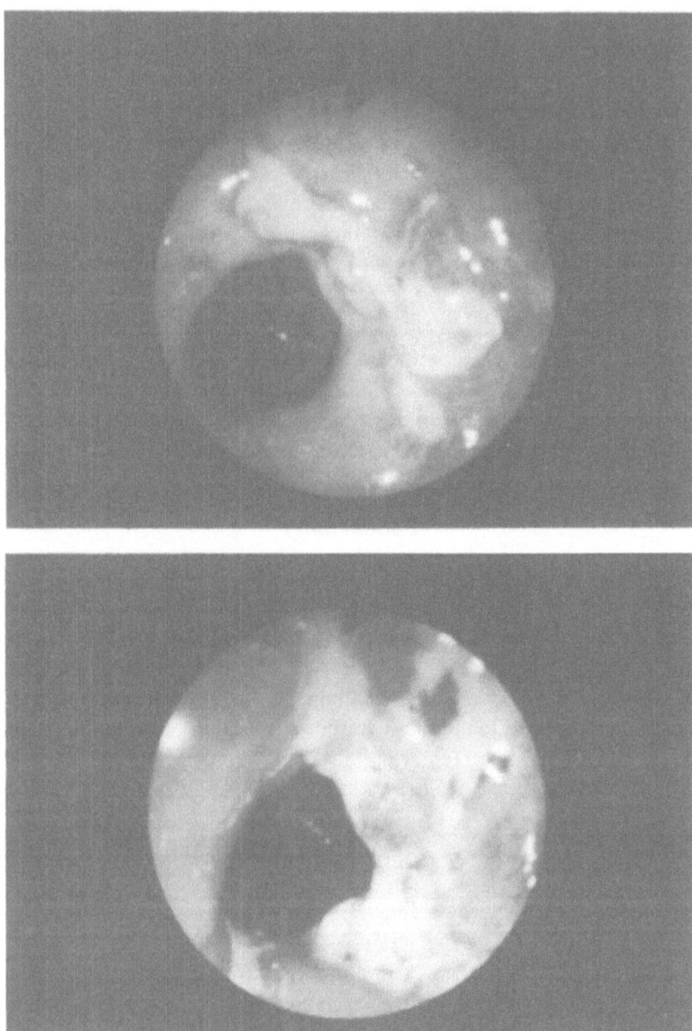

Figure 3. Solitary ulcer of the rectum. Coating with sucralfate suspension (p 1 h) 2 g/20 ml enemas. (A color version of this figure can be found in the color insert following p. 6.)

medical therapy were treated with a 10% sucralfate suspension enema of 2 g in 20 ml water bid.[6] In four of the five patients, symptoms disappeared and ulcer size diminished by 50%.

Similar results were obtained in two patients with solitary ulcer resistant to conventional therapy using sucralfate enemas in 10% glycerine pH 5.2 tid.[13] The sucralfate suspension was shown to adhere to the ulcer crater for at least 4 hr. Apparently the alkaline pH of the rectal lumen did not adversely affect the binding of sucralfate to the ulcer crater.

Finally, six patients with solitary rectal ulcers were treated with topical sucralfate suspension 2 g in 30 ml water bid for 6 weeks.[14] Four patients had complete relief of symptoms and the remaining two had marked improvement. Macroscopic healing occurred in all and five remained in remission for an average of 8 months.

Commentary

It is intriguing that topical administration of sucralfate speeds up healing of solitary ulcers. Presumably coating the ulcer base and sealing the latter from the septic toxic colonic content favors healing. Whether other mechanisms (binding of growth factors, stimulation of mucus secretion, stimulation of angiogenesis, etc.?) are also involved is unknown but probable.

The optimum dose of sucralfate and the optimal vehicle for preparation of the suspension need to be determined. Whether sucralfate suppositories would be equally effective is also unknown. Finally, placebo-controlled and comparative trials with other pharmaceutical principles are necessary before topical sucralfate therapy can be considered established for this indication.

Efficacy of Sucralfate in Ulcerative Colitis (UC)

The rationale of evaluating sucralfate in UC is mainly based on its capability of coating inflamed and denuded surfaces, thereby protecting the mucosa against the damaging effects of luminal irritants, and injurious toxins. Furthermore, stimulation of mucus secretion, improvement in epithelial cell renewal and repair, or changes in mucosal prostaglandin levels and blood flow may also be of potential benefit.

Studies using labeled sucralfate provided evidence in favor of the concept of specific adherence to inflamed or ulcerated areas. Dawson *et al.*[11] evaluated [^{99m}Tc]sucralfate in 34 patients with inflammatory bowel disease and 29 controls. Adult patients drank 250 mg sucralfate containing 130–200 MB_9 ^{99m}Tc suspended in 200 ml iced water followed by 500 ml 10% mannitol to hasten gastric emptying and intestinal transit. Serial isotope scans of the abdomen were obtained between 2 and 6 hr and after 20 and 24 hr. Positive scans were obtained in all ten UC patients. These initial promising results were, however, not confirmed in several later studies. Deveaux *et al.*[15] found a poor correlation between [^{99m}Tc]sucralfate scan and ^{111}In-labeled leukocyte scans and questioned whether separation of technetium from sucralfate was responsible for the discrepancy. Several others were unable to correlate [^{99m}Tc]albumin sucralfate scintigraphic findings with the presence and site of inflammatory lesions.[16,17]

A second reason to embark on clinical evaluation of topical sucralfate in UC was the apparently beneficial activity that had been observed in experimental colitis, induced by instillation of 10% acetic acid in rats.[18]

At first, several open trials were performed. Carling *et al.*[19] used a 10% sucralfate suspension in 100 ml water or propylcellulose solution bid and found improvement in 11 of 13 UC patients. Similar uncontrolled results were obtained by Bennani[20] in 55 UC patients using 8 g sucralfate in 200 ml water bid. In contrast, such improvement was not confirmed by other authors.[21]

Surprisingly, no controlled trial of sucralfate versus placebo has been carried out in UC so far. Instead several studies compared sucralfate with either topical steroids or mesalazine. Riley *et al.*[22] compared a daily 100-ml enema of 4 g sucralfate in 5% methylcellulose solution with 20 mg prednisolone metasulfobenzoate in 44 patients with distal UC for 4 weeks. In the sucralfate group there was clinical improvement in 77% and endoscopic improvement in 59%. Of the 37 evaluable patients there was greater resolution of rectal bleeding and more marked histological improvement in the prednisolone-treated group.

Boniface *et al.*[23] compared 20 g sucralfate in 100 ml to 20 mg methylprednisolone in a 100-ml enema bid for 1 week and uid for 3 weeks. Of the evaluable patients with distal UC, 7 of 16 sucralfate- and 11 of 20 prednisolone-treated patients improved or went into remission.

Campieri *et al.*[24] compared 100-ml enemas with either 10 g sucralfate, 2 g mesalazine, or placebo uid in 50 patients with distal UC. A 94% clinical, 88% endoscopic, and 83% histological improvement was observed in the mesalazine therapy compared with 22, 28, and 17% respectively in the sucralfate group, the latter values comparable to those obtained with placebo.

Commentary

Overall the results of sucralfate in inflammatory bowel disease are not very exciting. Perhaps the premises on which the putative applicability was based are erroneous. The electrostatic binding forces between sucralfate and free proteins in damaged mucosa are said to be pH-dependent. A low-pH environment favors sucralfate binding. The possibility exists in the colon that a relatively high pH minimizes these binding forces and that (labeled) sucralfate remains mixed with luminal contents instead. Furthermore, the long-term stability of [^{99m}Tc]sucralfate–protein complex has been questioned to allow its visualization by scanning after several hours. Also the pharmaceutical aspects of sucralfate enemas should be considered. Sucralfate powder sediments rapidly in a nonviscous base. Therefore, sucralfate powder is usually suspended in 5% methylcellulose solution. The effects of the latter compound on the sucralfate–tissue interaction are unknown. It may be of value to reassess sucralfate's action in UC once the conditions of dose, vehicle, pH, dosing scheme, etc. have been optimized.

Future Potential Applicability of Sucralfate

Many gastrointestinal disease states, especially those associated with mucosal damage and ulceration, deserve further evaluation with sucralfate. Priority should be given to those diseases for which no other efficacious pharmacologic possibilities are currently available.

The conditions that could theoretically benefit from sucralfate therapy should be selected based on sucralfate's most important and firmly established modes of action, both within the lumen and at the level of the mucosal surface: adhesion to inflamed and denuded areas, reduction of diffusion of "irritating" substances, inactivation of proteolytic enzymes, binding of bile salts, targeting growth-promoting molecules such as EGF, stimulation of mucosal blood flow and angiogenesis, stimulation of prostaglandin synthesis, stimulation of bicarbonate transport, improvement of the structure and function of the mucus gel and of surface hydrophobicity.

Clinical conditions to be evaluated at the level of the esophagus may include drug-induced mucosal damage or pill esophagitis, caustic damage, postelectrocautery or postlaser ulceration and perhaps mucosal damage after photodynamic therapy. W. A. Webb advises that patients with moderate to severe caustic damage of the esophagus be treated with a sucralfate slurry of 1 g in 30–50 ml warm water tid and nocte in addition to a liquid H_2RA to help with esophageal healing.

There is a spectrum of diseases of the stomach which is currently resistant to therapy, where evaluation of sucralfate might be considered. This list includes: raised erosive/varioliform gastritis; hypertrophic hypersecretory gastritis with severe mucosal inflammation and severe coarsening of the gastric rugae pattern; congestive (entero)gastropathy in patients with cirrhosis of the liver; gastric antral vascular ectasia or telangiectasia (antral angiomatosis or watermelon stomach) in patients with portal hypertension. In addition, necrotic lesions after injection of necrotizing agents, laser, photodynamic therapy, upper abdominal radiation therapy, etc. should also be considered for evaluation.

At the level of the small bowel, sucralfate's potential usefulness in diffuse chemotherapy-induced mucositis and diffuse NSAID-induced damage deserves further evaluation. Also, patients with chronic or recurrent bleeding from diffuse vascular malformation should be eligible for a pilot trial with sucralfate therapy, in an attempt to decrease the bleeding rate. Mucosal inflammation of an ileoanal pouch after proctocolectomy is a common condition. Although this inflammatory condition appears to improve with antibiotic therapy (metronidazole), the overall results are often incomplete. It would appear worthwhile investigating topical application of a sucralfate suspension because of the ability to coat inflamed and ulcerated mucosa and its capability to bind proteolytic enzymes, perhaps bacterial toxins and (secondary) bile acids.

Indications for evaluation of sucralfate at the level of the colon are speculative: ischemic damage with prolonged ulceration? caustic colitis after accidental or intentional injection of caustic fluids? indolent ulcers related to vasculitis? postlaser ulceration? NSAID-induced ulceration?

Commentary

It would appear that we might expect a widening of the spectrum of therapeutic applicability of sucralfate in the near future at least in some of the above-mentioned disease states. If sucralfate would appear to be truly efficacious, then it would be necessary to precisely determine its mode of action. This will help to broaden our understanding of sucralfate's pharmacotherapeutic profile, to improve the characteristics of the pharmaceutical composition, and to optimize the design of the necessary clinical evaluations.

References

1. Tarnawski A: Sucralfate. Is it more than just a barrier? Cytoprotection–future direction in prevention and treatment of gastrointestinal mucosal injury. *Curr Concepts Gastroenterol* **1**:5–8, 1984. Superb comprehensive overview of the various mechanisms that are involved in mucosal protection.
2. Tobiasson P, Stenstam M: Effects of sucralfate and cholestyramine on bile acid absorption. *Gastroenterology* **88**:393–396, 1985. This study illustrates the bile acid binding capacity of sucralfate.
3. Scherlacher A, Beaufort-Spontin F: Strahlentherapie von Kopf-Hals-Malignomen: Entzündungsprophylaxe der Schleimhaut durch Sucralfatbehandlung. *HNO* **38**:24–28, 1990. Oral sucralfate suspension was shown to protect against radiation-induced mucosa injury and symptoms.
4. Henriksson R, Arevärn M, Franzén L, *et al*: Beneficial effects of sucralfate on radiation induced diarrhea. An open randomized study in gynecological cancer patients. *Eur J Gynaecol Oncol* **11**:299–302, 1990. This is one of the first studies on the usefulness of sucralfate in ameliorating the acute radiation effects on the small and large bowel.
5. Henriksson R, Franzen L, Litbrand B: Effects of sucralfate on acute and late bowel discomfort following radiotherapy of pelvic cancer. *J Clin Oncol* **10**:969–975, 1992. This is one of the rare placebo-controlled studies in a substantial number of patients, supporting the efficacy of sucralfate in acute and late intestinal radiation damage.
6. Kochhar R, Mehta SK, Aggarwal R, *et al*: Sucralfate enema in ulcerative rectosigmoid lesions. *Dis Colon Rectum* **33**:49–51, 1990. Sucralfate enemas allow coating of the injured and inflamed mucosa, protecting from luminal irritants and facilitating healing.
7. Dietrich PY, Forni M: Prévention des mucites chimio-induites grâce au sucralfate per os. *Bull Cancer* **77**:613, 1990. Oral sucralfate improves chemotherapy-induced mucosal lesions.
8. Pfeiffer P, Madsen EL, Hansen O, *et al*: Effect of prophylactic sucralfate suspension on stomatitis induced by cancer chemotherapy. A randomized, double-blind cross-over study. *Acta Oncol* **29**:171–173, 1990. Radiolabeled sucralfate was shown to adhere to chemotherapy-associated injured buccal mucosa for over 2 hr.
9. Kotzmann H, Gisslinger H: Treatment and prophylaxis of chemotherapy-induced gastrointestinal complaints. Results of a pilot study. Proceedings of the Sucralfate Symposium at the European Digestive Disease Week, Amsterdam, 1992. Substantial improvement in nausea and heartburn was obtained with sucralfate in a large number of patients, treated with chemotherapy.
10. Shenep JL, Kalwinsky DK, Hutson PR, *et al*: Efficacy of oral sucralfate suspension in prevention and treatment of chemotherapy-induced mucositis. *J Pediatr* **113**:758–763, 1988. In this study sucralfate failed to improve chemotherapy-induced discomfort but produced colonization of the alimentary tract with pathogens.
11. Dawson DJ, Khan AN, Miller V, *et al*: Detection of inflammatory bowel disease in adults and children: Evaluation of a new isotopic technique. *Br Med J* **291**:1227–1230, 1985. This is the first study in IBD where coating of labeled sucralfate of inflamed, denuded intestinal segments was evaluated.
12. Batman F, Arslan S, Telatar H: Effect of sucralfate in the treatment of solitary rectal ulcer. *Endoscopy* **20**:128, 1988 (Letter). One of the first attempts to improve/heal solitary rectal ulcers is described.
13. Spilladis C, Skandalis N, Emmanouildis A: Treatment of solitary rectal ulcer syndrome with sucralfate enema. *Gastrointest Endosc* **35**:131–132, 1989. Two patients with solitary rectal ulcer were successfully healed with a sucralfate/glycerine enema.
14. Zarger SA, Khuroo MS, Mahajan R: Sucralfate retention enemas in solitary rectal ulcer. *Dis Colon Rectum* **34**:455–457, 1991. In this study sucralfate enemas were beneficial in healing solitary rectal ulcers.

15. Deveaux M, Macaigne O, Lecouffe P, *et al*: Radioisotopes et entérocolites cryptogénétiques: sucralfate marqué au technétium 99m et granulocytes marqués au tropolonate d'indium 111. *J Med Nuc Biophys* **13**:139–146, 1989. A poor correlation was found between labeled sucralfate and labeled leukocyte scans.
16. Mortensen PB, Lech Y, Møller-Petersen J, *et al*: ^{99m}Tc-sucralfate scintigraphy in inflammatory bowel disease. *Scand J Gastroenterol* **24**:1126–1128, 1989. Labeled sucralfate scintigraphy is a poor indicator of disease location.
17. Zeijen RNM, Van der Pol HAG, Teule GJJ, *et al*: Sucralphate-technetium scintigraphy in inflammatory bowel disease: Experience in 23 patients. *Neth J Med* **35**:76–85, 1989. A poor correlation is described between labeled sucralfate scintigraphy and IBD location in the GI tract.
18. Zahavi I, Avidor I, Marcus H, *et al*: Effects of sucralfate in experimental colitis in the rat. *Gastroenterology* **92**:A1707, 1987. Topical administration of sucralfate ameliorates acetic acid-induced colitis in the rat.
19. Carling L, Kagevi I, Borvall E: Sucralfate enema (SUC)—Effective in IBD? *Endoscopy* **18**:115, 1986. In this open study, almost all patients with UC improved on topical sucralfate therapy.
20. Bennani A: Utilisation du sucralfate (Ulcar^R) par voie rectale dans le traitement des localisations distales de la rectocolite hémorragique. *M.C.D.* **20**:181–184, 1991. The treatment of solitary rectal ulcer with sucralfate enemas is described in detail.
21. Singal AK, Anand BS: Sucralfate in ulcerative colitis. *Gastroenterology* **95**:A1160, 1989. Topical administration of sucralfate is not efficacious in UC.
22. Riley SA, Gupta I, Mani V: A comparison of sucralfate and prednisolone enemas in the treatment of active distal ulcerative colitis. *Scand J Gastroenterol* **24**:1014–1018, 1989. Topically applied steroids are superior to sucralfate enemas in distal UC.
23. Boniface VA, Wright JP, Warner L, *et al*: Sucralfate enemas in the treatment of ulcerative proctitis. *S Afr Med J* **80**:40, 1991. In this study the usefulness of sucralfate enemas is compared with topical steroids in UC patients. The results are somewhat equivocal.
24. Campieri M, Gionchetti P, Belluzzi A, *et al*: Sucralfate, 5-aminosalicylic acid and placebo enemas in the treatment of distal ulcerative colitis. *Eur J Gastroenterol Hepatol* **3**:41–44, 1991. In this well-conducted Italian study, topical sucralfate was clearly shown to be inferior to topical mesalazine therapy in distal UC.

Index

www.ingramcontent.com/pod-product-compliance
Ingram Content Group UK Ltd.
Pitfield, Milton Keynes, MK11 3LW, UK
UKHW041859190726
13854UKWH00002B/988

* 9 7 8 1 4 7 5 7 7 0 1 8 6 *